Counseling Individuals with Communication Disorders

Counseling Individuals with Communication Disorders

Psychodynamic and Family Aspects

Second Edition

Walter J. Rollin, Ph.D.

Professor Emeritus, Special Education, Communicative Disorders Program,
San Francisco State University, San Francisco

Foreword by
Audrey L. Holland, B.S., Ph.D.

Regents Professor, Speech and Hearing Sciences,
University of Arizona, Tucson

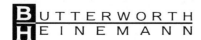

BUTTERWORTH
HEINEMANN

Boston   Oxford   Auckland   Johannesburg   Melbourne   New Delhi

Copyright © 2000 by Butterworth–Heinemann

 A member of the Reed Elsevier group

Every effort has been made to ensure that the drug dosage schedules within this text are accurate and conform to standards accepted at time of publication. However, as treatment recommendations vary in the light of continuing research and clinical experience, the reader is advised to verify drug dosage schedules herein with information found on product information sheets. This is especially true in cases of new or infrequently used drugs.

 Recognizing the importance of preserving what has been written, Butterworth–Heinemann prints its books on acid-free paper whenever possible.

 Butterworth–Heinemann supports the efforts of American Forests and the Global ReLeaf program in its campaign for the betterment of trees, forests, and our environment.

Library of Congress Cataloging-in-Publication Data

Rollin, Walter J., 1932–
    Counseling individuals with communication disorders : psychodynamic and family aspects / Walter J. Rollin ; foreword by Audrey L. Holland.—2nd ed.
        p. cm.
    Prev. ed. published as: The psychology of communication disorders in individuals and their families. Englewood Cliffs, N.J.: Prentice-Hall, c1987.
    Includes bibliographical references and index.
    ISBN 0-7506-7178-5 (alk. paper)
    1. Communicative disorders—Psychological aspects. 2. Communicative disorders—Patients—Family relationships. 3. Communicative disorders—Patients—Counseling of. 4. Psychodynamic psychotherapy. I. Rollin, Walter J., 1932—Psychology of communication disorders in individuals and their families. II. Title.

RC423 .R65 2000
616.85'50651—dc21   99-461973

British Library Cataloguing-in-Publication Data
A catalogue record for this book is available from the British Library.

The publisher offers special discounts on bulk orders of this book.
For information, please contact:

Manager of Special Sales
Butterworth–Heinemann
225 Wildwood Avenue
Woburn, MA 01801-2041
Tel: 781-904-2500
Fax: 781-904-2620

For information on all Butterworth–Heinemann publications available, contact our World Wide Web home page at: http://www.bh.com

10 9 8 7 6 5 4 3 2 1

Printed in the United States of America

One must not only think so much about
what we should do, but rather what one
should be. Our works do not enoble us;
but we must enoble our works.

Work and Being
Meister Eckart
c.1260–c.1327

Contents

Foreword

In this updated and revised second edition of his book, *Counseling Individuals with Communication Disorders: Psychodynamic and Family Aspects*, Walter Rollin makes a unique and important contribution to the professions of Speech-Language Pathology and Audiology. To describe its comprehensive nature, it is revealing to note what the book is *not*. It is *not* a book about specific disorders of speech, language, or hearing—*it is about all of them*. It is *not* a book about counseling children and their families nor counseling adults and their families—*it is about both*. It is *not* a how-to book, nor is it a review of the relevant literature—*it ties these features together*. What emerges as a result of Dr. Rollin's principled and extensive review of the literature relating to the psychology of language, coupled with his years of experience, is a unification of Speech-Language Pathology and Audiology, at least in terms of their counseling challenges and responsibilities. In this time of professional divergences, it is indeed refreshing to find the common ground.

It should come as no surprise that this common ground is the psychological underpinning of the disorders Dr. Rollin discusses in his book. But it is, in fact, a necessary reminder that none of us treats disorders. Rather, we treat individuals whose communication problems affect every aspect of their lives. Dr. Rollin gives us a model for providing counseling to them and their families, provides abundant examples, outlines techniques, and throughout this book, encourages us to take our counseling responsibilities extremely seriously. Walter Rollin and I were students together many years ago. As I read this manuscript, I was consistently reminded of old conversations. I even occasionally heard his voice, reminding our fellow students and me of the importance of putting a disorder into the context of the person who had it. This book embodies Walter Rollin's lifelong commitment to that principle.

Audrey L. Holland, B.S., Ph.D.

Preface to the Second Edition

When the first edition of *The Psychology of Communication Disorders In Individuals and Their Families* was published in 1987, our profession already was making considerable inroads in the expansion of its role within the realm of neuromuscular disease processes; namely, that of deglutition disorders. So much so, in fact, that dysphagia therapy has now become the mainstay of therapeutic practices in many hospitals, rehabilitation centers, home health care agencies, and skilled nursing facilities. I therefore believed it was necessary to include the very significant psychosocial ramifications of such a disorder in the present edition. It seemed appropriate to discuss these generically and in the context of neurogenic disorders. In this regard, the present edition gave more emphasis to Parkinson's Disease and some relevant discussion of HIV/AIDS.

Of no lesser importance over the last 10 years, at least, has been greater attention by our profession to factors unique to our growing multiculturally diverse population. In particular, I include research on our current understanding of specific familial aspects and how these impinge on those children and adults with communicative disorders. Consequently, I included counseling concepts unique to specific cultures attempting to cope with so-called traditional American values.

While traditional psychotherapeutic strategies have maintained a common denominator, I thought it necessary to update these, consistent with philosophic, pragmatic changes that have occurred over the last 10 to 12 years. It was appropriate, then, to incorporate these within the context of counseling-interview methods with the communicatively impaired and their families.

To those familiar with the first edition, I retained much, particularly the real-life anecdotes from my own professional experiences and added several others that I believe have relevance for those practicing in varied settings, but in particular, home health care. Also, I did not alter the present edition to suit any one audience. Indeed, I attempted here to include physical and occupational therapists as well as the students enrolled in communicative disorder programs and, of course, the practicing professionals in our field and other ancillary professionals.

It is impossible to avoid discussion of the effects of managed health care and reductions in Medicare on treatment modalities and consequent implications for families of the older patient. I trust I contributed material you, the reader, might find useful in helping them cope with the psychosocial ramifications.

In each chapter, I attempted to update those references that I believed most relevant to the continuing theme of the manuscript. Thanks to my last eight years as a speech-language pathologist in a major home health agency, the final chapter on the proper use of *therapeutic power* required a more expansive view.

Finally, without restating the final paragraph of the Preface to the First Edition, this edition is merely a continuation of a theme with which more professionals in the field are becoming comfortable. I trust that the next 10 years will bring an even greater interest in, commitment to, and reassurance in the use of counseling.

W. J. R.

Preface to the First Edition

This book was written for two major reasons. The first was to share with the reader the current state of knowledge regarding the psychological and social dynamics of the communicatively disordered population with whom we work. The second was to present counseling strategies that the reader might use to assist that population in coping more successfully with emotional factors accompanying these disorders.

During the course of my investigations into the psychological processes that constitute the various disorders, I was intrigued by the extent of contributions made by many other diverse academic disciplines, including linguistics, neurology, psychiatry, psychology, sociology, laryngology, and social psychology. It was a formidable challenge to try to bring them all together in order to establish a common frame of reference for fully understanding the needs of the communicatively disordered individual. I hope I have made a start in that direction. Even then it was plainly clear that subjective clinical data far exceeded the rigor of empirical evidence, in terms of quantity at best. The questions are certainly there for the asking and I attempted to raise some research issues in several chapters.

An even greater challenge was posed by the myriad counseling theories and therapies available to us as counseling speech-language-hearing professionals. I attempted, therefore, to establish a counseling base upon which counseling strategies could evolve for each of the various disorders. Although some overlapping was unavoidable, I believe also it was an essential factor toward reinforcing my discussion of the counseling processes common to the remediation of each of the disorders. In this regard, my intention was essentially to describe the counseling process as necessary for the development of the ideal client-therapist relationship in communicative disorders therapy.

For those who desire or require comprehensive descriptions of various counseling approaches, I have provided a substantial list of pertinent references. I discuss my own counseling approach for each of the disorders in an essentially generic fashion, as it was my intention only to introduce basic concepts and processes.

I wrote this book with consideration for several different groups of readers. For those readers at the undergraduate level it is an opportunity to arouse interest in generic psychodynamic processes associated with the major communication disorders and stimulate further reading and investigation. It will probably be most helpful if this group reads each chapter in sequential order so that a gradual understanding of psychotherapeutic processes can emerge and thus better prepare these readers for the impact of Chapter 9.

Those who are now in graduate studies should also benefit from the above, but beyond that as well. It is hoped that interest in developing counseling skills will be enhanced and that at the same time the reader will be inspired to challenge the many premises raised by myself and other authorities cited throughout the text.

For practicing professionals, regardless of work setting, it is hoped that a greater clarification of the counseling boundaries in speech-language pathology and audiology is accomplished. Whether a clinical researcher or research clinician, such a reader will be provoked into either solidifying previously held assumptions and beliefs, modifying them, or questioning even further the premises made throughout the book. No doubt my text should force the recognition of what it may mean for counseling to continue to be neglected as an intervention strategy among our more traditional ones.

There is a final group of professionals for whom I have written this book. They are the wide variety of practicing psychotherapists, many of whom I have known personally and professionally through the years, and who, because of their unfamiliarity with the complex dynamics of the communicatively disordered population, encouraged me "to get it all on paper."

There were several tangential topics I was tempted to explore. These were touched upon only generally. One of them concerns our evaluation of the therapy we do. There is very little we do to evaluate the outcome of our therapeutic interventions beyond superficial measurable linguistic units of discourse. Less is known of how our clients change and to what degree, particularly in regard to interpersonal communicative behavior. Hopefully, others will take up this challenge.

Although I may not have provided the definitive answers to all of the issues raised, I hope I have at least pointed in the direction for our profession to come to terms with all that is implied in the title of this book. The guidelines are there in order for readers, so inclined, to follow so that they may formulate their own counseling model and develop approaches unique to their own personal and professional needs and the special needs of their clients.

Acknowledgments

This book is essentially the product of the direct and indirect contributions of the many communicatively disordered individuals with whom I have worked over my professional lifetime of more than 45 years.

I extend my gratitude also to the many speech-language pathologists and audiologists who have long recognized the importance and significance of considering the psychosocial elements that are part of their patients-clients' struggles in coping with their communicative impairment.

I am grateful also to many of my former graduate students who are now practicing professionals, who served as critical referees throughout the development of my conceptualization of the ideas expressed in this text.

I am most thankful to my dear friend Molly Rannells, who has extensive experience as a major editor in the publishing industry and carefully scrutinized my writing as she proofed, corrected, and advised throughout the writing process.

Finally, I am deeply indebted to my wife, Bonnie, whose loving support, encouragement, patience, and critique based on her own professional expertise were vital elements in bringing this book to fruition.

1

Prevalent Counseling
Theories and Practices

Introduction

To many speech-language pathologists and audiologists the terms *counseling* and *psychotherapy* provoke a skeptical reaction, likely related to attitudes that have characterized the speech-language-hearing profession since its formal initiation in 1926. Until the 1950s, therapeutic practices were characterized essentially by symptom-related strategies with minimum attention to the dynamics of the client-therapist relationship. Some therapists and major authorities, such as Charles Van Riper, Wendell Johnson, William Perkins, and Jon Eisenson, were beginning to value the significance of the interpersonal communicative needs of the communicatively impaired person. Other therapists, adopting the behavioral model of B. F. Skinner (1971), began using *operant* approaches to eliminate or modify communication "deficits." Ironically, while many clinical professionals recognized then, and still do, the importance of treating the *person*, in practice, this is too seldom typical. As Backus (1960) cautioned in her timeless essay:

> The great risk now appears to be that the increasing numbers of people entering the field, the greatly expanded body of knowledge, together with the growing prestige of the profession—will produce an increasing dedication to subject matter and to the professional (I-It) rather than dedication to the person (I-Thou). Such a trend would inevitably bring serious consequences to clients, therapists, and to the profession. (p. 525)

Backus does not refute the implementation of our knowledge of the complex mechanisms of speech, language, hearing, and traditional treatment modalities necessary to bring about communicative change. She does insist that, by the very nature of what we do as therapists, however, we enter into relationships with our clients. Truly, as therapists, we *cannot not* relate. Since this reality exists, it therefore is appropriate to expand our understanding of psychological processes underlying relationships in the therapeutic environment.

Unfortunately, Backus's admonition still has failed to gain serious recognition by our profession. In a study by Culpepper, Mendel, and McCarthy (1994), counseling training and experiences in academic programs accredited by the American Speech Language Hearing Association had not changed substantially since the publication of our first edition in 1987. Neither departmental nor nondepartmental coursework and training in counseling had increased. Even though interest in counseling has increased considerably, as evidenced by more publications dealing with counseling in communicative disorders, we have yet to see substantial representation at national conferences or in seminars sponsored by the American Speech Language Hearing Association.

We understand that differentiating psychological dynamics related directly to various communication disorders from deep-rooted psychopathologies may fall outside the realm of our central professional expertise or purpose. It may be very difficult, in fact, to ascertain at times. Nonetheless, we believe it possible to establish a counseling framework with which students can begin to feel comfortable and professionals can integrate successfully in their practices. To do so, it will be necessary for us to describe the relation of psychotherapy to counseling.

Relation of Psychotherapy to Counseling

If we were to merely define *counseling* lexically as meaning "advise, recommend, guide, and exchange ideas and opinions," there would be no reason for attempting to relate the term to psychotherapy. Then, as clinicians, our task would be simple, in that we would have no further responsibility to our clients than to impart to them the store of knowledge, expertise, and good sense with which presumably we have been trained. If, on the other hand, we are to define *counseling* more realistically, in its connotative form, we would say that counseling is a dynamic process that involves a complex interaction between and among people. To insist that professionals, such as lawyers, vocational counselors, high school counselors, physicians, speech-language pathologists, audiologists, and other professionals, adhere only to imparting information to their clients would be naive. Communication (and who should know better than we) involves an active and reactive interrelationship between helper (counselor) and the one being helped (client). Furthermore, we need to recognize that, because informational content and people vary obviously from profession to profession, the quality, degree, and context of the counseling interrelationship will differ as well.

Practices in our profession involve one further process, somewhat akin to counseling, that requires identification and discussion. Over the last 10 years, several authorities in our field have written extensively on the value and necessity of fine-tuning the *interview* of the client, parent, caregiver, or combination thereof, to facilitate therapy (Shipley, and Wood, 1997; Cormier, Cormier, and Cormier, 1991; and Crowe, 1997; among others). Generally, these experts tend to weave interviewing within the coun-

seling fabric. In some instances, this is very appropriate, as we shall discuss later. But, if we turn again to lexical meaning, the interview is a face-to-face formal meeting or conversation between one or more individuals in which one individual is attempting to obtain information from or provide information to another individual or individuals. This, in some instances, actually could impede the interpersonal communicative process by erecting a static barrier between speakers and perhaps impede the flow of necessary etiological or clinical information. It also could create or contribute to a subservience factor, which will be addressed further in later chapters.

Regardless, it is important first to define *psychotherapy* and examine it more closely. By lexical definition alone, *psychotherapy* is the psychological treatment of emotional, mental, and nervous disorders. Viewed in a more abstract way, interpretations and applications have been made by various schools of thought and differing helping professionals, such as psychiatrists, clinical psychologists, clinical social workers, family and child therapists, clergy, and by rehabilitation counselors. Intrinsic to psychotherapy, regardless of the school or disciplines that represent the process, is the concept that the interrelational dynamics determine the ultimate outcome. The complexity of the dynamics depends not only on the theoretical framework but also on the nature, severity, and degree of pathology or dysfunction. For further appreciation of the extensive range of disorders, the reader is referred to the DSM-IV criteria established by the American Psychiatric Association (1994). Although the professions representative of psychotherapeutic practices still abide by nosological criteria and rules (disease classifications), they recognize that the vast diversity of people troubled by the demands and complexities of life do not always *fit*. Fortunately, we are not so eager now to compartmentalize those who suffer emotionally or who are *different*, into vacuous categories of "neurotic," "maladjusted," or "abnormal." Even the term *dysfunctional*, according to some practitioners, has become somewhat vague, misleading, or plainly irrelevant. For this reason, our task in differentiating between psychotherapy and counseling becomes more challenging and difficult.

Viewing Counseling and Psychotherapy on a Continuum

In attempting to differentiate between counseling and psychotherapy, it would appear obvious to consider these processes along a continuum, but this is not as simple as it might appear. Hansen et al. (1993) explore the theory and process of counseling from classical analysis to cognitive-behavioral counseling. Earlier writers in the field attempted to differentiate counseling from psychotherapy along a continuum. One group viewed the continuum relative to degrees of normalcy versus neuroses, and others viewed the continuum relative to process, or the manner with which the counselor or psychotherapist works with clients (Hansen, Stevic, and Warner, 1977). They point out that, because people vary in their ability to deal with role problems in their environment or with deep-seated intrapersonal conflicts, it would be better to consider the *degree* to which, or the intensity with which, people suffer from their problems. Complementing their earlier work, Hansen and colleague's more recent perspective stresses the importance of counselors developing a personal approach to their work and encourages would-be counselors to develop a "personal theory of counseling," regardless of theoretical orientation. We would agree with this combined perspective. First, it helps us to avoid the use of labels to categorize individuals, urging us instead to focus on *how* they cope uniquely with their difficulties. Further, it suggests that we need not feel committed to any one theoretical orientation.

As we see it, a counselor works with individuals who may function at least minimally in daily living activities but who are troubled emotionally by either internal or external circumstances that interfere with maximal functioning. In contrast, the psychotherapist works with individuals who are overwhelmed by either internal or external circumstances, be it a role conflict, deep-seated psychopathology, or both, and who need to restructure major attributes of their personality in order to function maximally. That is, they are individuals who may be affected profoundly by adverse circumstances, regardless of an identified neurosis.

A further differentiating feature justifying either counseling or psychotherapeutic intervention is that of the therapeutic relationship itself. Our position is that psychotherapy requires an intense and complex relationship between therapist and client in which the relationship itself becomes the instrument for change. The therapeutic relationship in counseling also is intrinsic to helping the individual learn new means of coping with and adjusting to life. But, as we discuss later, the concept of compliance by the client becomes a significant factor, regardless of theory, orientation, or complexity of therapeutic process.

It is obvious the distinctions between counseling and psychotherapy may be equivocal and that, by the nature of any therapeutic process, overlap can occur. Nonetheless, as we see further on, it is possible to establish boundaries, allowing the clinician to function effectively, securely, and ethically as counselor during communication therapy. Now, though, we need to identify more closely the distinctive elements of both psychotherapy and counseling.

Distinctive Elements of Psychotherapy

Typically, the psychotherapist focuses on intrapersonal conflicts characterized by anxieties, depression, guilt, anger, and ambivalent behavior that, although real to the individual, may have little basis in objective reality. The psychotherapist is concerned with the following questions about the client's personality characteristics.

1. What has been its course of development?
2. What factors have impeded its growth?
3. What factors are impeding growth now?

With the medical model as a referent, the psychotherapist typically has viewed the individual as sick and requiring major reductions in psychopathological behavior. In the last 30 years, however, several schools of psychotherapy, including those representative of eclectic approaches, have emerged that lean toward a so-called well model, in which the individual is not viewed as *sick* but as *behaviorally dysfunctional*. While a few of the more classically oriented disciplines, such as the Freudian and Jungian schools, continue to practice deep psychoanalysis, the trend has been toward a combination of approaches or a more eclectic practice dependent on the client and the nature of the problem. Still, with the major advances in drug therapy, particularly for clinical depression, the medical model persists. In essence, though, psychotherapy is characterized by the reorganization and reinterpretation of destructive behavior patterns or unresolved conflicts within the personality pattern of the individual.

Distinctive Elements of Counseling

The essential task of the counselor is assisting individuals work toward an understanding of themselves in order to learn new ways of coping with and adjusting to either negative life situations or those to which they may respond negatively or unrealistically. Individuals need not restructure or reorganize their personality to cope with their traumatic brain injury (TBI), cerebral vascular accident (CVA), or psychogenically induced vocal dysfunction, unless, of course, such individuals are guided by deep-seated psychopathological conflict. Indeed, such individuals would require the psychotherapeutic intervention discussed earlier. But we are concerned now with individuals whose problems relate directly to role definition; that is, difficulty in adapting in a unique way to a particular life situation or event (the stuttering child, the hearing-impaired adult, the linguistically impoverished child, the vocal abusing adult, etc.).

The counseling process is characteristically supportive, insight re-educative, and usually short term. It is used to help individuals make practical changes in their lives without necessarily modifying established personality patterns. Represented by distinctive or blended schools of thought, counseling is based on a well model and uses some methods not unlike those of psychotherapy. The methods would include cognitive-behavioral, client centered, rational-emotive, informational-educational, or variations and combinations of these. Let us now consider these in depth, toward developing a model we may apply in our work with the communicatively impaired and their families who require counseling assistance.

Major Counseling Theories

The Self Theory or Client-Centered Approach of Carl Rogers

Probably the most influential figure in the field of counseling has been Carl Rogers, whose first publication in 1942, *Counseling and Psychotherapy*, has served as the seminal source for counseling theory practices as they evolved over 58 years. Rogers, in his ever-growing wisdom, modified his theory, consistent with the dramatic changes that occurred over that span of years, in all aspects of society and in a variety of different professional settings. From his earliest publication (1942) in which he states that the "self is a basic factor in the formation of personality and the determination of behavior" to his thesis in 1959 that the self is "the organized, consistent, conceptual Gestalt composed of characteristics of the 'I' or 'me' and the perceptions of the relationship of the 'I' or 'me' to others and to various aspects of life, together with the value attached to these perceptions" (p. 20), Rogers views change in the client to be the direct result of the dynamic way in which the client and therapist experience their relationship.[1] According to Rogers, the structure of personality is based on three major elements, which he describes as the phenomenal field, the organism, and the self.

The Phenomenal Field, the Organism, and the Self

According to Rogers (1951), people always are in the center of an ever-changing phenomenal field that is continuously being experienced either consciously or unconsciously. How we respond depends on how we perceive reality, whether it be internal or external. Therefore, when our perception of reality changes, so do our reactions to that reality. More recent writers have expanded on Rogers's original concepts and developed research models to further validate his earlier concepts. They also have developed both person-centered and family-

---

[1]Those readers who wish to read more fully on the derivation and essence of the (I-Thou) relationship may refer to Buber (1958).

centered paradigms, which is described in later chapters (Levant and Schlien, 1984).

As might be illustrated in speech-language therapy, if aphasic adults perceive their disability as the essence of their reality, it becomes that alone on which they focus and to that which they react negatively. If, on the other hand, they perceive positively their other traits or personal qualities as their essential reality, they are likely to contribute more effectively to their overall recovery. We do not wish to imply that an *either-or* perception is desirable because aphasic individuals must perceive the reality of their disability. But if the person can perceive realistically both realities, positive change is more likely.

Rogers considers the organism as a total individual who acts as a complete, organized system in which modification of any part of that system produces changes in any other part or parts. The organism consists of all the thoughts, behaviors, and physical attributes that make up the individual.

As humans we never function in separate parts but holistically or as a total entity, in order to have our needs expressed or satisfied. Achieving what some refer to as *self-actualization* or personal dynamic and continuous growth, Rogers clearly advises, does not occur without struggle and psychic pain. It always is easier to maintain the status quo or take the pathway of least resistance. As we see later, in our discussion of stuttering, it is very difficult to relinquish that with which we have been familiar. Conversely, the organism desires to develop as fully as possible without the constraint of external controls. But positive change can occur only by altering our perception of reality and our reaction to it. Rogers implies that, the more we are willing to acknowledge our reactions and identify them consciously, the more likely we are to grow positively.

Rogers's most important principle is that of the self. As an individual strives to maximize his or her potential, that person must differentiate and discriminate the object of one's feelings and perceptions—personal environment, experiences, the self—and the interrelationship among them. In doing so, the individual becomes less fixed on and more open to his or her perceptions, or stated differently, the individual's experiences are symbolized more accurately. The person comes to understand the incongruity between certain experiences and how they are interpreted in personal reactions. Feelings that previously were denied or distorted are experienced more fully, resulting in a reorganization of the individual's self-concept. As the structure of the self continues to reorganize, the concept of self becomes more congruent with the individual's experience, with the self now including experiences that previously would have been too threatening to recognize or acknowledge (Rogers, 1959).

In their discussion of the self, Avila, Combs, and Purkey (1977) provide evidence to support the thesis that human behavior is not determined so much by life situations per se as "by the individual's perception of the situation" (p. 56). Hence, it is particularly important to recognize that there may be a discrepancy between the actual reality and the way the individual perceives that reality. The relationship between the two realities is dynamic, however, and influenced by the complex interrelationships among the individual's experiences, life environment, and unique constitutional or genetic factors.

In summary, the personality evolves around the self, which is the nucleus or center. As the individual interacts with his or her environment, the self develops. In doing so, the values of other people, (family members in particular) are either integrated, modified, or distorted. Phenomenologically, individuals integrate experiences that are consistent with how they tend to conceptualize themselves. If the experiences are inconsistent or incongruent, they are perceived as threats. Worse, is that the individual begins to function in a dysfunctional way or inappropriate manner. Of crucial importance to self-concept is that it always is in process and, as a function of its dynamic interaction with the phenomenal field, changes and grows. The reader is encouraged to investigate the work of Kurt Lewin for the genesis of the concept of phenomenology (Stivers and Wheelan, 1986). It is obvious that, although each of us is unique in fulfilling the values necessary for self-actualization (Maslow, 1968), our basic needs are essentially similar. Rogers hypothesizes that each individual has the ability and capacity to settle personal conflicts or overcome obstacles through the enhancement of his or her own value system as well as through the value system of their particular social milieu (Rogers, 1959, 1961).

The essential therapeutic process for Rogers is the use of reflection, whereby the therapist mirrors feelings expressed by the client with the intention that the latter begin to recognize the true nature of what that person is experiencing. Rogers tends to equate reflection with empathy, a concept that has been explored with greater interest the last several years, but as we discuss later, more recent writers tend to make a very clear distinction between the two (Bozarth in Levant and Shlien, 1984). Having examined Rogers's basic self theory of personality, we can consider appropriately how his principles may be understood in the context of our work with communicatively impaired individuals.

Application to the Communicatively Impaired

We already noted that an aphasic individual may focus on the disability to the exclusion of other aspects within his or her phenomenal field (the person's unique perceptual reality). For this person and others with different communicative disorders, how they perceive their subjective realities depends on the nature and quality of their own interrelated past experiences. Included among these are their familial, social, cultural, and physical background or environment. We further would add such inherent elements as native intelligence and constitutional nature and predilections that contribute to people's uniqueness as individuals. Each of us, then, like the communicatively impaired, responds every waking moment to those figures or significant features perceived uniquely or that stand out from the *ground* or from our entire perceptual environment. Because the phenomenal field includes perceptual experiences that are both internal and external to the individual, the communicatively impaired may misperceive how others respond to them, may distort perceptually the reality of their own disorder, or both. Thus, the totality of the person's particular perception becomes fixed within his or her personal phenomenal field. We also pointed out Rogers's belief that the organism acts in a total way to the phenomenal field and changing any aspect of the organized system that has been established will bring about changes in other aspects. Therefore, the

communicatively disordered individual who fixates only on the disorder itself will tend to identify the disorder as representing the totality of his or her own being or nature. Such individuals not only will have difficulty recognizing the potential for changing their attitude about their disorder but also may inhibit opportunities for developing a more positive attitude toward themselves. Of major importance, however, is that the potential does exist, because as humans we are constantly striving "to expand, extend, develop, mature" (Rogers, 1961, p. 351). It entails, however, the opportunity, the motivation, the will, and the courage to become more fully aware of self-being and self-functioning. As part of this process, which was described earlier as self-actualization, communicatively impaired individuals must be helped to recognize that, regardless of the disorder, they are worthy, they have capability and potential not only to modify or eliminate the disorder but also to remove the distorted, destructive, and limited perceptions of other aspects of their life. In sum, these individuals need not continue to symbolize all continuing life experiences in terms of only the disorder itself.

A Behavioral Theory

We shall now look at behavioral theory—considered by many to be antithetical to Rogers's self theory model—and how it may serve as a counseling strategy for the communicatively impaired. B. F. Skinner (1953), the chief proponent of behavioral theory, believes that human behavior is determined essentially by the environment and that the way humans react is in response to external events that occur around them. The basic assumption underscoring behavioral theory is that behavior is learned when that behavior is followed by an event in the environment that brings satisfaction to the individual. The probability of that behavior being repeated is thereby enhanced. The satisfaction to the individual may be brought about by events either external or internal to the individual. An example of Skinner's assumption is the babbling infant. Through maturation and likely external influences, the infant discovers pleasure by babbling, and it is therefore rewarding. The probability for that behavior to recur is increased. Thus according to Lattal (1992), operant conditioning occurs as a result of a specific behavioral event, the behavior shaped by the consequences of the environmental events that follow. In this way babbling is reinforced, paving the way for higher levels of speech development.

Most learning theorists would contend that learning also will occur through imitation or by identifying with the model copied, without the necessity of receiving a reward. As cognitive psychologists, DeBell and Harless (1992) acknowledge that individual uniqueness, internal states, vicarious learning, and observation by another individual are not inconsistent with Skinnerian theory and address instructional implications involved in learning. They also contend, of course, that reinforcement may be necessary for the observer's performance of the behavior.

A Learning Theory Position

We have already recognized that behavior operates to produce the reinforcement. Each is dependent or contingent on the other. That is, behavior that is rewarded or given positive reinforcement can be increased in frequency or maintained, whereas behavior that is punished by the removal of positive reinforcers or the addition of negative reinforcers can be extinguished or decreased in frequency.

Establishment of new behaviors depends on the immediacy of the reward. New behavior may be extinguished if a reward is terminated abruptly or presented infrequently. Partial reinforcement, however, or a schedule of reinforcement may help to maintain behavior once it has been learned. According to Hansen et al. (1977), reinforcement schedules consist of "ratio reinforcement" and "interval reinforcement." For the former, a reward is given after a certain number of responses have occurred. For interval reinforcement, a proper amount of time must pass before a reward can be given. Generally, learned responses are retained longer on intermittent schedules than on a continuous schedule. Complex behaviors are developed through processes of extinction, generalization, discrimination, shaping, and mediating.

Extinction.   Our ability to change our behavior continuously depends on the frequency of the inter-

mittent reinforcement and our ability and recognition of what is appropriate to any one stage of our development. To grow from childhood to adulthood, reinforcement of earlier behavior is withheld so that the behavior will decrease and eventually be eliminated. What is yet mysterious is how most parents intuitively know to do this, notwithstanding extraneous factors impinging on development.

Generalization.   A second important principle of learning is generalization. In essence, a stimulus that is accompanied by a reinforcement produces a particular response, but it also transfers to other stimuli as well. It is important for the two stimuli to be related in some way, however, if the response is to recur. We are familiar with the child who vocalizes when the mother appears and who transfers the same response when the father appears. Without generalization, it would be difficult to explain the rapid development of language during the early formative years.

Discrimination.   Our uniqueness no doubt results partly from the way we generalize but also from the way we learn to discriminate between situations or events. Thus, we also make small changes in behavior when exposed to similar situations. Relative to discrimination, relationships between stimuli and responses that are initiated through generalization may be distinguished separately. Through the interaction of extinction and reinforcement, the appropriate response to a stimulus is reinforced, whereas an inappropriate response to a similar event is not reinforced. The infant learns early to respond similarly to both parents but differently to strangers because the stimulus given is likely to be qualitatively or quantitatively different.

Shaping.   Moving from simple behaviors, which are gradual approximations of the final behavior to be expected, and ultimately to the final behavior itself is known as *shaping* (Hansen et al., 1993). This is a process in which specific behaviors that come close to the desired behavior are reinforced. Any extraneous behaviors receive no reinforcement. It is crucial that, at each level of the process, successive approximations of the behavior are expected before any reinforcement is provided. Infants apparently learn this process as they move through the highly complex evolution of speech and language development. Parents tend to reinforce those sounds and words that approximate the desired final product and typically do not reinforce those behaviors that remain static. How parents seem to know when to recognize the appropriateness at each level of development is unclear and not our purpose to discuss at this time. Similarly, we do not know if the infant makes adjustments of vocal and verbal behaviors by responding to their own internal time clock of appropriateness. Certainly, as we develop, we reinforce ourselves for behaviors that are rewarding, but exactly when this begins also is uncertain.

Mediating.   As humans, we distinguish ourselves from other animals by our ability to develop mediating responses that permit us consciously to plan, evaluate, and react to our environment through the use of language and symbolization, labeling, stimuli, and reconciling our effects. Behaviorists believe that as humans we have not only the capacity to sort out the effects of environmental events but also the ability to become aware of that capacity.

As a direct result of Skinner's formulation, during the last three decades, we have seen the emergence of an evolution of counseling and psychotherapeutic strategies based on behavioral-cognitive principles (Schoenfeld, 1993). It therefore is appropriate for us now to consider how these principles may be applied generally in counseling those who are communicatively disordered.

Application to the Communicatively Impaired

Mowrer (1977) has made one of the most important contributions to our understanding of how behavioral strategies can be employed in counseling the communicatively impaired. Citing Menacker (1976), Mowrer emphasizes the importance of the client being an active participant with the therapist in removing barriers to more effective communicative interaction with others. Both work together to achieve favorable environmental conditions, conducive to positive behavioral change. The process essentially is directive rather than reflective, and

uncharacteristic of self theory. Mowrer describes it as an empirical-rational approach; it is assumed from the beginning that the client will derive the greatest benefit by using an instructional and very direct attack on the problem. Use of the intellect is key to desired change.

Although they do not address the communicatively impaired directly, Zeiss and Steffen (1996) recommend cognitive-behavioral intervention techniques using a collaborative relationship between client and therapist in treating elderly patients. They suggest explicit goal setting and acknowledgment of the client's personal strengths. They stress the importance of understanding changes in cognitive processing and learning that may be associated with aging. Modifications of therapeutic technique are made in response to differences in learning styles, sensory deficits, chronic health problems, and to capitalize on the life experience of the older adult. Operant or behavioral methods continue to be used today in the treatment of school-age children (Lincoln et al., 1996).

From the individual who desires a more effective way to manage the voice to the frustrated aphasic individual, the counseling process is a learning situation in which the individual is helped to define the specific behaviors that contribute to the major problem. The goals of counseling must be stated in specific terms and therapy directed toward one specific concern at a time. Therefore, if loud vocalization is seen as a behavior that must be extinguished, the therapist and client work together to reinforce vocal intensity that is more hygienic and balanced. That this may not occur immediately is apparent from our discussion of shaping. But any close approximation to the desired goal is to be rewarded through either therapist affirmation or client self-realization. In essence, the client is helped to develop whatever system of self-management is deemed appropriate for that individual to control his or her communicative future.

The Rational-Emotive Therapy Model

The fundamental assumption behind Albert Ellis's rational-emotive therapy (RET) model is that we essentially control our own destinies as long as we believe in and act on the values that are important and significant to us. A corollary to this assumption is the position that most emotional disturbance is a function of basic irrational beliefs that are "self-defeating and absurd." Ellis believes that we can learn to use RET as a self-help tool, and through the process, discover our irrational beliefs and learn how to use the logical and empirical methods of scientific inquiry. These include questioning, debating, challenging, and disputing irrational beliefs. The essential aim is to convince the individual to recognize the absurdity of his or her assumptions or beliefs and relinquish them. The individual then is instructed how to adopt new and adaptive attitudes (Ellis and Grieger, 1977; Ellis and Dryden, 1987; and Ellis et al., 1997).

The ABCs of RET

Ellis's contention is that, whenever an energizing experience or event (A) occurs and is followed by a consequence that is emotional or behavioral in nature (C), we have at least two major choices of belief (B). Say, for example, your stuttering client has been following a particular home assignment involving analysis of his *blocking* pattern and returns to therapy fully confident that his analysis has been accurate but learns during the session that it is not so. Your client is at point (A). The client reacts to the experience with an emotional or behavioral consequence (C), which follows almost immediately. The irrational response (B) would be the belief that (A) caused (C) and your client concludes that his home efforts were useless and that home practice is a waste of time. A more rational response would be for your client to acknowledge frustration and displeasure but then to analyze with you, the therapist, what factors may have impeded progress. Perhaps, your client simply did not do the assignment accurately. Now the two of you can work together to help create a more positive outcome for the next session.

In his later writings, Ellis expands his ABC framework to identify a more complex cognitive interrelationship, which includes genetic predispositions, prior interpersonal learning, and innately predisposed habit patterns (Ellis and Dryden, 1987).

Ellis also differentiates between preferential RET and general RET. The former encompasses long-range philosophical and ego developmental changes, while the latter is concerned with the alleviation of more immediate emotional problems, such as depression, anxiety, or addiction. It would be beyond the scope of this book to elaborate on preferential RET, since it tends toward more intense psychotherapy rather than counseling. Ellis (1962) contends that it is not events that upset us but rather our view of events. He lists many central illogical beliefs common to Western thought that contribute to emotional dysfunction. Several of these are summarized here:

1. It is of the utmost importance for an adult to be approved or loved by nearly everyone for virtually everything that adult does.
2. One should be completely competent, adequate, and achieving in everything one does.
3. Certain people are evil, bad, or wicked and therefore should be blamed severely and punished for their transgressions.
4. It is horrible, terrible, and catastrophic when things do not progress the way one would like.
5. Human unhappiness is caused by external events and we have minimal or no ability to control our sadness or eliminate those negative feelings.
6. If anything should be dangerous or scary, we should be overwhelmed with and distressed about it.
7. It is simpler to avoid confronting life's difficulties and our responsibilities than to take on more rewarding modes of self-discipline.
8. Past events in our lives determine our present behavior; they always have and cannot be changed.
9. Difficulties in life should not exist, and people and events should be different from the way they are; also, it is catastrophic if the perfect solutions to the grim realities of life are not immediately discovered.
10. We should be very concerned and upset by other people's problems and difficulties.
11. Maximum human happiness can be achieved by inertia and inaction or by passively and uncommittedly "enjoying oneself."

These are only a few of the 259 central self-defeating irrational ideas Ellis has collected. He contends, however, that, although such beliefs exist in virtually all of us, in varying degrees, some individuals tend to behave more irrationally.

Cognitive, Emotive, and Behavioral Techniques and the Counseling Process

Because RET essentially is a logicoempirical method of questioning, the most common technique used by therapists is *disputing irrational beliefs.* These include *detecting,* which consists of the *musts, shoulds, oughts,* and *have-tos* that characterize self-defeating behaviors. *Debating* involves asking the client questions geared to help the person to relinquish irrational beliefs; for example, *What evidence is there that this always happens to you?* The client is aided in acknowledging the fallacy of his or her irrational belief or beliefs and is helped to recognize rational alternatives. *Discriminating* is the process by which the client is helped by the therapist to distinguish between nonabsolutist values, such as wants, likes, and desires, and his or her absolutist values, such as needs and personal demands (Ellis and Dryden, 1987).

Far from neglecting emotive techniques, RET therapists offer their clients opportunities to express their emotions and offer "unconditional acceptance." While therapists accept their clients as fallible as the rest of us, they do not acquiesce to their client's negative or irrational behaviors. Some therapists indeed share with their clients their own experiences with irrational attitudes and behaviors. (Self-disclosure is discussed later in this text.) Like Rogers and other representative figures of the humanistic school of psychotherapy, Ellis (1962) believes that "one of the main functions of psychotherapy is to enhance the individual's self-respect (or 'ego strength,' 'self-confidence,' 'self-esteem,' 'feeling of self-worth,' or 'sense of identity') so that the person may thereby solve the problem of self-evaluation" (pp. 99–100). Ellis emphasizes the importance of understanding the way in which the client sees the world and considers the client's behavior from the client's point of view. The therapist refrains from getting immersed in the client's irrational belief system or behavior and must instead strip away the illogical ideas that are the basis of the client's anxieties and self-deceptions. Although Ellis recognizes the importance of being supportive and empathic and allowing the free expression of feelings, the therapist also must be confrontive, directive, and persuasive if the client is to be channeled into a more rational mode of thinking and behaving (Ellis, 1962; Ellis and Dryden, 1987).

Ellis's RET model has evolved also in the use of behavioral techniques (REBT), which include homework assignments, desensitization techniques that may be gradual or "flooded," and antiprocrastination exercises. The use of "rewards and punishments" is employed or negotiated with the client to reinforce taking on uncomfortable assignments in pursuit of long-range goals (Ellis and Dreyden, 1987). Earlier and even more recent writers (Hansen et al., 1977, 1993) describe Ellis's approach as a teaching process in which the clients learn to recognize rigid values that have dominated their thought processes and learn new ways of directing their lives in a more productive, healthy, and creative way.

Cognitive Counseling with the Communicatively Impaired

It would appear that REBT might readily be applied to self-defeating cognitive processes of various communicatively impaired individuals. Not unlike the behavioral approach discussed earlier, REBT could be applied as both an educational and a counseling tool to modify or eliminate irrational or unrealistic beliefs that may distort the quality or exacerbate the degree of some communicative disorders.

It is of some significance that Ellis should base several important aspects of his theory on the postulates of general semantics, among whose pioneers was Wendell Johnson, one of the most prolific authorities on stuttering behavior and whose theories continue to characterize treatment modalities for stuttering therapy today (Bloodstein, 1995). Other theorists, among them Williams (1957), have developed strategies that essentially attack the *linguistic insanities* (italics, my own) and irrational attitudes that appear to perpetuate stuttering behaviors and maintain the self-effacing and self-destructive attitudes of those who stutter. The work of more recent proponents of a cognitive-behavioral approach to the treatment of stuttering, such as Goldberg (1981), Ryan and Van Kirk Ryan (1995), and Onslow and Packman (1999), is discussed later in this text.

Use of REBT in counseling the vocal abuser misuser would appear appropriate because misuse or abuse of the voice can be eliminated by a conscious, rational decision to use the voice in a different manner. The speech-language pathologist would be the likely professional to educate and counsel the client toward that goal. Those who view vocal personality as an important dimension of continued vocal mismanagement (Cooper, 1973; Aronson, 1969) could readily apply REBT principles to a voice-disordered client, combining an objective analysis of the actual vocal possibilities, applying symptomatically based strategies with a rational acceptance by the client of his or her changing vocal image.

We presently will see how behavioral, cognitive, and self theory may be integrated or reconciled in the development of a counseling model appropriate for communicatively impaired individuals.

Developing an Appropriate Counseling Model for the Communicatively-Impaired Individual

Development of a counseling model for use by speech-language-hearing professionals must include not only the practical realities of the communicative needs of the client but also those elements of counseling theory and technique that may be readily applied regardless of type of communicative disorder.

The Essential Similarities Among Theories

Even the mildly interested reader of counseling theory immediately would recognize marked differences among the theories dictated by the various schools. But, because actual practices of counselors representing these schools bring them much closer together, we prefer to discuss the similarities in the counseling process. Implicit in our assumption is

that counselors are humans first and, regardless of theoretical orientation, are subject to the often mysterious forces that underlie their own personality processes and behavior. In particular is the attitude that *we, the professionals, know best what our clients need.* We explore these issues in the final chapter of the book.

Perhaps of even greater interest to the reader is that, during the last 15 years, there has been a gradual merging of therapeutic philosophies, emergence of eclectic thinking, and reassessment of long-held rigid principles. For example, the Rogerian concept of client-centered therapy has been transformed into a *person-centered approach* focusing more on the concept of the *well model* rather than the *sick* one (Schlien, 1984). Rogerian principles have been blended with the concept of boundaries to describe the ground rules, quality, and type of therapeutic relationship, albeit one still humanistic in nature (Owen, 1997). Some writers, notably O'Hara (1995) even go so far as to describe Rogers's transformation in his later years, bordering on a "mystical universalism" approach with his clients; that is, viewing individual behavior as inseparable from the rest of the world.

The Goals of Counseling

Fundamental to all counseling approaches is the common agreement that counseling is structured to facilitate changes in the client's behavior. Even though self theory counselors tend to be concerned with modifying and reorganizing the *total* behavioral or structural pattern of the individual's personality and behavioral counselors are more concerned with altering *specific* counterproductive behavior patterns, both groups recognize the significance of etiological factors that underlie all behaviors. In fact, Ellis and Dryden (1987), representing rational-emotive-cognitive therapy, also believe in assisting clients toward major changes in their personality and their life. Neither school, however, dwells solely on etiology, because changing present and future behavior is considered more important.

Common as well is the reduction of depression, anxiety, guilt, anger, and frustration, while discovering new ways to cope successfully with life. Although differences emerge in terms of degree, the self-actualization, positive self-regard, and person-in-process concepts of self theory certainly are compatible with the self-acceptance, self-direction, and choice-making concepts of rational-emotive-cognitive therapy and other approaches.

The Process of Counseling

In the self theory approach, the client is given total freedom to express his or her feelings. Regardless of the feelings expressed, the client is accepted unconditionally by the therapist and learns to examine those feelings and experience them in an objective manner. The client discovers the incongruity between distorted perceptions of experience and his or her concept of self. As experiences are more objectively examined, the client begins to reorganize concepts of the self, thereby leading toward congruency between both. As the client begins to take more responsibility for personal behavior, the possibilities for positive change are increased. The client soon realizes the limitless opportunities for taking charge of his or her life while minimizing the effects of external events, situations, and other people. The individual now adapts more readily to new and changing life circumstances with positive feelings of worthiness and infinite capabilities for growth.

While not representing themselves as strictly *Rogerian* in their approach, Duncan, Solovey, and Rusk (1992) present a client-directed approach that has as its main framework an eclecticism that includes a selective application of techniques borrowed from all schools but adapted to the specific needs of the client. Also related to the paradigm is the application of different theoretical models based on the client's own idiosyncratic combination of various approaches presented by the therapist. Underlying this approach is a technique in which factors that cut across theories are operationalized to bring about a successful therapeutic outcome. Thus, there is an integration of cognition, affect, and behavior. It should be noted here that much of the model just described evolved from the strategic model of family therapy developed at the Mental Research Institute (MRI) by Watzlawick, Weakland, and Fisch (1988).

Scales to develop more objectively the dynamic aspects of the counseling process related to self the-ory have been developed by Carkhuff (1969a, 1969b, 1971,1977). A major extension of self theory, Carkhuff's model includes not only the need for client self-exploration and self-understanding but also the need for client action. Understanding alone without action is seen as essentially unproductive. Carkhuff's research appears to represent an attempt to shift self theory toward a position in which the counseling process can be more effectively objectified, as is characteristic of cognitive-behavioral therapy. Moreover, his eclectic position reminds us of the action-oriented position of rational-emotive therapy.

In rational-emotive-behavioral therapy, the client also is given the opportunity to express personal feelings and attitudes. Like other behaviorists who would be more concerned with changing specific attitudes, however, REBT views the client as able to make rational decisions based on thought processes. Although this may appear to differ from self or client-directed theory and does not appear to allow the client to work through feelings toward self-realization, REBT encourages clients to discover the irrational and destructive emotional behaviors that have interfered with their personal growth. They are helped to recognize the incongruities between their irrational attitudes and the realities of their self-potential. As in other forms of counseling, clients learn that it becomes unnecessary to continue to blame external issues or events on their maladaptive behavior and that they have the power and choice to make whatever decisions in their lives that are deemed rational and necessary.

Although classic behavioral counseling emphasizes and uses reinforcement and shaping schedules, with greater attention given to behavioral than attitudinal change, the actual process does not differ that much. Wright and Davis (1994) explore in detail the working relationship that must develop as an essential part of any psychotherapy. Follette, Naugle, and Callaghan (1996) describe how the therapeutic relationship itself may be enhanced by specified behavioral mechanisms that will mediate change but also imply that the client-therapist alliance need not require extensive contact. The implication is that the client must take on more extensive self and social responsibility for change.

In REBT, the self-perpetuating irrational attitudes and behaviors are attacked and ultimately extinguished, even though behaviors may not be changed immediately. Clients certainly differ with regard to their timelines for change and the gradual withering away of self-indoctrinations.

We recognize that, although many significant distinctions may be made among the various behavioral approaches and even more between them and the self theory approach, in terms of therapeutic process, they all share, but in differing degrees, the importance of insight. (It would be inappropriate to delve into a philosophical debate regarding insight as an emotional versus intellectual process, a combination of both, or perhaps indistinguishable; of more importance for the clinician is the consistency and ultimate permanency of change). Weiner (1975) supports this latter contention, adding that insight essentially is both therapist and client generated through the psychodynamic interaction of both parties and prefers to describe the process as "the conscious experience, integration, and modification of unconscious conflicts and past influences so that a change occurs in the person's general framework, enabling a reorganization of information processing and the belief about oneself." Duncan and Solovey (1989) further elaborate on the concept by clarifying the distinctions between client-ascribed meaning and therapist-ascribed meaning as they relate to the emergence of insight; that is, the gradual emergence of meaning based on the accumulation of many interpretations made by both the client and therapist.

The Client-Counselor Relationship

Regardless of theory, probably the most important attribute of counseling therapy is the dynamic interplay of client and counselor. Crucial to this process is the counselor's belief that the client has the ability to cope successfully with all those experiences brought into conscious awareness. A further assumption is that the counselor respects the client and must feel totally nonjudgmental toward and empathic with the client and his or her thought structure. The concept of empathy, in particular, has undergone considerable change within the paradigm of self theory. Rogers's earliest style appeared more as an intellectual restatement of feelings expressed

by his client, as represented in his now classic filmed interview of "Gloria" in 1964 (Rogers and Wood, 1974). Other and more recent writers examine empathy from many perspectives and view the concept as a vital therapeutic ingredient in its own right (Bohart and Greenberg, 1997). What we often found lacking in most of the literature surveyed is any description of empathy as a true feeling-level response by the therapist to feelings expressed by the client. The therapist's response too often is shaped in a cognitive-intellectual and in some cases insincere or inauthentic manner or *coming from the therapist's own beliefs*. It should be noted, however, that Farber, Brink, and Raskin (1996) likely would argue with us that Rogers indeed demonstrated a high degree of empathy with his clients. Duncan and colleagues (1992) describe what they consider the ideal: "empathy is therapist attitudes and behaviors that place the client's perceptions and experiences above theoretical content and personal values" (p. 35). (This assumes, of course, that the therapist is fully conscious of his or her own attitudes, biases, etc.) Mearns and McLeod, (1984) come close, however, in mirroring our concern. Rogers (1995) himself admits, in his final years, that acting as though he were something he was not did not contribute to his relationships. In fact, he found that *acceptance and understanding reduced a desire to rush in and fix things*.

Ideally, an atmosphere is established whereby the client can perceive unconditional regard and true empathic understanding. As these conditions are initiated through the two persons being in contact, the client feels freer to express feelings verbally and motorically. What is most important now is the ability of the counselor to authentically reflect back to the client those feelings expressed. We emphasize here no restatement of content but an expression of actual feelings felt by the therapist manifested in his or her own speech, voice, bodily movement, and other meta-linguistic elements. Crucial to the process is an understanding of another individual without the projection of one's own personality. (Any misinterpretation made of this complex process is clarified more carefully in the final chapter of the text.)

As noted earlier, the client soon begins to express feelings that refer to the self rather than to the nonself or to the feelings and attitudes of others. In doing so, the client differentiates the objects of these feelings and perceptions. They include the environment, other people, perceptions of self, experiences, and how all of these interrelate. The more able the client feels in receiving empathic feedback, the less threatened the person feels in revealing previously feared material. As the client's feelings of vulnerability and anxiety diminish, the therapeutic relationship becomes more congruent, resulting in greater self-regard and more positive changes in behavior. Also engendered are new meanings for the client, so that the context of both their therapeutic and changing real life experiences are enhanced (Duncan et al., 1992).

Although REBT and other behavioral-cognitive approaches are not primarily concerned with motivating clients to express feelings per se, they stress the value in learning about clients' feelings and attitudes that perpetuate their self-defeating behavior. Like self theory, REBT emphasizes the importance of an effective client-counselor relationship and the engendering of trust by the client in the counselor. Behavioral counselors also recognize the importance of being authentic, genuine, and honest with their clients and avoiding coldness, aloofness, and self-righteousness.

Also included is the establishment of a therapeutic atmosphere in which the client feels accepted and recognized as a person who has the potential for change. The key intention is to change the behavioral pattern and not the person. As we discuss later, this has significant implications for those who are communicatively impaired and for counselors who must modify their usual methods regardless of theoretical counseling orientation.

REBT and other behavioral approaches rely more on "teaching" clients new attitudes and behaviors, including the use of confrontation. It then would appear that the empathic aspect might be imperiled, but not if both counselor and client are "in tune" with each other as the therapeutic process develops and unfolds.

The research literature clearly indicates unique differences among the various approaches to counseling, but it also reveals marked similarities, particularly in actual practice. Albeniz and Holmes (1996), in a meta-analysis of over 250 articles on psychotherapy integration found a rapprochement among different theoretical models, a convergence of ideas and methods, eclectic selection from many different schools, and appropriate integration of therapies. They concluded that, at the level of theory, clarification and creative conflict are essential but also that different therapeutic approaches should work closely together yet retain their separate identities. According to Lambert, Shapiro, and Bergen (1986), the outcome literature suggests that, aside from spontaneous remissions accounting for 40% of outcome variance, common factors account for 30% and placebo and specific technique account for 15% of the variance. They reviewed decades of outcome literature, dealing with a wide range of clinical populations in diverse settings, using a variety of research designs. Lambert (1986) asserts, however, that common factors such as genuineness, empathy, and mutual respect likely may account for most psychotherapeutic successes. Patterson (1989) concurs that an eclectic approach, whereby nearly all schools of therapy accept these factors, is most significant toward achieving therapeutic success. Also apparent from the literature reviewed is that the client's positive perception of the relationship itself is a key element in any espoused approach.

What Is and What Is Not Applicable in Counseling the Communicatively Impaired

In the Preface and in the introduction to this chapter, we stated the overall value and necessity of interacting with communicatively impaired individuals on an interpersonal basis. This implies a counseling relationship. The justification for such a relationship with many such individuals and their families has been well documented by Rollin (1988), Mowrer (1988), Klevins (1988), Luterman (1996), Shipley (1996), and Crowe (1997), among others. We believe that, before we can substantiate the efficacy of counseling and which approach is appropriate to use with which communicatively impaired person, we need to discuss those factors that warrant the use of counseling and those that do not. Bear in mind, however, these factors are not mutually exclusive and the uniqueness of the individual disorder, client, counselor, and clinical circumstance often will dictate a course not initially indicated. Our discussion will consider the contrasting principles generally, thereby serving as an introduction to the analysis and application to the pertinent disorders presented in later chapters.

Origin of the Disorder

The decision to intervene psychotherapeutically[2] cannot be determined solely by etiology. Just as communicative disorders that are psychogenic in origin may not necessarily require counseling intervention by the clinician, neither may communicative disorders that etiologically are genetic, neurogenic, or otherwise organic require such intervention.

As speech-language pathologists and audiologists, we place great value on our assessment and case-history-taking procedures in order not only to differentiate among etiologies but to determine also which specific aspects of communication performance are impaired, which are variable, and which are intact. Here is where interview technique is crucial in determining the direction intervention should proceed. Other authors, including Shipley (1996, 1997), Cormier, Cormier, and Cormier (1991), and Cormier and Cormier (1997), have thoroughly described the process and it needs no further elaboration now. Based on the information learned from our clients and their families, we plan pertinent treatment strategies. Because our assessment also informs us of the factors in the past that maintained or continue to maintain the disorder, we consider their significance in the overall treatment plan. What do these premises suggest, what are the parameters, and where might they lead us?

First, it is obvious that, theoretically at least, we tend to regard each individual uniquely, albeit with a tendency toward some generalization and comparison with others. We assume that, as professionals in the field, we view the individual in a holistic manner or as a composite of mind and body and affirm to treat the *person* and not the *disorder*. If this is so and if we are to act consistently within our philosophical and theoretical beliefs, our decision to intervene psychotherapeutically should be based on specific indicators, regardless

of disorder or etiology. The following represent the major indicators:

1. *Present environmental stress related to organicity.* This includes the wide range of neurological, neuromuscular, oral-maxillary-facial-esophageal-laryngeal, and physiological disorders that, either congenitally or adventitiously, create stress for the individual.
2. *Previous physical disability.* Any of the physical disabilities just described is not apparently present but the individual persists in the perception that it is or distorts the reality of its extent.
3. *Previous environmental stress.* This includes the previously listed disorders, as well as continuous or intermittent pressures that the individual experienced earlier but that no longer exist in objective reality.
4. *Present environmental stress.* Here, we refer to the continuous or intermittent pressures or influences of varying degrees from family members, peers, school, job, and so on, related or unrelated to speech, language, and hearing, with which the child or adult client must cope.
5. *Nondescript stress.* The individual cannot identify or describe any external pressures but is stressed by continuous or intermittent undefined self-actuated pressures.
6. *Persistent abuse or misuse of the mechanism for speech and language.* These would include the articulatory, respiratory, phonatory, and resonatory functions. The individual denies any reason for the persistence of the disorder.
7. *Effect on the family.* In this instance, a family member or members are having difficulty or are stressed by the individual's disorder and concomitant features, thereby unintentionally affecting or stressing the individual further.
8. *Multicultural factors.* Cognizant of the dynamics that may be characteristic of varying ethnic families, therapists must be attuned to unique factors that could mitigate, negate, or enhance counseling intervention.

It is obvious that these indicators may overlap and any one should be considered with any other. We further note that each may vary in quality or degree. We also recognize that individuals differ in how they respond to the multidimensional forces in their environment. Most significant, however, is the

---

[2]The use of the term *psychotherapy* henceforth shall be used contextually and synonymously with the term *counseling* where the two tend to overlap.

element of psychological stress that may permeate a personal response to the disorder. Finally, we need to be cautious that we not intervene in a pronounced way, psychotherapeutically, if any indicators do not relate to a communication disorder. It should be apparent, however, that maladaptive behaviors, aside from clearly discernable communicative disorders, will be reflected in these indicators. With this understanding, we turn our attention to how the speech-language pathologists and audiologists, as counselors, decide to intervene psychotherapeutically.

Dealing with Related Issues

The major determining factor that must guide us along the counseling path is the establishment of a definitive relationship between the client's disordered communication and maladaptive psychological behavior or interpersonal dysfunction. This is not as simple as it appears. One obvious consideration is the motivation of the client. Assuming we have established the connection, does it follow that the client will follow suit? Not necessarily, if the client's agenda does not allow psychological probing. In addition, can we assume that psychotherapeutic intervention is appropriate at the time, regardless of verifiable cause-effect relationships and client motivation? No, not if the major overriding element, such as the disorder itself, demands our traditional therapeutic attention..

Second, we need to remember that the initial referral was made for speech-language therapy and not for psychotherapy. This consideration takes on greater significance in the case of young clients whose parents must participate in the therapeutic process. Can we expect these parents to share in a psychotherapeutic approach that may involve probing into their possibly dysfunctional family life?

The reader may now be wondering why we should complicate our professional duties and not follow the traditional practices in which we have been trained. Perhaps this is true, but we might do our clients an injustice in not providing them the best we truly have to offer in terms of a holistic approach to communication competence.

Let us, therefore, identify several guidelines to use in facilitating the decision to intervene psychotherapeutically, assuming that the disorder is related in part at least to psychodynamic issues and recognizing as well the possible obstacles involved. We need to be cautious, however, and refrain from doing so should we have any doubt about our decision.

1. Determine, indirectly, the extent to which environmental influences impinge on the perpetuation of the disorder. Such influences may be revealed during the gradually developing therapeutic relationship.
2. Be sensitive to overt client disclosure of emotional stress, troubled feelings and attitudes about self or toward others.
3. Be alert to undisclosed indicators of emotional distress as revealed through physical illness, moodiness, anxiety, or pronounced depression in the client.
4. With respect to children, in particular, be sensitive to those who are hyperactive with poor attention span, withdrawn, passive, uncooperative, disruptive, inconsiderate, sad, hostile, undisciplined, angry, demanding, rejecting, or fearful.
5. Be cognizant of the child client's relationship to the parents and siblings in terms of mutual disrespect, uncaring, negative verbal or nonverbal communication, and other inappropriate interactions.
6. Recognize excessive parental concern, anxiety, depression, defensiveness, denial, rejection, self-effacement, or inappropriate affect. In the case of adult clients, recognize excessive spousal concern, anxiety, depression, denial, overprotectiveness, mothering or fathering, anger, rejection, or inappropriate affect.

This list certainly is not exhaustive, and we must be cautious not to overinterpret but rather to interpret to the best of our ability those behaviors that are apparent in the client, parents, spouses, and significant others. We must be mindful that the behaviors we describe, in and of themselves, are not necessarily contributory to or manifestations of the communicative disorder with which we are dealing. Only if we gather together all the clues available to us can we decide on an appropriate course of action.

Going Beyond Related Issues

We already inferred that, when there is no apparent link between the communicative disorder and the client's emotional disturbance or dysfunctional psychological behavior, generally it is wise for the clinician to refrain from intervening psychotherapeutically. This rule, although obvious and more clearly justified than in the previous section, nonetheless presents some difficulty. Three questions emerge.

First, can we be certain that there is no underlying connection, and in our avoidance or ignorance of that, may we not be practicing somewhat shortsightedly? Second, how do we cope with the client who insists either consciously or unconsciously on using us and the relationship to ventilate feelings about him- or herself and other life issues unrelated to the disorder? The latter question should not be difficult for the self-assured, sensitive, and empathic clinician, who can gently guide the client back to the initially referred complaint. But, do all of us have the necessary competence to do that effectively? We address this issue later. The answer to the first question is somewhat implied in our answer to the second one, but it demands even greater scrutiny. The third question relates to the client who may resist either symptomatic or psychotherapeutic treatment. How do we define our role in circumstances where we may be interfering with client choice? In any case, our task becomes even more complex when we work with children and their parents.

Speech-language therapy, by its very nature, is interpersonal, unless of course we believe it is necessary to treat only the disorder. Even so, we still are in a relationship with our clients, whether we admit it or not. As Backus (1960) so clearly stated 40 years ago and which is so relevant today,

> In the field of speech disorders we are exhibiting conflicting attitudes regarding a decision to reckon squarely with psychological pressures in human behavior. We are interested and at the same time we are afraid, both for the professional and for personal reasons. There is a threat professionally because we are not trained in this area; and personally, as our own anxiety is stirred. Since most of us have been well integrated enough to pursue successfully our educational aims and to engage productively in professional work, it may be inferred that we have well-developed defenses against anxiety; hence the conflicting attitudes show up less as overt anxiety than as responses of defensiveness against the idea of delving into unconscious processes. There are the commonly heard responses which reflect irritation and then attempt to belittle the idea: "Why do we always have to go around poking around in other people's insides?" "Why

on earth must you make everything psychological?" The defense may take the form of an extreme position in either direction: on the one hand, a pseudo-positive position of intellectualizing about psychological processes, talking about them in clients with studied casualness; on the other hand, an out-and-out negative position, that no one but psychiatrists should be concerned with the depths of human existence.

> The latter attitude is easily recognized as being discrepant when we consider that of necessity we deal with unconscious processes in ourselves and others, both personally and professionally. Our own emotional responses to others together with the ways in which we deal with their behavior, have an impact on them for good or ill. These constitute our own private system of "psychotherapeutic" measures whether we are aware of them as being that or not. So it is not a question of whether we will use psychological tools or not, but rather of the extent to which the psychological tools we are using are in accord with those broad principles which promote or hinder growth. (pp. 507–508).[3]

Determining the Need for Referral

It is clear that the emotional needs of clients demand that we develop our intellectual and personal abilities so that we may make appropriate clinical decisions. Although the task may be formidable and not always carried out successfully, if we at least can attempt to ascertain what is and is not appropriate and in our professional domain, our decision to refer to other mental health professionals will be more reliable.

If we are unable to determine how to proceed, it would be more appropriate to consult with more knowledgeable colleagues who could assist us. We might also decide that we can help our clients through traditional methods regardless of their emotional needs. Whatever our course of action, we need to defend the decision made.

An Eclectic Approach to Counseling the Communicatively Impaired

Earlier, we described several essential similarities among self and person theory, behavioral, and

---

[3]Reprinted with permission from O. Backus, The Study of Psychological Processes in Speech Therapists. In D. Barbara (ed.), *Psychological and Psychiatric Aspects of Speech and Hearing* (Springfield, IL: Charles C Thomas, 1960).

rational-emotive-cognitive approaches to counseling. We also acknowledged that, despite intrinsic differences, in actual practice there appears to be a merger. With this in mind, we wish to take an eclectic position in presenting a counseling approach to be used with the communicatively impaired that is systematic, practical, and realistic.

There are those who view eclecticism as a somewhat amorphous process, akin to grabbing indiscriminately bits of techniques from the widest array of therapeutic schools of thought. We prefer to view eclecticism differently. Albeniz and Holmes (1996) found many effective psychotherapeutic treatments to be integrative or a rapprochement between different theoretical positions. Goldfried and Newman (1986) identify eclecticism in terms of how divergent approaches complement each other; the interactive significance of cognition, behavior, and affect; the need for a common theoretical language; the elaboration of universal meta-theoretical principles of human change; and the desire for an empirically based procedure.

The obvious implication is that all psychotherapeutic relationships are unique and therefore different. Hood (1974), in discussing the client-therapist relationship in communication therapy, declares: "There are quite possibly as many different approaches to the clinical management of communicative disorders as there are therapists who have ventured forth into the arena. Much of whatever skills we possess results from our unique ability to recreate the form to meet a wide variety of clinical cases" (p.46).

We certainly do not advocate the simplistic utilization of ideas taken from several positions without integrating them or endorse the counselor for whom theory has no relevance. Counseling is too complex a process to be conducted in an indiscriminate fashion or treated unidimensionally from one rigid viewpoint. We need to consider, then, how an eclectic approach can best be used in counseling clients.

Counseling as a Relationship

Those of us who have chosen the profession of helping those with communicative disorders as a lifelong career often have been admonished that

"we should not get too involved with our clients." If we stop to consider that warning, we might raise several important questions:

1. What is meant by *involved*?
2. How can we avoid a relationship with our clients?
3. Are we essentially teachers rather than therapists?
4. What is communication therapy without therapist-client communication?
5. How far do we enter a therapeutic relationship within ethical boundaries?

In response to the first question, we understand it to mean that we must refrain from becoming "emotionally" involved with our clients; that is, we must prevent our personal feelings from impinging on our client. Our answer is that few of us can escape being affected emotionally when we respond to the needs of others, unless we are automatons. What is of utmost importance, however, is that we learn to distinguish those feelings that belong to us from those that belong to our clients. Empathizing with our clients is quite different from identifying with them. The not infrequent occurrence of burnout in the helping professions, we believe, in part is due to our inability to distance the integrity of our own emotions from that of our clients, by absorbing their stresses or pain.

We once treated a young woman with bilateral vocal nodules. Although the nodules had been excised surgically, her hoarse voice persisted. During the course of voice therapy in which symptomatic techniques and vocal hygiene instruction were used, she began to express her intense dislike of her voice. Apparently, the feelings were long standing. During one therapy session she asked me, "Will you get into my feelings?" I replied, " No, but I'll help you get into yours." What was most significant is that she understood exactly what I meant, whereupon the path toward reconciling her feelings with a more balanced and effective use of her voice was taken. A revealing footnote to this case was a comment she made toward the close of our final session: "You know, I was always afraid to get into psychotherapy because it meant getting too involved with a complete stranger. But what's been strange about these last six months of therapy is that

I have been involved and yet I haven't. Do you know what I mean?" Although a verbal response may have been unnecessary, I replied, "Yes, and in a sense, it's been the same for me." The point here is that we were able to work together with all of the dynamic factors affecting her use of the voice, yet I refrained from probing too deeply into personal elements that affected other aspects of her life. Interesting, however, was her revelation that her life in general had improved.

Our answer to the second question is that we cannot help but relate whenever we come in contact with another person. It is unlikely that any one of us in our profession would disagree. Yet, the difficulty arises when we attempt to define the process by which we relate and entrap ourselves in analyzing, intellectualizing, and classifying. Kennedy (1977) and Kennedy and Charles (1990), in books written for the " nonprofessional counselor," focus clearly on the meaning of relationship, particularly in terms of the presumption that it is easily understood. They argue that one cannot merely theorize about it but must actually do or perform it. The relationship is interactive, requiring an often complex interaction of stimuli and responses that change moment to moment among the parties concerned.

The field of communicative disorders fortunately has progressed to the point where many of us, including those who practice strictly traditional symptomatic strategies, are less likely to actively *do* something to our clients. We would rather enter into a reciprocal relationship whereby both therapist and client share the responsibility for effecting communicative change.

In answer to the third question, we believe that therapy is teaching, but in the most dynamic sense of the word, whether we are counseling or eliminating /w/ for /r/ substitutions. It does not consist of two people sitting opposite each other separated by a desk or table but of two people alongside each other, attempting to take on a challenge to solve a problem together. Therapy is learning as well, for both client and clinician, in that it is a sharing of information whereby neither person has more power than the other. Even though the knowledge may differ, we have as much to learn about our clients as they do from us. Thus, relieved of the burden of having to come up with all the answers, we

are free to experience something very different with our clients. Certainly, that may include their painful feelings and frustrations. And, if we begin to understand our work as sharing instead of performing, we are less likely to feel intellectually and emotionally pressured and more likely to experience greater self-confidence, more excitement with our client's progress, and a distinct feeling of having contributed something of value for both of us.

We do not suggest that what we have just described is necessarily simple, but neither are personal nor family relationships. They, too, have their highs and lows, like the relationships with our clients. We, therefore, need to be prepared to cope with all of the unexpected therapeutic situations in which we find ourselves. This brings us to question four.

By definition, the communicative interaction we have with our clients is the essence of what our profession is all about and the core of the counseling process. Those of us who have taught in communicative disorder programs are familiar with students who, when confronted with a new and perhaps minimally verbal client, exclaim in panic, "But I don't know what to say to him." As teachers and clinical supervisors, we must admit that spoon-feeding simplistic directives to such students will do little to enhance their relationship with their client and will not contribute toward developing greater competence and confidence in using therapeutic skills effectively. It is better that we ask the student, first, what exactly he or she is anxious about and, second, what is being disclosed by the client's nonverbal communication. Helping the student be responsive to the nonverbal aspects of communication and having that student verbalize what already is known about the client will put the necessary responsibility on that student's attempt to initiate a meaningful relationship.

The fifth question requires considerable self-analysis, which goes beyond the ethical principles very clearly defined by Shipley (1997) and not to be minimized with respect to professionalism. Shipley, however, fails to include what we believe to be of primary value; that is, for the clinician to be able to recognize and objectify to the best of his or her intellectual ability and own emotional awareness, virtually every moment of the therapeutic process taking place, without influencing negatively the client's concept of self and that of the clinician.

Knowing Ourselves in the Relationship

Probably one of the most difficult aspects in all our personal relationships is to be fully aware of what we are, who we are, and what we are feeling when in the presence of others. Kennedy (1977) describes it as the "willingness to listen to what is taking place within ourselves" (p. 6). It means relinquishing for a time our own personal attitudes and ideas so that we can attend fully to the other person. It means opening ourselves to our clients so that they will be less afraid to share the thoughts, ideas, and feelings that trouble them. Bohart and Greenberg (1997) provide us with a plethora of descriptions of the concept of knowing oneself, depending on the school of therapy. We would add this to the process: critically being in tune with what we feel is taking place within the client as well.

In this way we are enabled to learn as much as possible about the client and formulate an objective but not insensitive impression of that person. As the relationship continues, there is a reciprocal flow of communication involving feelings and ideas in which not only the client thrives but the therapist as well.

Transference   An important aspect of the client-therapist relationship is the transference phenomenon, which Freud found to be necessary if therapy is to have a successful outcome. Because we are not concerned with deep psychoanalytic therapy, however, and because many disavow themselves of the concept as posited by Freud (namely, Cooper, 1987, and Gill, 1982), we prefer to describe it in terms of a therapeutic alliance. Luborsky and Crits-Christoph (1998) describe this alliance as consisting of two elements. First, the client must experience the therapist as a warm, caring, and supportive person. The second depends on the idea of working together jointly in a struggle with the elements that are impeding progress. This includes coping with the emergence of feelings directed at the therapist that can be viewed objectively in terms of unresolved and unrecognized attitudes stemming from childhood. Therapists must not misinterpret these as feelings the clients are having toward them

as individuals but as an essential aspect of the ongoing alliance. A naive therapist certainly will distort the alliance by making a personal response. The following excerpt from a clinical interview with a stuttering client illustrates one aspect of transference:

CLIENT: I kept thinking about what you said about my avoidance of speaking situations last time.

THERAPIST: I get a sense you were preoccupied with it?

CLIENT: Yeah, but it was like your voice was always there, telling me that I needed to focus on what I was afraid of.

THERAPIST: Like, somehow, I must have made a very distinct impression on you?

CLIENT: That's right! The way my father was always telling me to speak more slowly when I was a kid.

THERAPIST: Then you've been feeling like that same child again?

CLIENT: In a way, but that's ridiculous because you're not my father.

This abbreviated protocol suggests that the rapport established between therapist and client has provoked considerable feelings that the client is assigning to her therapist. It is as though the therapist may have become somewhat of a father figure for the client, who perhaps is denying the impact of her aroused feelings. Nonetheless this valuable interaction can be enhanced to help the client understand that her feelings are quite natural and to be expected, considering the history of her stuttering.

Ellis and other cognitive-behavioral therapists are unconcerned with transference per se. Ellis views it as an irrational belief that the client feels the need for the therapist's approval and without it is unable to accept him- or herself. Consistent with this approach, the therapist distances and separates personally from the projection (Ellis and Dryden, 1987). We wonder though if, in actual practice, this is indeed possible, particularly when we consider the concept of countertransference.

Countertransference   Opposite to transference, countertransference consists of feelings in the therapist triggered in response to something said or unsaid by the client. These feelings are based on personal past experiences or external events activated within the therapeutic relationship. These feelings are likely to be activated when the client is transferring but also may occur independent of the client's projections. (We discuss this further in Chapter 9.) The important element to understand about countertransference is that it describes something about ourselves. Whether that consists of feelings of powerful attraction, antipathy to the client, or sadness related to our own personal experiences, it reveals aspects of ourselves, our value systems, and therefore we must be conscious of it before we can move ahead therapeutically.

Cognitive-behavioral therapists discount the concept of countertransference, claiming that their therapeutic relationships essentially are thought processes rather than emotional in nature. We do not believe this is possible. Even for symptomatically inclined speech-language-hearing clinicians, it is not unusual to fall prey emotionally to psychodynamic events experienced by client and clinician. These are as likely to occur while teaching language to a five-year-old as while helping an aphasic individual retrieve language. We do not wish to imply that, in such cases, we should attempt to analyze or interpret these feelings to our clients or manipulate their life relationships but only to recognize and understand them so that they do not interfere with ongoing traditional therapy.

The following is an excerpt from a later session with the client discussed earlier, in which an aspect of countertransference may be occurring:

THERAPIST: I get the feeling that you're holding yourself back from that job interview, because you feel you'll fail.

CLIENT: It's not that; it's just that I don't feel ready for it.

THERAPIST: Or that you don't feel you're good enough for the job?

CLIENT: Maybe that's it. But I feel like I'm being pushed into it.

THERAPIST: By me?

CLIENT: Well, that's part of it.

This interaction suggests a very subtle inclination by the therapist to want more for the client than the client can handle at the moment. What is difficult for the therapist is to separate his own expectations for the client from those the client may be uncertain about for herself. Is this my own personal agenda? Do I want her to do it for me or do I want her to do it for herself?

Brammer, Abrego, and Shostrom (1993) provide us specific guidelines to handle transference in counseling relationships and keep it from developing into a deep transference that lies outside the domain of the speech-language-hearing professional. They may be summarized as follows:

1. The client is permitted to feel free to live out projected feelings while being unconditionally accepted by the therapist.
2. Transference feelings may be interpreted directly by the therapist but presented to the client for confirmation.
3. The focus is on feelings expressed in the present without any exclamation as to *why?*
4. The client may respond defensively to the therapist, calling attention to feelings and these should be discussed.
5. Projection by the client should be discussed and the client asked to reverse the projection and encouraged to repeat it, to arrive at the genuine feelings.
6. Finally, the counselor needs to distinguish transference that may emanate from the past from that which may relate to present environmental influences. Should the relationship develop to the degree where the therapist feels overwhelmed, appropriate referral should be made without traumatic rejection of the client.

Active Listening and Understanding

One of the most fundamental principles to learn while training for the field of communicative disorders is the ability to listen critically and objectively to clients' speech, language, and hearing patterns. Typically, the emphasis has been on the "how" of communicating, with less focus placed on the "why" of what is being communicated. This unbalanced approach restricts our ability to understand fully the communicatively disordered person, unless of course we are interested in only the disorder. But, can we really separate the disorder from the person? It is doubtful many of us would reply affirmatively to the question.

We maintain, therefore, that, if we are to be consistent with our belief in treating the individual from a holistic perspective, we need to attend to the entire communicative process of that person. In doing so, we not only help our clients learn to manage their communicative abilities more effectively, we as well learn to be more competent as helpers. In a very real sense, our clients become our teachers, and what we allow ourselves to learn from them could be applicable in dealing with other clients. No academic course could teach us as well. While Shipley (1997) describes aptly the many components of listening and cites various authoritative sources, our approach is to compartmentalize the process less; we prefer a more individualized approach based on the therapist's ability to listen to him- or herself first.

Learning to listen actively and critically is not accomplished faultlessly. Who among us would deny that "to err is human," but we would add that "to err is professional" as well. Frustrating, annoying, painful as that might be, we have the potential for learning much from the errors we make as long as we can tolerate them in ourselves. REBT therapists who must dispel the perfectionistic, catastrophic attitude of the client would most likely agree the same is necessary for themselves, should the client be listened to incorrectly or inaccurately. Self or person theory therapists also would take responsibility for inaccurate active listening and, should clients be thus misunderstood, attempt to understand each client more clearly and precisely. Let us examine a case in point. Mrs. B. is the 55-year-old wife of a minimally aphasic client. She complains of her husband's lack of attempts at communicating:

MRS. B: I don't understand. I try to get him to talk to me—I know he can—but he just seems to be thinking of something else when I talk to him. It's like he really doesn't want to be with me, but I know that isn't so.

THERAPIST: It sounds like you really need nurturing from your husband.

MRS. B (looks at therapist quizzically): No. That's not it at all. I feel frustrated because I hear him talk to his friends on the telephone, and if we're to have any kind of relationship, we need to communicate with each other.

Obviously, Mrs. B. is trying to communicate her frustration about her relationship with her husband. She doesn't know what to do about it and is genuinely worried. The therapist's response is an interpretation and not based on what the client has actually communicated. It is as if the therapist is putting the burden on the client rather than listening to her frustration and her search for a more meaningful relationship with her spouse. In a very real sense, the client is assisting the therapist to understand.

The reader may wonder how and why the therapist has responded to Mrs. B in this way. We submit that the therapist is tuned in to something else not immediately present. Perhaps it is the therapist's own projection or expectations of what the wife's problem *should* be. This agenda is different, apparently, from that of Mrs. B. The therapist obviously has insufficient data to judge, based on the information given. Not only must the therapist listen to the client more attentively but must also listen to himself more acutely and objectively. A more appropriate response could have been as follows:

THERAPIST: It's so confusing to you, yet you know his difficulty really has nothing to do with the affection he feels for you. It's just that you don't want him to cut himself off from you even though he has difficulty in communicating.

An effective way to learn how we listen is to audio- or videotape a full counseling session so that we may sit back and objectify or even feel humiliated about what is occurring. Better yet, ask a supportive colleague to join you. This is difficult to do, because it means learning something of ourselves we may not wish to acknowledge, particularly before colleagues. But, if we are to be effective change agents, we need to be prepared to accept the faux pas we make, learn from them, enlighten our colleagues, and in a real sense allow the client to help us.

A difficulty novice therapists, and perhaps a few professional ones, frequently have is not only listening actively but understanding what their clients are communicating. Instead of focusing on the feeling state expressed, they attend to only the content or the problem being communicated. Our concern, as counseling clinicians, is not to solve the client's problem per se but to attempt to understand the feeling state underlying the problem. Naturally, if the client is struggling to adjust to the output of a hearing aid, it is incumbent on the audiologist to provide the necessary informative guidelines. But, if that same client complains of difficulty in adjusting to wearing the aid—embarrassment, feelings of inadequacy—the counseling therapist must be prepared to switch gears and attempt to understand and reflect the feelings expressed.

This is what we mean by being in relationship to the client—putting oneself into the same life space as the client and remaining totally open to receive whatever the client has to offer, without judging the adequacy, effectiveness, or emotionality of the message. Putting oneself in the place of the client to experience vicariously, what the client may be experiencing or suffering, is not always easy. Certainly we would not wish to trade places, yet we must somehow allow ourselves that sense of "what it must feel like," recognizing our own vulnerabilities. In doing so, we clear our own feelings and thoughts of subjectivity and prepare, more or less, an open slate for the client to bounce feelings off or, as the case may be, scribble on. By its very nature, a relationship is reciprocal and allows therapists to freely offer themselves uncontaminated by egoistic or absolutist "professional edicts." In essence, we are speaking of being authentic, and if we are authentic, the likelihood increases for our clients to feel accepted and authenticated as well. Our chief danger, however, is to lose sight of ourselves as we enter the life space of our clients.

*The Values of the Therapist
and Client Rather Than the Technique*

We have attempted to identify active listening as fundamental to the ongoing client-therapist relationship and a major determinant toward the enhanced well-being of the client. Having done so, we wish to clarify active listening as a process, not a technique. That is, active listening is independent of rigid sets of rules that must be followed in an exact fashion with every client. On the contrary, it is a transaction that occurs between at least two people and is subject to the distinctive nature of each clinical relationship. It further implies that the therapist must be

the determining factor in the dynamic way in which that person responds to the client.

It is not our intention to imply that technique has no place in counseling. We merely maintain that it should not be the focus of what we do or an end in and of itself, but a flexible and creative guide that makes the clinical relationship viable.

Albeniz and Holmes (1996), Hansen et al. (1993), and Avila et al. (1977) present powerful arguments to support the thesis that the clinical interrelationship, and not representative techniques of the various schools, contributes more to helping. They contend that effective and ineffective helpers cannot be distinguished on the basis of methodology but rather in the way they perceive themselves, others, and their clients and the authenticity with which they relate to them.

Guidelines for Facilitating
the Counseling Relationship

We propose a series of general guidelines that speech-language-hearing professionals might follow in facilitating the counseling relationship. Consistent with the eclecticism discussed earlier, we include several aspects of self or person theory and behavioral and rational-emotive-cognitive approaches that lend themselves to appropriate blending. The reader should be aware that the selection of any one or combination of these principles is determined by the unique circumstances of each clinical relationship. We have omitted family systems and existential theory for the moment but include these in later chapters, where applicable.

*Developing the Appropriate
Attitudes Necessary for Critical Listening*

This guideline implies being open to the client's expression of feelings and thoughts and trusting that the client has the capacity to work through problems and the ability to solve them. Although these feelings and thoughts may not necessarily be consistent with the therapist's perception of reality of the situation, they nonetheless represent the client's own way of struggling with his or her own perception of reality. It further implies viewing the client separate from the therapist as a person. McKay, Davis, and Fanning (1983) and Shipley (1997) list several ways in which active listening may be facilitated. Included in their discussions are the use of paraphrasing and clarifying and providing feedback to the client. Total listening implies listening with empathy, openness, and awareness. It implies the necessity for the therapist to verify with the client the accuracy with which the communicative message is being perceived. Nothing should be assumed or taken for granted and, if the therapist has any doubt, questioning should be pursued to better understand what and how information is being communicated.

Viewing the Client as a Person

As clinicians, we need to separate the disorder from the person, in the sense that the disorder is only one aspect of the total behavior of the client and does not represent the true essence of the person. Our perspective, then, implies avoidance of such categorical labels as *stutterer* or *aphasic* as the only means to identify these persons. In this way, we can better respect the total integrity of the individual while attending to the handicapping behaviors as manifested in communication. (At an ASHA national convention many years ago, during a symposium on stuttering, one of the younger speakers alluded to "stutterers," as if to imply they were lepers to be feared. Wendell Johnson, with whom most readers should be familiar, yelled out angrily from that same panel, "we are not stutterers; we are human beings who just happen to stutter.") Respecting the integrity of the individual demands our attention to the following clinician attitudes: (1) respecting the client's need to conceal self-threatening emotional material, (2) being open to and accepting emotional material the client feels a need to express, (3) responding to the client rather than making a "good" response, and (4) responding to the client nonjudgementally.

Being Aware of the
Obstacles to Active, Critical Listening

Because clients are helped through what they experience in relationship with their therapists, barriers

erected to interfere with that knowledge must be brought to conscious awareness. Such barriers would include personal insecurities regarding the clinician's own competency, personal feelings activated by the client's communicative material, and attending to content issues rather than the client's affectual state being communicated. An example of the last is the clinician's unawareness of the dysphagic patient's unsaid terror of suffocating as the clinician attempts in all good faith to feed the patient, even in small quantities. McKay and colleagues (1983) describe 12 blocks that interfere with the therapist's ability to listen effectively. They are identified as:

> (a) comparing the client to oneself; (b) mind reading based on intuition, hunches, and attempting to figure out what the client is *really* thinking and feeling; (c) rehearsing how to respond for the client; (d) filtering out some messages from others; (e) judging statements and behaviors before all the information is available; (f) daydreaming; (g) identifying with the client; (h) advising and not attending to the feelings being communicated; (i) sparring, which includes arguing and debating with the client; (j) being right and rejecting criticism; (k) derailing by avoiding the discomfort or anxiety provoked by the client; and (l) placating. (pp. 16–19)

Viewing Ourselves Realistically

Our own self-understanding as therapists can significantly affect the interpersonal elements that occur in therapy and contribute to the success of the relationship and therapeutic outcomes. It implies self-recognition of the following needs: (1) the need to be liked or appreciated by our client, (2) the need to be perfect or successful in everything we do, and (3) the need to have all the knowledge and answers that are conceivable. Obviously, to have these expectations places an impossible burden on ourselves and our attempts to relate freely to our clients.

Our own struggles as therapists and as human beings require that we strive to accept our limitations, know that we may not necessarily be liked by all our clients, and understand that we may not succeed with all of them. To act otherwise is to present an unreal model to our clients, impossible for them to emulate; further, it places an inordinate amount of stress on ourselves. Our goal, then, is to be authentic with ourselves and clients so that we may be freer to enhance the relationship and therapy.

Valuing Client Choice

The notion that we must do something to our clients in order to facilitate real change is self-aggrandizement, which denies them opportunities to use their own potential for change and growth. We are mere agents who provide the opportunities, possibilities, and means by which they can choose to move in more positive directions for themselves. We need to be prepared also to allow them to struggle with their resistances, uncertainties, and indecisions; yet, at the same time, gently guide them toward the goal they have chosen for themselves. This, obviously, is not so simple when we stop to consider the difficulties we all have in life's choice-making decisions. To do otherwise is to project what we think is best for ourselves onto the other person and thus negate their own values. That the attained goal may not always be consistent with our own expectations is the reality we need to learn to accept as helping professionals. Birdsong (1985) states one aspect of the process very succinctly:

> The more an individual manifests his decision-making abilities the less frantic the world appears to be, the more he becomes involved, the more his creativity is restored to life, the more the individual is encouraged through his own responsibility and performance, the less fervent his world seems to be. As a result, the individual gains, in his sense of power, to keep his energy, creativity, and presence in a constructive mode for making a living creating a life for himself. (p. 151)

Using Client-Therapist Contracting

The use of contracts between client and therapist in counseling and psychotherapy is not new. It consists of a negotiated agreement between both parties in which desired behavioral changes are specified. Clients are taught to analyze and modify their own behavior (Mahoney and Thoresen, 1974; Derisi and Butz, 1975; Moursand, 1990). Contracting allows the therapist and client to decide jointly what goals and expectations are desired, with a clear and objective statement of what the requirements are. It also

consists of an agreement regarding the degree to which a certain behavior will result in a positive consequence. Also, opportunities must be provided to scale downward any expectations or goals the client may choose not to pursue during a particular period of time. Of key importance is setting goals that the client realistically can achieve. Failure to follow through with mutually agreed-on behaviors should be openly discussed so that the client takes full responsibility for the choice in not doing so (Hansen et al., 1977, 1993). The astute clinician will discover that, regardless of psychotherapeutic school of thought, contracting can be applied appropriately and even eclectically.

Using Confrontation

Use of confrontation by the therapist is necessary when incongruency occurs in the following ways: (1) discrepancies between verbal and nonverbal messages, (2) inconsistency between communication and action, (3) discrepancies among a series of messages, (4) variances between statements and feelings, and (5) irrational modes of thinking and behavior.

Here, again, it is necessary for the clinician to use caution in bringing discrepancies out in the open. We may not be certain if the client is unaware of them or consciously is behaving in such a manner as a means to resist exploring certain material. The key is to share with your client the difficulty you are having in understanding the discrepant event. This should be done without judgment, but the client must take responsibility for clarifying exactly what was intended in the message communicated.

Carkhuff and Berenson (1967) aptly describe the use of confrontation on a continuum:

> from a light challenge to direct collision between the therapist and client. It constitutes a challenge to the client to mobilize his resources to take another step toward deeper self-recognition or constructive action in his own behalf. Frequently it will precipitate a crisis that disturbs at least temporarily the client's personal and social equilibrium. Again crises are viewed as a series of self-confrontations. Confrontation is a vehicle that ultimately translates awareness, and insight into action, directionality, wholeness, and meaning in the client's life. A life without confrontation is directionless, passive, and impotent. (p. 172)

Although the counseling clinician may be somewhat skeptical and uncertain about using confrontation, we would point out that, as long as clinicians are clear in their own minds about what may be ambiguous in communicative messages from their client and do not communicate from their own position of self-involvement or projection, confrontation can be a useful tool in aiding the client to become integrated within the totality of his or her experiences.

Understanding Denial and Noncompliance

Somewhat related to confrontation are the concepts of denial and, in particular, noncompliance. The author views the latter as client resistance to following through with contractual arrangements made with the clinician; in particular, the lack of carry through with outside of office assignments originally agreed on. These often get manifested in the form of excuses such as "I forgot about it," "I was too busy," "The wife didn't remind me," "I didn't understand the assignment," "We had a lot of visitors." (The reader surely could come up with even more choices.) McFarlane, Fujiki, and Brinton (1984) and Shipley (1997) provide abundant examples of behaviors that relate to the "difficult" client. Here, again, objectivity and empathy is demanded of the clinician so that the behavior manifested is considered in the context of the overall personality and behavior reflected by the communicative disorder present.

Acknowledging the Value of Therapist Self-Disclosure

Self-disclosure essentially is the sharing of personal information of the self with others. It is apparent that self-disclosure by the client is a necessary condition for the successful consummation of therapy. First defined by Jourard (1958), self-disclosure has been determined to be effective and important for the therapist also (Jourard and Jaffe, 1970). Although classical psychoanalysis theory strongly opposes its use by the psychoanalyst practicing depth therapy, many so-called neo-Freudians today find the practice useful. It appears, though, that the counseling literature defends its use. Apparently, there is a reci-

procal effect in the client-therapist relationship in that clients are more likely to increase disclosure of themselves when their therapists do so as well. It helps to strengthen the empathic attitude, helps to remove artificiality from the relationship, and fosters an "equality among equals" (Weiner 1998; Hackney and Cormier, 1993).

Unfortunately, the speech-language-hearing professional has no definitive guidelines to follow in determining its use, but we do suggest that it is appropriate when there is a mature partnership between client and clinician and when no transference or countertransference is occurring. At best, it is most useful when the therapist can share personal or professional experiences that relate directly to the client's communicative impairment. It has been found to be most helpful when counseling parents of communicatively impaired children or families of brain-injured or aphasic adults who require specific information about the impairment. We are not ruling out the disclosure of material that may be only indirectly related to the impairment. Ultimately, therapists must trust their own mature and professional judgment, but if in doubt about sharing, refrain from doing so.

Blending Symptomatic Strategies with Counseling

The role of speech-language-hearing counselor differs significantly from the role of the typical counselor in the management of therapy. We consider it unwise to focus on the client's emotional struggles unless (1) the client clearly indicates a desire to do so, (2) use of symptomatic strategies is being impeded by covert or overt emotional resistance, or (3) the client requires information necessary for the successful execution of speech-language-hearing therapy. If the therapist is unable to obtain a clear perspective on whether or not to proceed with counseling, it might be necessary to confirm with the client its appropriateness. If clinical rapport already has been established, it is unlikely for the client to feel particularly threatened, since a state of trust already exists. However, if threatened still, the clinician can refrain from any further emotional probing without risk to the relationship. Once there is mutual agreement, though, it is legitimate for the therapist to incorporate both strategies within and among therapy sessions. Such an approach is useful during the formulation, putting into practice, and appraisal of therapy contracts, but it is certainly applicable in less structured clinical environments as well.

Most knowledgeable therapists are keenly aware of the inherent emotional components in most symptomatic strategies used. Not only are clients emotionally affected by the techniques they experience but also by the means with which they are introduced. Most often, encouragement and empathic support are sufficient to neutralize any negative attitudes or responses that may be incurred. Naturally, if such behaviors persist, the therapist should deal with the client patiently and genuinely.

Attending to Body Language and Paralinguistic Cues

We already described how we cannot not communicate with others when in their presence. Therefore, as professionals, we need to be sensitive to and aware of the way our clients communicate through body movements and gestures (kinesics). It is believed by most writers that body language accounts for more than 50% of a message's impact. For this reason it is especially important for us to attend clearly to the facial expressions, gestures, and posturing of our clients, as these will reveal information that may not be derived from the verbal message alone. It is particularly important that, as communication experts, we need to attend critically to the use of vocal components of speech (paralanguage), which includes articulation, phonation, resonation, timing, and rhythm, as they relate to the message being conveyed. We include these irrespective of deficiencies in one or several aspects, which indeed presents a formidable task merely to analyze, much less change. Those who protest that "we know all that" should not confuse their vast knowledge of the basic mechanics of these components with the necessary knowledge of how they interact with each other and with the psychodynamic process of the individual.

Paralinguistic cues refer to the intonational, prosodic, inflectional, and melodic features that are characterized by pitch, length, and loudness, as well as by such vocal qualities as breathiness, thinness, hoarseness, jitter, shimmer, and whining. These cues, along with body language, provide us with the fine nuances of our client's communication, which frequently may be incongruent with the actual words spoken. They also bring to our awareness the actual feeling state of our clients before, perhaps, their own consciousness of it. Possibly, that which we assign to subjective or so-called intuitive judgment are phenomena that can be described objectively and measured scientifically. Several important writers on the subject have already made such significant attempts, among them Birdwhistell (1970), Grinder and Bandler (1976), and Labov and Fanshell (1977).

Conclusion

In this chapter, we draw on the many valuable contributions to the fields of counseling and psychotherapy and begin to apply eclectically the theories and processes to our work with communicatively impaired persons. Those readers who desire or require a more thorough background on the many salient issues raised are referred to the extensive bibliography in the chapter's References section.

Note further that the counseling guidelines presented apply to both children and adults, and although several issues may not be appropriate for each or every case, we assume the astute clinician will modify them as is seen fit and necessary. We also did not distinguish between counseling the communicatively impaired client and that client's spouse, parents, and other family members. Obviously, the perceptive clinician will be able to apply appropriately the principles outlined and discussed to individual situations and circumstances. Subsequent chapters address these and other concerns and answer many of the specific questions raised here.

Of major significance to subsequent discussions on interaction with the family is the research of Bruce, Divenere, and Bergeron (1998), who describe the shift from a client-centered interaction to a more family-centered delivery approach. They describe an innovative approach, involving the training of students in speech-language pathology, to work with parents. While the techniques used were not family-systems-oriented in nature, the students felt the partnership with families were of significant value in fostering meaningful relationships toward resolving communicative impairments in their children. The authors conclude, "In preparing professionals to deliver services to our families, our academic programs have an ethical obligation to create training experiences that instill a philosophy of family-centered intervention" (p. 92).

References

Abravanel E, Sigafoos AD. Exploring the presence of imitation during early infancy. *Child Development.* 1984;55:381–392.

Albeniz A, Holmes J. Psychotherapy integration; its implications for psychiatry. *British Journal of Psychiatry* 169. November 1996;169:563–570.

American Psychiatric Association Task Force on Nomenclature and Statistics. *Diagnostic and Statistical Manuel of Mental Disorders,* 4th ed. Washington, DC: American Psychiatric Association; 1994.

Aronson A. Speech pathology and symptom therapy in the interdisciplinary treatment of psychogenic dysphonia. *J of Speech and Hear Disord.* 1969;34:321–341.

Avila DL, Combs AW, Purkey WW, eds. *The Helping Relationship Sourcebook,* 2nd ed. Boston: Allyn and Bacon; 1977.

Backus O. The study of psychological processes in speech therapists. In: Barbara D, ed. *Psychological and Psychiatric Aspects of Speech and Hearing.* Springfield, IL: Charles. C Thomas; 1960.

Birdsong SJ. *Decision Making: A Component of Learning* [doctoral dissertation]. Ann Arbor: University of Michigan Abstracts; 1985.

Birdwhistell, RL. *Kinesics and Context: Essays on Body Communication.* Philadelphia: University of Pennsylvania Press; 1970.

Bloodstein, O. *A Handbook on Stuttering,* 5th ed. Baltimore, MD: Lippincott Williams and Wilkins; 1995.

Bohart AC, Greenberg LS. *Empathy Reconsidered: New Directions in Psychotherapy.* Washington, DC: American Psychological Association;1997.

Brammer LM, Abrego, PJ, Shostrom EL. *Therapeutic Counseling and Psychotherapy,* 6th ed. Boston: Allyn & Bacon; 1993.

Bruce MC, Divenere N, Bergeron C. Preparing students to understand and honor families as partners. *Amer. J. Sp Lang Path.* 1998;7(3):85–94.

Buber M. *I and Thou,* 2nd ed. New York: Charles Scribner Sons; 1958.

Carkhuff RR. *Helping and Human Relations: A Primer for Lay and Professional Helpers,* Vol. 1: *Selection and Training.* New York: Holt, Rinehart and Winston; 1969a.

———. *Helping and Human Relations: A Primer for Lay and Professional Helpers,* vol. 2: *Practice and Research.* New York: Holt, Rinehart and Winston; 1969b.

———. Helping and human relations. A brief guide for training lay helpers. *J of Research and Dev in Education.* 1971;4(2):17–27.

———. *The Art of Helping.* Amherst, MA: Human Resource Development Press; 1977.

Carkhuff RR, Berenson BG. *Beyond Counseling and Therapy.* New York: Holt, Rinehart and Winston; 1967.

Cooper AM. The transference neuroses: a concept ready for retirement. *Psychoanalytic Inquiry.* 1987:7569–7585.

Cooper E. *Modern Techniques of Vocal Rehabilitation.* Springfield. IL: Charles C Thomas; 1973.

Cormier WH, Cormier LS. *Interviewing Strategies for Helpers: Fundamental Skills and Cognitive Behavioral Interventions.* Pacific Grove, CA: Brooks/Cole Publishing Co.; 1997.

Cormier B, Cormier LS, Cormier WH. *Interviewing Strategies for Helpers: Fundamental Skills and Cognitive Behavioral Interventions.* Pacific Grove, CA: Brooks/Cole Publishing Co.; 1991.

Crowe TA, ed. *Applications of Counseling Speech-Language Pathology and Audiology.* Baltimore: Williams and Wilkins; 1997.

Culpepper B, Mendel LL, McCarthy PA. Counseling experience and training offered by ESB-accredited programs. *ASHA.* 1994;36:55–57.

DeBell CS, Harless DK. B. F. Skinner: Myth and Misperception. *Teaching of Psycholog.* 1992;19(2):68–73.

Derisi WJ, Butz G. *Writing Behavioral Contracts: A Case Simulation Manual.* Champaign, IL: Research Press; 1975.

Duncan BL, Solovey AD. Strategic brief therapy: an insight-oriented approach? *J of Marital and Family Therapy.* 1989;15:1–9.

Duncan BL, Solovey AD, Rusk GS. *Changing the Rules: A Client-Directed Approach to Therapy.* New York: Guilford Press; 1992.

Ellis A. *Reason and Emotion in Psychotherapy.* New York: Lyle Stuart; 1962.

Ellis A, Dryden W. *The Practice of Rational Emotive Therapy.* New York: Springer; 1987.

Ellis A, Gordon J, Neenan M, Palmer S. *Stress Counseling: A Rational Emotive Behaviour Approach.* New York: Springer, 1997.

Ellis A, Grieger R. *Handbook of Rational-Emotive Therapy.* New York: Springer-Verlag; 1977.

Farber BA, Brink DC, Raskin PM, eds. *The Psychotherapy of Carl Rogers.* New York: Guilford Press; 1996.

Follette WC, Naugle AE, Callaghan GM. A radical behavioral understanding of the therapeutic relationship in effecting change. *Behavior Therapy.* Fall 1996;27(4).

Gill M. *Analysis of Transference* (vol 1). New York: International Universities Press; 1982.

Goldberg SA. *Behavioral Cognitive Stuttering Therapy.* Tigard, OR: C.C. Publications; 1981.

Goldfried MR, Newman C. Future directions in psychotherapy integration. In: Norcross JB, ed. *Handbook of Eclectic Psychotherapy*. New York: Brunner/Mazel; 1986:463–484.

Grinder A, Bandler, R. *The Structure of Magic II*. Palo Alto, CA: Science and Behavior Books; 1976.

Hackney H, Cormier LS. *Counseling Strategies and Interventions*, 4th ed. Boston: Allyn and Bacon; 1993.

Hansen JC, Stevic RR, Warner RW Jr. *Counseling: Theory and Practice*, 2nd ed. Boston: Allyn and Bacon; 1977.

Hansen JC, Rossberg RH, Cramer SH (contributor), Hansen JH. *Counseling: Theory and Process*. Boston: Allyn and Bacon; 1993.

Hood SB. Clinicians and therapy. In: Emerick LL and Hood SB, eds. *The Client-Clinician Relationship*. Springfield, IL: Charles C Thomas; 1974.

Jourard SM. *Personality Adjustment: An Approach Through the Study of Healthy Personality*. New York: Macmillan; 1958.

Jourard SM, Jaffe PE. Influence of an interviewer's disclosure on the self-disclosure behavior of interviewees. *J of Counseling*. 1970;17:252–257.

Kennedy E. *On Becoming a Counselor: A Basic Guide for Non-Professional Counselors*. New York: Seabury Press; 1977.

Kennedy E, Charles SC. *On Becoming a Counselor: A Basic Guide for Non-Professional Counselors,* rev. ed. New York: Continuum Press; 1990.

Klevins DR. Counseling strategies for communication disorders. In: Curlee RF, ed. *Seminars in Speech and Language*. New York: Thieme, 1988;9(3):145–208.

Labov W, Fanshell D. *Therapeutic Discourse: Psychotherapy as Conversation*. New York: Academic Press; 1977.

Lambert MJ. Implications of psychotherapy outcome research for eclectic psychotherapy. In: Norcross JC, ed. *Handbook of Eclectic Psychotherapy*. New York: Bruner/Mazel; 1986:436–462.

Lambert MJ, Shapiro DA, Bergen AE. The effectiveness of psychotherapy. In: Garfield SL, Bergin AJ, eds. *Handbook of Psychotherapy and Behavior Change,* 3rd ed. New York: Wiley; 1986:157–212.

Lattal KA. B. F. Skinner and psychology: introduction to the special issue. *Am Psychologist*. November 1992;47:1269–1583.

Levant RF, Shlien JM, ed. *Client-Centered Therapy and the Person-Centered Approach: New Directions in Theory, Research, and Practice*. New York: Praeger; 1984.

Lincoln M, Onslow M, Lewis C, Wilson, L. A clinical trial of an operant treatment for school-age children who stutter. *Am J Sp Lang Path*. 1996;5:73–84.

Luborsky L, Crits-Christoph P. *Understanding Transference: The Core Conflictural Relationship Theme Method*. Washington, DC: American Psychological Association; 1998.

Luterman DM. *Counseling Persons with Communication Disorders and Their Families*, 3rd ed. Boston: Little Brown; 1996.

Mahoney MJ, Thoresen CE. *Self-Control: Power to the Person*. Monterey, CA: Brooks/Cole; 1974.

Maslow AH. *Toward a Psychology of Being*, 2nd ed. New York: Van Nostrand Reinhold; 1968.

McFarlane SC, Fujiki M, Brinton B. *Coping with Communicative Handicaps: Resources for the Practicing Clinician*. San Diego, CA: College Hill Press, 1984.

McGinn LK. Interview: Albert Ellis on rational emotive behavior therapy. *Am J of Psychotherapy*. Summer 1997;51(3):309–316.

McKay M, Davis M, Fanning P. *Messages: The Communication Book*. Oakland, CA: New Harbinger Publicaions; 1983.

McWhirter EH. Empowerment, social activism, and counseling. *Counseling and Human Development*. April 1997; 29(8):1–14.

Mearns D, McLeod J. A person-centered approach to research. In: Levant RF, Shlien JM, eds. *Client-Centered Therapy and the Person-Centered Approach; New Directions in Theory, Research, and Practice*. New York: Praeger; 1984.

Meltzoff AN, Moore MK. Newborn infants imitate adult facial gestures. *Child Development*. 1983;54:702–709.

Menacker J. Toward a theory of activist guidance. *Personnel and Guidance Training*. 1976;54:318–321.

Moursand J. *The Process of Counseling and Therapy*. Englewood Cliffs, NJ: Prentice-Hall; 1990.

Mowrer DE. *Methods of Modifying Speech Behaviors: Learning Theory in Speech Pathology*. Columbus, OH: Charles Merrill; 1977.

———. *Methods of Modifying Speech Behaviors: Learning Theory in Speech Pathology,* 2nd ed. Prospect Heights, IL: Waveland Press; 1988.

O'Hara M. Carl Rogers: Scientist and mystic. *J of Humanistic Psychology*. Fall 1995;35(4):40–53.

Onslow M, Packman A. The Lidcome Program of Early Stuttering Intervention. In: Ratner NB, Healy CE, eds. *Stuttering Research and Practice: Bridging the Gap*. Hillsdale, NJ: Lawrence Erlbaum Associates; 1999.

Owen IR. Boundaries in the practice of humanistic counseling. *British Journal of Guidance and Counseling*. 1997;25(2):163–174.

Patterson CH. Foundations for a systematic eclectic psychotherapy. *Psychotherapy*. 26(4):427–435.

Rogers CR. *Counseling and Psychotherapy*. Boston: Houghton Mifflin; 1942.

———. *Client-Centered Therapy*. Boston: Houghton Mifflin; 1951.

———. A theory of therapy, personality, and interpersonal relationships as developed in the client-centered framework. In: Koch S, ed. *Psychology: A Study of a Science, Formulations of the Person, and the Social Context*. New York: McGraw-Hill; 1959.

———. What understanding and acceptance means to me. *J of Humanistic Psychology*. Fall 1995; 35(4):7–22,23–39.

———. *On Becoming a Person: A Therapist's View of Psychotherapy*. Boston: Houghton Mifflin; 1961.

Rogers CR, Wood JK. The changing theory of client-centered therapy. In: A Burton, ed. *Operational Theories of Personality*. New York: Brunnel/Mazel; 1974.

Rollin WJ. Counseling spouses of the communicatively impaired. In: Curlee RE, ed. *Seminars in Speech and Language*. New York: Thieme; 1988;9(3):269–282.

Ryan B, Van Kirk Ryan B. Programmed stuttering therapy treatment for children. Comparison of two establishment programs through transfer maintenance and follow-up. *J of Speech and Hear Research*. 1995;38: 61–75.

Schlien J. *Client-Centered Therapy and the Person-Centered Approach*. New York: Praeger; 1984.

Schoenfeld WN. The Necessity of "Behaviorism." *Educational-Technology*. October 1993;33(10):5–7.

Shipley KG. *Interviewing and Counseling in Communicative Disorders: Principals and Procedures*, 2nd ed. Boston: Allyn and Bacon; 1996.

Shipley KG, Wood JM. *The Elements of Interviewing*. San Diego, CA: Singular Publishing Group; 1997.

Skinner BF. *Science and Human Behavior*. New York: Free Press; 1953.

———. *Beyond Freedom and Dignity*. New York: Knopf; 1971.

Stivers E, Whelen S, eds. *The Lewin Legacy: Field Theory in Current Practice*. New York: Springer-Verlag; 1986.

Walsh F. The concept of family resilience: crisis and challenge. *Family Process*. 1996;35(3):261–281.

Watzlawick P, Weakland, JH, Fisch, R. *Change; Principles of Problem Formation and Problem Resolution*. New York: W. W. Norton; 1998.

Weiner IB. *Principles of Psychotherapy*, 2nd ed. New York: Wiley; 1998.

Williams D. A point of view about stuttering. *J of Speech and Hearing Disorders*. 1957;22:390–397.

Wilson L. A clinical trial of an operant treatment for school-age children who stutter. *Am J of Speech Lang Path*. 1996;5:73–84.

Wright JH, Davis D. The therapeutic relationship in cognitive-behavioral therapy: patient perceptions and therapeutic responses. *Cognitive and Behavioral Practice*. 1994;1.

Zeiss AM, Steffen A. Treatment issues with elderly adults. *Cognitive and Behavioral Practice*. 1996;3(2).

2

Psychological Considerations
for Aphasic Adults and Their Families

Introduction

The field of aphasiology has long recognized the traumatic and devastating impact on the family and on the individual who has suffered a cerebral vascular accident. The neurological, physical, and linguistic effects have been and are still investigated by neurologists, psychiatrists, psychologists, neuropsychologists, speech-language pathologists, and psycholinguists, among others. Considerably less attention has been given to the study of the etiology, nature of, and treatment for adult aphasia from the perspective of psychosocial dynamics. Unfortunately, the research often has been characterized by the methodological problems associated with descriptive studies and the subjectivity of anecdotal accounts. The experimental studies also have suffered from difficulties with diverse population variances, measurements of personality behavior, and well-meaning speculative conclusions. Even the outcome studies related to therapeutic success raise more questions than the answers found. Skillbeck (1996) contends that too little research has been devoted to the psychological aspects of CVA and provides us with a rationale for psychological services. Nevertheless, it is hoped that readers will consider the intrinsic values to be gained from the research already done and add to their knowledge and understanding of the real world of aphasia. Birkett (1996) provides us current clinical data on the

psychiatry of stroke and attempts to link neuropsychiatry's emphasis on the physical correlates and social psychiatry's focus on interpersonal and socioeconomic consequences of CVA.

We confine our discussion to psychological aspects, with only tangential references to purely neurological, cognitive-linguistic correlates, assessment, and typical treatment procedures. In doing so, we can explore better the many psychosocial dimensions, from the psychogenesis of aphasia, through personality and behavioral changes, to psychotherapeutic treatment strategies.

Psychogenesis of Cerebral Vascular Disease

During the last 30 years, medical science gradually has begun to consider the multiple elements—invasive, genetic, and psychosocial—that, combined, can change the human organism and create an internal environment conducive to pathological alterations. Our discussion first centers on the psychogenic aspects; namely, psychosocial stress. This we define as a psychophysical reaction characterized by agitation or physiological changes, or both, in response to provocative environmental stimuli. While some stress is healthful and necessary to keep us alert and occupied, when too intense it overtaxes our adjustive capacity, dampens our mood, and has harmful effects (Eckenrode, 1984).

Stress as the Hidden Precursor

Goldberger and Breznitz (1993) in reviewing the literature on stress first describe *stressors* as conditions or external events that affect human organisms. What they describe realistically and clearly is that particular stressors do not necessarily affect individuals similarly and, in fact, may have little or no adverse effect on some. McEwen and Mendelson (1993) describe evidence suggesting important structural and neurochemical features of the brain are modified by stress and the concomitant glucocorticoids or adrenal steroids found in the hippocampus and other brain areas. The very complex interrelationships among these and other biochemical and morphological changes that occur may likely have a deleterious effect in the onset and development of degenerate disease processes. In a later study, McEwen (1999) confirms earlier investigations, demonstrating that high levels of stress hormones can weaken hippocampal brain cells, or neurons, leaving them more likely to die if their oxygen supply is interrupted, which happens during a CVA.

Hans Selye, perhaps the most noted stress researcher, was the first to describe the *general adaptation syndrome* (GAS) in his research with animals. *Alarm* is the initial response to a stressor, with the body having a generalized stress arousal. Since no organism could sustain the alarm response, it later moves into the *stage of resistance*, wherein other biophysiochemical changes occur. The final stage is *exhaustion*, where either adaptation occurs (assuming the original stressor is no longer present) or the organism is adversely affected, with the body "just worn out" (Selye, 1976).

While stress can be viewed as a factor triggering an array of organismic reactions leading to illness, coping reactions actually may lead to physical recovery involving adaptive behavior and personal growth. Felton, Revenson, and Hinrichsen (1984) found that cognitive restructuring or learning new behaviors was associated with good adjustment patterns in patients with hypertension, diabetes, and rheumatoid arthritis. The implication, while not conclusive, is that these individuals were more likely to improve physically or, at best, become better stabilized. Other research has revealed that positive confrontive responses to stress and an optimistic attitude can exert direct control over an illness (Scheir, Weintraub, and Carver, 1986; Burgess, Morris, and Pettingale, 1988; Affleck et al., 1987).

The relationship of cardiovascular disease and the Type A behavior pattern—"excessive drive, aggressiveness, ambition, involvement in competitive activities, frequent vocational deadlines, and enhanced sense of time urgency"—has been well documented (Jenkins, Rosenman, and Friedman, 1967; Jenkins, 1976). Their early research has evolved into the development of the JAS (Jenkins Activity Scale), a self-report screening instrument to measure a specific pattern of behavioral thought that would relate to an inclination toward coronary disease (Williams et al., 1980). More recently, Matthews (1988) using meta-analysis demonstrated that Type A behavior was associated significantly with coronary heart disease when data was drawn from studies using the SI (Stress Interview) developed by Friedman and Rosenmann (1959). Throughout the literature surveyed has been the suggestion that hostility and anger are strongly related to coronary artherosclerosis.

Virtually little stress research has been done, however, relating coronary stress patterns to hypertension and cerebral vascular disease. House et al. (1990), in a study involving 113 patients who first were interviewed regarding the year prior to their stroke and reinterviewed a year later, found that at least 24% of the sample group had experienced stressful life events extending back over 6 months. Ormel et al. (1997) obtained data from a population-based cross-sectional survey of 5078 noninstitutionalized, late middle-aged and older Dutch persons. Although a variety of major medical conditions and sensory impairments were studied, they found cerebral vascular disease and cardiovascular disease had particularly strong associations with stress. They determined that not only the nature of the condition determined psychological distress but the psychological characteristics of the patient. Bjorntorp (1997), based on his research and reviewing the work of others, helps to confirm that noxious factors such as psychosocial and socioeconomic handicaps may lead to a defeatest reaction in individuals who have suffered a stroke or heart attack. This reaction is described in terms of how these patients perceived stress with associated endocrine abnormalities.

Kim et al. (1998), in the most recent research of type A behavior, administered a questionnaire developed by Eysenck and Faulkner (1982) to 224 patients with acute stroke without aphasia. Using multiple logistic analysis, ruling out other precursors of infarction, they found a significant relationship between psychological tension and large vessel infarction.

Researchers at the University of Cincinnati Medical Center estimated that more than 700,000 first-ever and recurrent strokes occur each year in America—40% more than the usually quoted figure of 500,000. The researchers say that their study reflects the country's racial and economic diversity. They confirm other studies that identify strokes occurring in African-Americans at almost twice the rate it does in whites. Statistically extrapolating their findings to the U.S. population, the researchers estimate that, during 1996, there were 138,000 strokes among African-Americans and 593,000 among all other people (Broderick et al., 1998). Our earlier discussion regarding the relationship among stress factors and lower economic status would tend to support the findings of the Cincinnati group.

While the relationship between stress and hypertension continues to be subject to complex study, little doubt remains that stressful situations will alter the homeostatic state in certain individuals and thereby compromise those persons physically, neurologically, and further physiologically (Obrist, 1981). We cannot ignore the possibility that cerebral vascular disease, stress, and hypertension come together in a yet undefinitive paradigm. Implied in this analysis would be a breakdown in the organism's immune system. Any further discussion of the latter, however, would go beyond the scope of the present text.

Individual and Family Life Factors

Our present understanding of risk factors associated with cardiovascular disease has led us to identify those factors relating to cerebral vascular disease. These include high serum cholesterol, smoking, obesity, high-saturated-fat diet, lack of exercise, and drugs. The frequent use of mind-altering drugs has been found to be a major contributor to stroke, which might explain its growing incidence among the 45-year-old and under population.

Because few longitudinal studies, like the Framingham study on cardiovascular disease (Kannel, Sorlie, and Gordon, 1980), have been conducted, we can only speculate on the significance of individual and family life factors and how these relate to hypertension. In doing so, we need to bear in mind that the Type A behavior pattern does not equate with personality and emotional factors per se. It appears more likely that the interplay of certain behaviors and emotional responses within the work and home environment bear greater examination. The Psychiatric Epidemiology Research Interview Life Events Scale developed by Dohrenwend et al. (1987) has been a major contribution to the measurement of stressful life events. Although the authors admit to the scale's technical weaknesses, it is nonetheless methodologically rigorous. Among the major stressful circumstances studied were physical exhaustion from illness or injury, loss of social support, and ominous negative events.

While the research relating psychosocial factors (namely, stress) has been far from abundant with respect to cerebral vascular disease, some social stressors require attention:

1. *Marital status:* Divorce, separation, death of a spouse, marital conflict.
2. *Job:* Loss or change of job, greater responsibilities, fewer responsibilities, forced or unforced retirement.
3. *Finances:* Diminished, increased.
4. *Parenting:* Rejection by or conflicts with children; death of an adult child.
5. *Aging and illness:* Depression or anxiety associated with these factors.

It is obvious from the extensive research on stress that a mere combination of reported stressful events is insufficient to account for incipient disease processes. A more fruitful approach has been for researchers to consider not only the role of particular combinations of events within specified periods of time but to relate these to personality and constitutional components.

We believe, however, that the dynamic way or the style with which the organism, effectively or ineffectively, copes with stress will determine, in part, vulnerability to certain disease processes. This is not to suggest that specific traumatic events like the death of a spouse would not induce a high degree of stress in the significant other, but *how* that person adapts to the stress is of crucial concern. Goldberger and Breznitz (1993) emphasize the importance of individual differences and view personal cognitive appraisal as playing a major role in the interaction between the individual and the potentially stressful environment.

Specific Behavioral Indicators and Measures for Prevention

Regardless of the uncertainties about stress-induced hypertension and its connection to CVA, we have to consider the specific behavioral indicators, if any, that would move us to predict infarctions. Frequently, prior to a massive CVA, the individual may suffer a minor or little stroke that does not handicap seriously the person nor is brought to the attention of others, family or physician. Such an episode may be a temporary interruption of the blood supply to a vessel or vessels within the brain, commonly known as a transient ischemic attack (TIA). This sometimes is referred to as a *silent stroke*, since there may be no apparent or overt physical symptoms. More typically, though, it may be characterized by a temporary drooping of the corner of the mouth, brief tingling or numbness in an arm or leg, transient blurring or loss of vision, dizziness, or temporary disturbance of speech.

Nagaratnam and Pathma (1997) describe several psychiatric and behavioral symptoms in relation to silent cerebral infarctions. They identify four symptom clusters including affective, paranoid, delusional, and confusional states. Also included in their findings are mood disturbances. While the researchers are uncertain of the mechanisms involved, they theorize biochemical alterations involving neurotransmitter mechanisms, vascular changes, or structural damage. They clearly point out, however, that cause and effect relationships are yet unclear. Lawlor and Anderson (1995) found that minor cerebrovascular lesions, such as deep white matter lesions, lacunar infarcts, and silent cerebral infarction, can be demonstrated in some late-onset depressives and may be relevant to the development of depression or associated with the persistence of symptoms and the emergence of treatment resistance. They advise treatment strategies to address underlying vascular risk factors to reduce the likelihood of fatal strokes.

We have interviewed, in 45 years of practice, countless numbers of family members of patients who had suffered a stroke and who reported the following uncharacteristic changes to have occurred during the months or weeks prior to the infarction:

1. *Moodiness and depression:* Withdrawal from other family members and unwillingness to speak as frequently as usual for that person; disinterest in activities typically enjoyed.

2. *Anxiety and tension:* Uncharacteristic outbursts of inappropriate anger, agitation, or restlessness; profuse frustration over minor or major like events that are unpleasant and over which they may have little control, such as a toaster that does not work or a well that goes dry; more typical might be the overreaction to adult children's behavior that is unacceptable to the victim.

3. *Preoccupation with insignificant details or objects:* Characterized by staring off into space, inattentive to spouse; contemplating or gazing at generally uninteresting objects, such as a bowl of fruit, perhaps even attempting to ingest artificial fruit; watching a TV program the person typically dislikes.

4. *Short-term memory loss:* Characterized by forgetting such events as driving home from work when indeed they had done so only one hour before.

5. *Long-term memory loss:* Forgetting a grandchild's birthday for the first time; forgetting a personal wedding anniversary or a visit to an adult child the previous month.

6. *General forgetfulness and disregard of bodily needs*: Failure to wash themselves or brush their teeth unless reminded by the spouse; wearing the same clothes day after day; confusion with numbers, day of the week, month of

the year; getting lost in otherwise familiar surroundings.

7. *Emotional flatness:* The person's countenance
   appears masklike, uncharacteristically unex-
   pressive verbally, phlegmatic or lethargic,
   physically inactive and unresponsive to others,
   including immediate family members.
8. *Denial:* The person denies any need to be conscious of changes or correct any of the behaviors just identified, particularly by the spouse or
   other family members; feels rejected or
   negated, testy, defensive, sometimes becoming
   infuriated to the point of rage.
9. *Subtle physical or soft signs:* Intermittent light-
   headedness and distortions of vision unilater-
   ally or bilaterally; loss of balance and bumping
   into objects or falling; brief moments of memory lapses and confusion; occasional inappropriate word usage or word distortions.
10. A *general feeling of uneasiness:* The person
    complains of "just not feeling like myself" or
    "something's going on I can't put a handle on."

Conceivably, such behavioral indicators may be
related to one or several TIAs or cognitive regression related to concomitant early generalized
dementia or Alzheimer's disease and need to be
brought to the attention of a physician. Too often,
however, the family is brushed off with the
response: "What can you expect at his age? We'll
all get like that!" Such a response demands another
medical opinion. What needs to be examined is the
possibility that these behavioral changes may occur
in conjunction with the stress-inducing life events
previously discussed, regardless of, or connected
to, our earlier comments. Because any one or combination of these behaviors may be a warning signal for an imminent thrombosis or hemorrhage, a
neuropsychiatric examination including magnetic
resonance imaging (MRI); computerized tomography (CT), single photon emission tomography
(SPECT), or positron emission computerized
tomography (PET) scans; or carotid endarectomy
may be necessary. Included perhaps could be anti-
coagulant medication, hypertension control, and
nutritional counseling. Ideally, a cardiovascular
specialist should be included in the comprehensive
workup. We hope that a skilled and sophisticated
physician will recommend individual and or family counseling, particularly if stress factors appear
evident.

Psychological Factors Subsequent to Cerebral Vascular Disease

The neurological, physical, physiological, and psycholinguistic changes produced by a CVA have
been well documented by empirical and clinical
research conducted over the last 60 years and are
reported in Sarno (1991), Kirschner (1995), Brookshire (1997), Ferrand (1997), Visch-Brink and Bastiaanse (1998), and especially Geschwind (1997).

Changes of Affectual State: Neurological versus Psychological

We already stated that only recently have
researchers and therapists begun to acknowledge
the significance of the psychodynamic effects on
individuals who have suffered a CVA. As early as
1942, Goldstein (1942) held the view that many of
the symptoms of brain damage are manifestations
of the patient's changed personality "and also an
expression of the struggle of the changed personality to cope with the defect and with the demands it
can no longer meet." He also believes that the corti-
cally impaired individual would have a "catastrophic reaction" or sudden and pronounced
change in behavior when confronted with tasks he
or she was unable to perform, resulting in "disordered behavior and anxiety" (1942, 1948). Goldstein, representing a holistic perspective, believes
that the patient's psychological instability is an
essential aspect of neurobiological changes. We
consider these latter factors first.

Neurological Changes

Lamendella (1977), in an extensive review of the
role the limbic system plays in human communication behavior, considers this system responsible for
most nonpropositional speech and language as well.
Evidence is presented that connects the communication and social function in primates to the limbic
system. According to Lamendella, the dominant left
hemisphere in some way inhibits affective function.

He sees automatic speech to be relatively unaffected when there is damage to the left hemisphere, with resultant disordered propositional language. A major reason is that automatic speech derives from areas within the limbic, thalamic, basal ganglia, or midbrain structure. He refers specifically to automatic speech of the scatological type, which he believes to originate in the limbic system.

Examining patterns of regional cerebral blood flow (RCBF) in 18 patients with major depressive disorder in late life, found using SPECT and hexamethylpropylenamine oxime (HMPAO), Awata et al. (1998) found dysfunction of the limbic system, the cerebral association cortex, and the caudate nucleus. They speculate that such findings may be implicated in late-life depression and that hypoperfusion, especially in the anterior cingulate and the prefrontal regions, may relate to persistence and exacerbation of depression.

Sackeim and Weber (1982), after reviewing earlier studies, suggest that, in many cases, affective changes subsequent to brain lesions may be secondary or psychological reactions to deficits in other areas:

> It would not be surprising, for instance, to observe depression in a patient with left-side damage who is paralyzed and aphasic. Second, even if mood change in many of these cases is produced directly by changes in brain functioning, linking side of damage to type of mood change does not explicate the role of each side of the brain in subserving the altered emotional state. Unilateral destructive lesions may disinhibit emotional behavior subserved by the same or opposite side of the brain. (p. 85)

Sackeim and Weber (1982) also found that both hemispheres of the brain differ in subserving contrasting emotional states. In Wernickes-type patients they found euphoric behavior, particularly in the acute phase. They suggest that mood changes are perhaps secondary reactions to associated sensorimotor and cognitive deficits rather than a direct result of brain mechanism disruption. In the same study, they found laughing and crying to be evident in 16 of 22 patients with bilateral damage.

Among their conclusions are that indifferent-euphoric reactions and uncontrollable laughing are consequences of right-side lesions. Dysphoric reactions and uncontrollable crying are consequences of left-side lesions. They further add that emotional behavior is "subserved by integrated networks comprising cortical and subcortical regions." They finally conclude with the possibility that the expression of positive and negative emotions may reflect asymmetries in the content of, or responses to, particular neurotransmitters in the two sides of the brain.

More recently, Heilman (1997) theorizes that the cortex is critical in regulating activities of the limbic system, basal ganglia, and reticular system. He sees the frontal lobes mediating both positive and negative experiences. The right hemisphere, particularly the parietal lobe, is important in activating arousal systems and motor activity; and the left hemisphere modulates inhibition of these systems. While not addressing cerebral infarctions per se, it would be difficult to rule out unique emotional experiences as sequelae to disturbed patterns of neural activation in the modular network described by Heilman. Mega et al. (1997) present a model of limbic function in which there is an implicit integration of affect, drives, and object associations involving thought, feeling, and action. Understanding the complex development and organization of the system becomes especially important if the system breaks down and should help to inform us how best to care for patients who are neuropsychiatrically impaired.

Cummings (1997) reveals a wide variety of neuropsychiatric syndromes associated with right brain dysfunction, including bipolar manic-depression, psychosis, hallucinations, personality changes, anxiety, dissasociative states, and altered sexual behavior. It should be noted that Cummings's work is based mainly on individuals and case study. What is interesting to note, however, is that he found most neuropsychiatric syndromes associated with damage to the limbic system. (It should be noted, however, that Cummings's research includes cases with traumatic head injury, which will have greater relevance in the next chapter.)

Spencer, Tompkins, and Schulz (1997), in their comprehensive study of depression in poststroke victims, found the methodological limitations involved that contribute to conflicting outcomes and conclusions when attempting to assess depression. They offer suggestions for improving the specificity, consistency, validity, and reliability of assessment methods and procedures when investigating depression.

Probably one of the more significant philosophical and illuminating positions, based on years of research, is posed by Geschwind (1997), who for many years, until his death, held the belief that organicity could not be separated from functionality and that any disease of the brain is an important and a frequently treatable cause of behavior disorders. He cautions us, however, that specific sites of lesions of the brain do not necessarily dichotomize the affected individual into specific acting behaviors. He clearly emphasizes the importance of careful use of differential diagnosis before designing a program of treatment.

Psychological Changes

In discussing the psychological changes that manifest themselves following a CVA, we need to bear in mind the difficulty of isolating such changes from neurobiological alterations. Goldstein (1959) recognizes the complexity of such a relationship by associating the loss of abstract attitude or cognitive processing with personality deviations. Eisenson (1984) reinforces Goldstein's findings that personality changes accompany impairment of the abstract ability and states that "our clinical impression is strong that many aphasics who become predominantly concrete and ego-oriented in their behavior were premorbidly so inclined" (p. 90).

Consistent with the psychobiological reactions discussed previously, several writers have examined the emotional lability factor. *Emotional lability* may be defined as the uncontrolled expression of emotions, characterized chiefly by inappropriate crying or laughing. Although emotional lability often has been described as lacking true emotional significance, Jenkins et al. (1975) believe that it does occur in an environmental context and that it relates directly "to something the patient has deep feelings or acute anxiety about" (p. 278). As Eisenson notes:

The persistence of catastrophic emotional lability is a negative indicator for recovery. In the early, post-onset stages, however, such behavior is a response to disability and frequently a manifestation of the patient's awareness of his or her linguistic-communicative impotence. In the early post-onset period the expression of emotion—the reactions—should be accepted by the therapist and by the family as behavior that is quite in order and to be expected. It is far better for the patient to feel that he or she has the right to cry than to be discouraged from crying by any suggestion that crying is for children and not for an adult. (1984, p. 94)

In comparing catastrophic reactions to emotional lability, we prefer to describe the former as an extreme response and the latter as a moderate or subdued one. Whether the concept of emotional lability can be considered a secondary reaction to associated sensorimotor and cognitive deficits or a direct result of brain mechanism disruption of the limbic system, as discussed earlier, therapists have observed the quality and intensity of the behavior to diminish in time in many patients. Moreover, it would be naive indeed for any investigator to suggest that the patient does not experience some direct emotional reaction to the physical, physiological, and social consequences of their CVA. Let us, therefore, examine several representative studies.

Horenstein (1970), in his summary of the effects of cerebrovascular disease on the emotional behavior and personality changes of the patient, equates depression with a grief reaction. Horenstein, among others (Baretz and Stephenson, 1976; Ullman, 1962; Weinstein and Kahn, 1955), discuss the patient's denial of illness in terms of a psychodynamic reaction related to the premorbid personality. Adler (1980) developed a six-stage model based on the psychoperceptual disorientation of stroke patients during the acute postonset period. Citing stage 4 (psychoperceptual disorientation) as the most significant, he suggests that the most disturbing to patients and family members are the schizoid symptoms reported. In light of the neurological evidence discussed earlier, however, any definitive statement about a purely psychological reaction must await further empirical study.

Personality and Behavior Changes

The research concerning the psychodynamic factors associated with cerebral vascular infarctions has not clearly differentiated the neurobiological from the psychological in terms of primary or secondary determinants. Nor has significant data been added to the professional literature since the late 1980s regarding persistent specific personality and behavioral changes that occur as patients react to their trauma. More recent investigators, such as Krishnan, Ranga, and Gadde (1996), using MRI, have found considerable evidence in their studies of older depressed patients that cerebrovascular pathology plays a major role in etiology and found imaging studies of stroke patients to clarify neurosubstrates for the emergence of late-life depression. Previously, though, many investigators and therapists have written about or observed profound emotional responses. Ulman (1962), in his three-year systematic study among 300 stroke subjects, found that feelings of depression, hopelessness, and futility were directly related to the duration and severity of the physical disability. He observed that, although depression was associated with the premorbid personality, it could also be attributed to the reality of the physical trauma. Friedman (1961) studied a group of aphasic patients in a Veterans Administration hospital and found all of them suffering diminished self-concept, loneliness, and feelings of isolation. Projecting feelings of rejection on others, they tended to exaggerate their own deficits and withdrew even in the group therapy setting. Perhaps most revealing was the sense of loss of their biological and psychological integrity, contributing to their alienation from other aphasic patients as well as other patients. Although unexplored by Friedman, we would propose that, by the very nature of a Veterans Administration hospital, patients there would be less likely to have the support system of family members, thereby exacerbating the degree of abandonment and loss.

Horenstein (1970) also describes the effects of stroke on the personality by specifying depression as a manifestation of grief. He discusses the degree and quality of the depression relative to the patient's self-awareness and sense of self-worth, the type and severity of the neural deficits, intellectual level, and premorbid adaptive ability. Horenstein alludes to the profound sense of loss felt by the patient, particularly in regard to the personal and family situation. Probably the most extensive discussion of loss

and grief in aphasia, explained in terms of mourning theory, is provided by Tanner (1980). He reviews the states in the grieving process as variously outlined by Bowlby (1970), Engels (1964), Moustakas (1972), and Kubler-Ross (1969, 1975). With respect to the loss of self-respect, Tanner writes:

> The loss of some aspect of the self can involve changes in the individual's health, body function, sense of worth, self-concept, attractiveness, and family loss. Loss of self is a broad dimension and includes functions which the individual can lose or perceive as lost. . . . Loss of some aspect of the self can have both an extra-dimensional and an intra-dimensional spreading of effect. Extra-dimensional spreading of effect can occur when the individual is placed in a nursing home or institution; as a result, loss is experienced in other dimensions such as security, loved ones (symbolic), and loss of external objects. Intra-dimensional spreading of effect experienced as a result of paralysis could involve loss of feeling of self worth, role, libido, and general reduction in self-concept.

> Aphasia is perhaps the most significant disorder seen by the clinician which results in the dimension described. In aphasia, loss is not limited to verbal expression; aphasics often have difficulty in reasoning, memory, and comprehension. General reduction in ego, swallowing deficits, hemiplegia, and visual deficits are also common. In addition, many aphasics are institutionalized; grief can be expected not only relative to loss of speech but also as a result of the concomitant disorders and subsequent placement. (p. 92)

Coping and Defense Mechanisms

While not pathological by definition, aphasic individuals, either consciously or unconsciously, employ coping and defense methods to protect themselves against the frustrations and demands of the reality with which they are faced. Individually, every person responds differently: Some attempt to avoid the reality, others find some means of adapting to it. Among some typical responses are withdrawal and overconcern for the patient's spouse. Depending on personal feelings of adequacy, the individual may use a positive or negative strategy in coping with the reality. Our own preference is to view the struggle as a means of attempting to achieve "homeostasis"; that is, to achieve a steady state of being so that the organism, the patient, can survive. First suggested by Cannon (1939), it is the individual's attempt to maintain a constancy and stability in his or her internal environment, which involves a complex interrelationship among physiological, hormonal, and neurological components.

Roskies and Lazarus (1979) describe coping as a dynamic process whereby the individual is actively involved in responding to what *has* happened but coping also determines what *will* happen when reacting to an event. Meichenbaum and Turk (1982) believe that either improving a situation (if it is at all possible) or escaping from one that is intolerable may be sufficient. They further note that rationalizing, being detached, or avoiding thinking about things, under some conditions, may be effective ways of coping.

While few investigations have systematically examined coping strategies among chronically ill patients, much less, aphasic individuals, Lazarus and Launier (1978) describe the denial, withdrawal behavior, rationalizations, and overprotectiveness often seen in patients as a timely, if not appropriate, response to a seemingly intolerable situation. Eisenson (1984), in fact, believes that, although a patient's euphoria may be inconsistent with truth or reality, it could be viewed as a means of self-defense. Eisenson (1984) and Sarno (1981) present anecdotal accounts of patients who were able to describe the emotional impact of their experience with aphasia. Among the coping strategies described were euphoria, attention to only optimistic things, and denial of the disability. What was most revealing is how the premorbid personality often determined the method of coping.

It would appear that the reactive strategy or strategies used are unique to the individual and therefore should be considered when intervening therapeutically. It certainly could be argued that the defense and coping strategies employed by the patient are essentially psychobiological in nature. Although unique to the individual, they may reflect the structural and chemical changes in the brain. One might, in fact, support the notion of a psychological homeostatic reorganization, discussed earlier, although it would be difficult not to include the function or interactive effects of the sympathetic nervous system. Nonetheless, the therapist is faced with the patient's own perceptual reality and all of its implications and needs to be prepared to intervene therapeutically according to the patient's emotional and linguistic needs.

Depression

As noted earlier, the neurochemical changes induced by an insult to the brain is likely to result in profound emotional changes manifested by depression. Cummings and Sultzer (1993) report the incidence of depression ranging from 0% to as high as 71%. While Boone et al. (1995) declare that the left hemisphere may exert a regulatory control of affect and the right hemisphere predisposing to depression, any definitive evidence to suggest one simple explanation still is lacking. Most investigators would agree, however, that depression has a direct and profound effect on clinical demonstration, functional recovery, and outcome. Not only are cognitive skills affected but also psychomotor skills, attentional control, memory, and learning (Brand, Jolles, and Gipsen-de-Wied, 1992; Boone et al., 1995; Sweet, Newman, and Bell, 1992, among others).

Although it may be difficult to differentiate depression in terms of a secondary reaction or as a direct result of brain mechanism disruption, late-life depression is one of the most common psychiatric disturbances. Salzman and Shader (1978) estimate that, of the 20 million individuals over 65 years of age, at least 1 million suffer from depressive illness. Because of the stresses, defenses, and adaptations related to age, depression manifests itself differently in older than in younger age groups. They also note, because society often isolates the aged and places them in dependency roles, their feelings of inadequacy, exacerbated by physical and psychological decline, are reinforced. Thus, symptoms of depression are further perpetuated by the loss of self-esteem and self-worth. Definitive evidence appears to be lacking that the location of the lesion and changes in biochemistry do not necessarily account for poststroke depression. Sarno and Gainotti (1998), in their survey of the literature, conclude that the patient's emotional reaction, regardless of site of lesion or even generalized pathology, most likely accounts for the depression. There appears to be sufficient conflicted evidence that keeps the organicity versus functional dichotomy unresolved. What indeed may appear to be likely in future research is the recognition that the two paradigms probably are inseparable.

Breslau and Haug (1983) provide the most comprehensive account involving the aged, citing the contribution of 17 of the foremost authorities. They predict that, with the increase of the elderly population, the incidence and prevalence of such depression could attain epidemic proportions. What also should be noted, however, is that several later investigators have found depression to be weakly related to age and that surveys of psychological well-being reveal that older individuals are just as happy and satisfied with life as younger individuals (Costa and McCrae, 1984; Costa, McCrae, and Locke, 1990).

It is obvious that contradictory findings make it presently impossible to make any accurate assumptions regarding the association of depression with cerebral vascular disease, since sampled populations under study appear to escape precise controls. Nevertheless, we would not be remiss in assuming depression, even though perhaps temporary, to be a direct psychological consequence to cerebral infarction and aphasia.[1] Herrman et al. (1998) assessed the prevalence of depressive symptoms, their clinical correlates, and the effects of depressive symptoms on stroke recovery in relation specifically to functional independence with a sample population of 436 patients at the beginning of the study. One year later, 150 patients were assessed with marked depression, 21–22%. Finding a direct correlation between depressive symptoms and functionality, they concluded that treatment of depression would optimize recovery.

Anxiety, Guilt, and Anger

Discussion of the psychological forces operating in the patient would be incomplete without mentioning the varying degrees of anxiety, guilt, and anger experienced during the course of the mourning

process. But, as Davis (1983) has noted, "The aphasic person is not always depressed and angry, or anxious. Though there may be some common phase of reaction to the condition and to interacting situations, people with aphasia are as different as people in general are different" (p. 294). Unfortunately, most therapists who treat the aphasic family are not always privy to their hidden thoughts and feelings. Many of us must often rely on intuition without attempting to break through the protective barriers the patient and or the family erect. Nonetheless, the various effects on the family have been observed and documented by most investigators, as we presently illustrate.

Ramifications for the Family and Patient

Webster and Newhoff (1981), in their comprehensive review of how families and family members are affected by the communication impairment of one family member, refer to a family systems model in explaining how the family balance is at first disrupted and how the family attempts to stabilize itself. Rollin (1984) developed a framework for understanding "aphasic families" within the context of a family systems approach and summarizes the literature describing the loss and devastation felt by the patient and the family.

Family Reactions

Shontz (1965) formulated four stages that family members experience in reaction to the sudden impairment in communication in one member—shock, realization, retreat, and acknowledgment. We discussed earlier this grieving or mourning process with respect to the patient. In either case, we should bear in mind that, whatever grief theory we may support, the varying stages are neither discrete nor orderly. Patients or family members actually may "get stuck" anywhere along the continuum or even skip stages. Moreover, the timeline during each stage may vary from patient to patient, family member to family member, and family to family. Unfortunately, few studies have made any definitive statements regarding representative family reactions,

---

[1]As a speech-language pathologist in a rural home health care agency for the past eight years, we have encountered depression in at least 80% of the more than 200 patients seen or treated. Most of these have been on antidepressant medications.

but several have made serious attempts. Kinsella and Duffy (1979), in their study comparing spouses of aphasic and nonaphasic CVA patients, found impaired areas of social adjustment, sexual satisfaction, interpersonal communication, and loss of partnership. Of particular note was the disruption of social and leisure activities. Christensen and Anderson (1989) also support earlier studies finding spouses of aphasic patients to be affected more negatively in areas such as adjustment to role change, and inability to communicate with their spouse.

The most recent research confirms earlier findings regarding spouses of chronic aphasic patients, particularly when compared to spouses of subjects with no physical or cognitive impairment. Santos et al. (1999) found the opinions of both husbands and wives of aphasic patients reflecting provocative disturbances within the family system. Most problems related to communicative and physical impairments. The authors stress the importance that adequate attention be given to the long-term psychosocial problems.

Shifting of Family Roles

Consistent with the family's initial disruption and attempts at reorganization or attainment of homeostasis, Lubinski (1981) stresses the importance of each individual within the immediate family developing mechanisms to cope with the consistent emotional drain associated with the redefinition of the family following the onset of stroke in one of its members. Following resolution of the immediate physical danger to the patient, the family, particularly the spouse, faces the task of integrating an impaired communicator into the group, including children, grandchildren, brothers, or sisters. Unintentionally, the aphasic patient becomes the family member around whom all changes and accommodations are being made. Others assume new roles in the face of the decrease in responsibility of the patient's role. This is especially significant for the spouse, who typically assumes the role of caregiver while also coping with a possible role reversal and the added responsibility of maintaining home, financial obligations, and family integration. Denman (1998), in his analysis of nine in-depth interviews with a selected group of spouses caring for their aphasic partner, concluded that these caregivers expressed needs mainly in areas of support, information, role change, training, and day or respite care.

The family of the aphasic patient is involved in a rehabilitation process made more demanding by the patient's sometimes antisocial behavior. Lubinski sees this as related to the patient's attempt to shun the "handicapped" role he or she must assume. Such a role includes relinquishing former responsibilities, becoming dependent, and looking forward (and not always positively) to rehabilitation therapy. Patients who are noncompliant may be "stigmatized as uncooperative, unmanageable, or hostile," compounding the problems the family must handle. More typical, though, we and other therapists have found resigned acquiescence, mood changes, insufficient effect of antidepressants, and other unpredictable behaviors. The presence of associated cognitive or memory deficits only exacerbate the situation. Malone (1969) found that, among 25 families interviewed, role changes were particularly traumatic when the male patient was the chief means of financial support. When the spouse assumed the role, she did so with either resentment or satisfaction. The latter is not so surprising when we consider how, even with the increased emancipation of women over the past two decades, many married women have not always been able, nor wished to, maximize their own life potentials.

Rollin (1988) finds that the quality of the premorbid marital relationship often determines the mode with which both patient and spouse learn to cope with their predicament and one another. For example, if the marital relationship was one in which the impaired partner, the husband, was the dominant person, his wife must now take control of the management of family affairs. Often, some spouses do this readily, regardless of prior experience. Others, however, feel helpless, unable to manage, attempt to seek help from their spouse or adult children. Should the impaired spouse be unable to assist, for any one of a combination of communicative or cognitive deficits, an already disturbed emotional stability may be jeopardized.

If the roles originally had been reversed, whereby the wife had previously enjoyed a domineering or mothering role, she may be tempted now to encourage a greater dependency in her impaired husband. Such overprotectiveness may impede his efforts toward independence but not necessarily interfere with all aspects of rehabilitation. In the extreme case in which the person has been profoundly impaired, such a role may be the only one feasible.

Wenz and Herrmann (1990) in a pilot study of 10 chronically ill aphasic patients and their relatives demonstrated clear emotional restraint of the patients and their relatives in the occupational, social, psychological, and communicative areas. While the patients were more burdened by restrictions of independence, their relatives gave more importance to emotional changes and family problems. Hemsley and Code (1996), while examining only five subjects at three and nine months post onset of stroke, employing a series of objective and subjective measures, found unique patterns of individual, emotional, and psychosocial adjustment in patients and their significant others regardless of aphasia type and severity. The authors conclude that, given the unique nature of factors and of individuals, the value of single subject investigation is strongly indicated.

Whatever the situation or circumstances, speech-language pathologists with the assistance, ideally, of physical and occupational therapists need to maximize the potential of both spouses, given the reality of the past marital relationship and the desire of the unimpaired spouse to work toward the reestablishment of the impaired partner's previous role. Counseling therapists need to be prepared, though, to cope with special circumstances in which the unimpaired spouse may be content with the new situation and gives only apathetic attention to the demands of rehabilitation. Counseling therapists, nonetheless, can play a significant role in minimizing the negative aspects associated with role changes and maximizing the positive outcomes. Among the helpful possibilities are the following:

1. Assist both spouse and patient in recognizing practical and positive aspects of the new roles to be assumed. Often, the mere strangeness of new roles may produce anxiety and distort the spouses' perception of them.
2. Stress the transient nature of a new role if it is likely to be temporary only, while redirecting attention toward improving the environmental situation at home.
3. Help the spouse assist the impaired partner in adapting positively to the newly assumed role. An individual may have viewed the previous role as a considerable burden and, in a real sense, now be relieved of previous anxiety-producing responsibilities but may not readily adapt to the new role.
4. Complete role reversals may not be appropriate and the unimpaired spouse should be aided in seeking other family or outside support to assist in taking on some responsibilities. Although a martyrlike role of the unimpaired spouse may satisfy deep-seated psychological needs, it may not be in the best present or future interests of either the spouse or patient.

Porter and Dabul (1977) used a transactional analysis model to conceptualize the role changes that may take place in both patient and spouse. Using examples, they describe how the three ego states of Adult, Parent, and Child shift in the patient-spouse interaction. No longer able to maintain the responsibilities as "head of household" and as the Adult, the male patient regresses to the Child state, feeling increasingly dependent and helpless. The female spouse, in turn, her own Parent state triggered, may respond by relinquishing her Adult state and take on a mother role. Obviously, the shifts in roles vary, depending on the premorbid family history, and become more complex when children are at home.

While Campbell and Patterson (1995) report that the research on family caregiving has expanded significantly over the past decade, particularly with regard to the elderly who are neurologically impaired, they provide no information or data regarding the use of family therapy with such a population, nor any reference to its use with stroke families. Our own exhaustive research of the literature in family therapy reveals virtually no evidence of such research. In two studies, Evans et al. (1988 and 1992) compared the impact of providing information about stroke to the family versus a comprehensive psychoeducational and patient counseling program and found the latter to have a positive effect on family behavior and consistently positive family functioning. Other authors, such as Van Amburg, Barber, and Zimmermann (1996), paint an even more dismal picture regarding the extent to which gerontological issues have been addressed in the family therapy literature and professional conferences. Only 28 articles focused on aging out of the more than 873 articles in the major journals of family therapy from 1986 to 1993. Of these, most deal with aging and dementia, which is addressed in a later chapter.

Despite the paucity of empirical and case analysis research, we prefer to draw on classical family systems theory as described by Satir (1967). Using her basic perspective, Satir believes that the aphasic family's homeostasis or stability has been disrupted. Although, typically, each family member's role may be defined and perceived in terms of an unspoken, assumed consensus by other family members, it is possible for one member to be perceived differently by another. In an "aphasic family" behaviors may be seen as disturbing by one or more family members. This distress then is translated to identify the family member, who is viewed as creating the problem and becomes the "identified patient" or "identified symptom." (See Satir, 1967, for a more comprehensive discussion of the identified patient and the dysfunctional family.)

Not only has the family reality changed, so has the perceptual reality of each family member. There no longer may be the consensus originally established, and therefore family members must struggle to satisfy a different perceptual reality, the latter being consummated with varying feelings of loss, helplessness, anger, rage, guilt, depression, and frustration. Webster and Newhoff (1981) describe it in the following way:

> This identified patient or scapegoat gives others a place to project family stress and/or blame for many of the family's failures. When the role of scapegoat or identified patient is essential to a unit's homeostasis, it may be impossible for other family members to participate in helping the impaired person to improve. (p. 230)

One must realize, however, that the aphasic patient may not necessarily be made a scapegoat, as long as the premorbid family system was functional or reasonably stable and the family continues to be governed by the previously established and acceptable rules. Nonetheless, because the trauma is experienced by all, we would expect a necessary, if not dramatic, shift in roles to occur to satisfy the drive toward homeostasis. The key factor is that a crisis has occurred and the family may be desperately searching for a means of psychosocial survival.

Each family member may develop different roles or ways of dealing with the new reality. For preadolescents and adolescents living in the home, whose world may also have been shattered, personal needs and expectations no longer can be fulfilled in the style to which they had been accustomed. Not only must they readjust to the impaired parent but to the unimpaired parent as well. The family alignment now begins to shift dramatically, each member, including the patient, struggling to discover a means to cope. Naturally, we do not assume that all families are as devastated as just described. Families that have functioned in an essentially healthy psychological manner have their own intrinsic mechanisms for coping, despite the suffering they might endure. Burns (1996) provides a very definitive family systems approach with ways change is both promoted and measured. A very succinct description of techniques provides the counseling therapist a clear direction to lead the aphasic family toward positive communicative change and family adjustment.

We also are alert to the fact that the effects of a stroke on the family may not emerge immediately. Only the competence, sensitivity, and careful scrutiny by those therapists assisting in the recovery process may bring to light the underlying struggles, through counseling intervention. We now turn to this subject.

Counseling Intervention

Because the entire family has been affected by the stroke, we would immediately want to intervene to assuage some of the powerful feelings surfacing, as well as to manage the continuing adjustment difficulties the patient and family members may have throughout the recovery and rehabilitation periods. In doing so, we also focus attention on the spouse, likely the most significant person in the patient's life now and the probable caregiver.

Initial Considerations

Malone (1969) proposes that family members cannot function effectively as part of the total rehabilitative effort until they have been advised of the many problems associated with aphasia and the various strategies for dealing with these problems. Conversely, to work meaningfully with affected families therapists must be knowledgeable regarding the pervasive effects of aphasia on the family constellation. Supported with this information, the therapist is better able to assist family members in appropriately avoiding certain situations, changing situations that have the potential for change, and accepting the unchangeable. In so doing, we would prefer to view the family actively, rather than labeling it *normal, neurotic,* or *psychotic.* Family therapists generally consider this preference more realistic in terms of a continuum of dysfunctionality than holding to traditional absolute labels as designated by medical manuals of mental disorders.

Importance of Providing Information

Skelly (1975), Linebaugh and Young-Charles (1978), Manuel (1979), and Goldberg (1980) concur that the most difficult problem for the family is their ignorance of the cause and effects of the stroke on the patient. Baretz and Stephenson (1976), in their description of practical management guidelines, highlight the importance of providing information about the disorder "to patient and family to allay fear, banish misconceptions, stress positive aspects, and provide the basis for a slowly developing recognition of the realities of the situation an renewable adjustment" (p. 56). Interviewing 50 aphasic patients who had attained a functional level of speech, Skelly (1975) found that many believed they would have experienced less fear and anguish had they been given reassurance and a basic explanation of what had happened to them. In his study of 20 hospital inpatients, Goldberg (1980) found that none of those patients nor their families had received any explanation from the attending physician of the language and concomitant problems before they met with the speech-language pathologist. He also found that interactions with family and staff reinforced patients' reactions that they felt they had "gone crazy." More recent writers such as Luterman (1996), Shipley (1996), and Crowe (1997), also stress the value of imparting information to the family.

While most authorities recognize the value of providing information to both patient and family members, it is equally important to recognize that any one of them may not be able, during the initial stages of posttrauma shock, to hear or understand the information given. The patient's cognitive-linguistic impairment or psychological state may prevent accurate processing of information. Similarly, family members may be too numb, confused, overwhelmed, or depressed to comprehend clearly what has occurred and what may be expected to occur in the future.

It appears to us, in these initial stages, what is important is that the medical and therapeutic providers give the patient and family basic information about CVA and, perhaps more valuable, that the family senses caring, support, and understanding from therapists and physicians. Representative testimony to this need comes from the spouse of a patient whom we interviewed: "If only they gave our family some information when he had the stroke, we wouldn't have felt so lost and frightened. We probably still wouldn't have understood everything that was going on, but at least we'd have some comfort in knowing that somebody cared, just by talking to us."

Ideally, we believe, all members of the rehabilitation team, including the physician, home health care nurse, physical and occupational therapists, and speech-language pathologist, would want to help in dealing with the multitude of problems the patient and family must face. Unfortunately, such an ideal event is less likely to occur now, given the strangling effects of managed health care and reduction of Medicare benefits (Boswell, 1999). Considering these problems, a more practical solution will need to be found. We address this issue later in the chapter.

Separating Premorbid from Postmorbid Issues

It has been noted that, because the spouse probably will have the greatest interaction with the patient, any counseling strategy employed should include a distinction between premorbid and postmorbid issues. This is all the more important for the speech-language pathologist, who has had minimal training in psychopathology and yet most often is the essential agent in rehabilitation efforts. The therapist will need to keep a clear perspective on only those issues that refer specifically to the stroke, whether they include the spouse's anxiety about her husband's withdrawal, her feelings of resentment and guilt about her newly assumed burdens or responsibilities, or her feelings of sexual deprivation. For the therapist to delve into elements involving the premorbid marital relationship, including money matters, lack of intimacy, and conflicts over adult children not only may be irrelevant but counterproductive and destructive. Bear in mind that, but for the CVA, the couple would not have sought psychological assistance in the first place. The therapist must then honor the spouse's possible need to conceal earlier conflicts, while remaining attuned to the nuances, expressed or unexpressed, of premorbid marital struggles.

Although it is conceivable for the spouse now to express pent-up feelings that refer back many marital years, given a willing and caring ear, the therapist will need to steer such verbalizations gently in the direction of what is happening in the present. We do not suggest the therapist invalidate these powerful feelings but at least acknowledge understanding of them and then deal in positive terms with ways of coping now. Ironically, in some cases, the current crisis may actually diminish, neutralize, or nullify elements of previous family conflicts. In some instances, though, powerful feelings of guilt may emerge and these too will have to be managed to proceed with traditional therapy. The reader may wish to consider any one or perhaps an eclectic counseling approach discussed in the last chapter. It is possible, though, that those couples who had been in constant turmoil may now put aside egocentric needs and unite to move forward together. This is one example of a more homeostatic state brought to reality.

Family Involvement in Rehabilitation Efforts

The question now arises of how the family should be involved in rehabilitation efforts. We already saw that, in a very real sense, the family must undergo its own rehabilitation regardless of the special needs of the patient. The extent to which the family should be involved directly in the rehabilitation process for the patient, however, depends on the following factors:

1. *Comprehensive analysis of the patient's linguistic abilities and communicative competence.* The therapist defines and determines the short- and long-range goals for the patient, consistent with the nature and quality of the deficits revealed.

2. *Psychological analysis of the patient and family.* Through formal counseling or testing, the therapist determines the interpersonal perceptions of the spouse, therapist, and, if possible, the patient (see the Code and Mueller protocols; Code and Mueller, 1992). Based on their analysis, the therapist may derive a clearer understanding of the attitudes that could hinder or facilitate the rehabilitation process and determine in specific ways how families may participate. The therapist also must be alert to changing family circumstances and attitudes that positively or adversely influence the process.

3. *Communication environment analysis.* The therapist determines the patient's opportunities for communication and hindrances to communication in their environment, as outlined in Lubinski "Profile of the Communication Environment of the Adult Aphasic" (1981). We would include in the analysis a premorbid psychosocial linguistic history with particular emphasis on the patient's prior communicative style; for example colloquial and slang usage, vocabulary, stereotyped expressions, and environmentally determined linguistic variations. Of utmost importance would be the use of multiculturally diverse language patterns, if appropriate

4. *Developing a rehabilitation plan.* The therapist formulates short- and long-term therapy plans consistent with the patient's abilities, deficits, and ever-changing needs and the flexibility to change goals when deemed necessary. Input from family members is desirable insofar as it may contribute positively to the total rehabilitation process. Once the level and degree of family involvement have been determined, the environmental goals for the entire rehabilitation program can be set.

Davis (1990) provides the reader a very basic but useful list of practical procedures family members and others can follow in helping the patient cope, during both the initial and later phases of rehabilitation. He also succinctly describes behavior changes that need to be addressed.

Spousal and Family Counseling

Thus far we have discussed the importance and ramifications of giving information to the patient and the family. We have also noted the delicate relationship of pre- and postmorbid issues and guidelines for the therapist to initiate with the family during the recovery process. We now consider the rationale and indications for continued spousal and family counseling.

The success of any rehabilitation program depends on the active cooperation of the professionals and the family. We concur with Lubinski (1981) that family counseling should be considered a reeducation process. Lubinski provides 18 definitive communication strategies that both family and hospital personnel may use to enhance communication with the patient. Naturally, any successful efforts necessitate full cooperation by the family. Implied is a willingness by the family to modify previous assumptions and behaviors and attitudes and to accept the necessity of defining different roles, if necessary, within the family constellation.

The presence of any hidden psychopathological precursors also could undermine rehabilitative efforts. Kinsella and Duffy (1979) report the incidence of minor psychiatric disorders in wives of aphasic patients (but apparently not in husbands of aphasics). One explanation for the latter might be the notion that men, even during this more enlightened time, try to maintain the proverbial "stiff upper lip," withholding their feelings, maintaining a state of denial of the actual reality. Regardless, either spouse not only must cope with the profound crisis of the stroke but also loses "the protective function of an intimate relationship or a supportive social network . . ." (p.129), thereby increasing the likelihood of psychological disturbance. With children living in the home, spouses feel even more overwhelmed, becoming impotent in dealing with the children's own "reactive behavior problems," while coping with the patient's variable and oftentimes

erratic state. Caution should be taken in generalizing from these data because of the limited population used, but it should be considered an important indicator for counseling, nonetheless. In their study of 65 spouses of CVA patients, Artes and Hoops (1976) emphasize that the communication problems of the patient are not always the major concerns of the spouse, that most wives were equally or more concerned about problems involving intrapersonal behavior and overall health care.

It is apparent from our discussion that family counseling in aphasia has two central goals: a reeducation process in which the family assists the patient and participates in those activities that will enhance the total rehabilitation effort and an opportunity to help family members cope with their own emotional responses to the trauma, modifying previous behaviors and establishing a different manner of living. Implicit are the assumptions that family counseling can satisfy both goals simultaneously and that the speech-language pathologist typically can fill this counselor role as long as enhancement of communication for the patient is involved.

Family Therapy

Thus far we have discussed the efficacy of traditional family counseling, which should not be confused with family therapy, a more systematic interactional approach to the treatment of families, even though the profession of family therapists admits to not having addressed the issue in treating the elderly, much less the aphasic family (see the discussion of this, earlier in the chapter). Nonetheless, we recognize not only the importance and significance of determining the family's premorbid communicative interaction but propose that a family systems approach can be an appropriate process to facilitate rehabilitation efforts.

Rationale and Value

Traditional family counseling often excludes the direct participation of the patient in the actual process, thus perhaps isolating and alienating the patient further from the immediate family and thereby impeding the rehabilitation process. The patient's mere physical presence during the interview or counseling session is insufficient. The tendency to ignore the patient, particularly if verbal communication is absent, too often is observed in professional clinical settings. We are suggesting that family counseling can be made more dynamic; the literature clearly has demonstrated its value in helping the patient recover and the family readjust. We suggest that the patient be induced to attempt interacting communicatively, from the beginning, to strengthen the notion that he or she still is part of the family. This is particularly crucial in the light of results found by Stein et al. (1992) in their examination of depression in the spouses of 41 stroke patients. First, they found that spousal depression was not correlated with the severity of the patients' physical, cognitive, or language impairment. Interestingly, they also found that spouses' perception of the aphasic partner was more accurate than that of the clinicians. It further appears obvious to us that it is far better to involve the patient, whenever or wherever practical, in changes deemed necessary for all concerned. Such participation would help validate the patient's role, albeit a different one perhaps, as an active member of the family. As the patient and other family members are provided the opportunity to explore areas of concern and conflict in an atmosphere of acceptance and safety, the patient may feel less singled out as the only problem or represented as being chiefly responsible for the family crisis. The patient's concern may now focus on the spouse's struggle to "make ends meet" adding to feelings of guilt and inadequacy. But these feelings can be dealt with as a family issue, with the potential for each member to assist the others in reestablishing family equilibrium. Although the patient will need to take responsibility for the personal reality of the disability, also recognized is that this is a family problem, too.

Family therapy motivates other family members, if only the spouse, to include the patient in all communicative interactions. They are aided in learning how to focus on the significant nuances and elements of the patient's communicative efforts, become more skilled in understanding aphasic messages, and adapt their own communicative efforts suitable to the patient. The patient, in turn, feeling

related to the spouse and more encouraged, is likely to feel more positive about him- or herself. All small gains in communicative competence are positively reinforced by the spouse or other family members, strengthening the person's available assets and reducing the liabilities, thus giving the patient a sense of real progress. Those patients unable to tolerate errors in their linguistic attempts, who have family support and understanding, are more likely to take the risk and experience communicative reward.

Finally, family therapy provides not only a linguistic environment for reacquiring communicative competence but also a rich source for the carryover of communicative skills gained through conventional speech therapy. It should be emphasized, however, that family therapy is not a panacea for all the difficulties the patient and family may be having. Its appropriateness and value will be determined by the application of several criteria.

Criteria for Family Therapy

Ideally, the patient or other members of the family should request help when they are unable to cope with the problems they are experiencing. Therapists have observed that many families do not require extensive counseling or family therapy but merely an exchange of information. These families apparently have their own healthy internal mechanisms for coping with crisis and adapt readily to the rehabilitation program prescribed by the professional staff. With other families, it may be only the spouse who requires counseling assistance.

We counseled the 60-year-old wife of a 62-year-old severely impaired aphasic patient who described their sexual relationship prior to the stroke as virtually nonexistent for the previous 20 years of a marriage characterized by his alcoholism and her own enabling behavior. Frustrated and resentful over his pronounced dependency needs, she sought permission from this therapist to ease her burden and have transient sexual relationships with other men. Recognizing also her profound sense of guilt, she needed to struggle with her conflict and arrive at some accommodation with which she could continue to be an effective caregiver to her spouse and herself. At her instigation, couples counseling was initiated to help her husband become more self-sufficient at home and provide her time off. It was felt inappropriate and counterproductive to raise the sexual issue during counseling with both parties, because this was the wife's problem and he could not be expected to cope with that issue as well.

Unsurprisingly, her need for sexual liaisons diminished when she found that she could adapt by taking time out for herself and he resumed his favorite hobby of oil painting. A more positive home environment came to fruition and soon both were able to enjoy getting out together more often. Letourneau (1993) examined several of the sexual issues, including the need for warmth and affection, the need for the patient to "perform," rejection by the spouse of the patient's sometimes increased sexual drive and certainly the patient's loss of sexual interest. Finger (1993) believes that disruptions in sexual functioning are due predominantly to psychological causes. He stresses the importance of dispelling the myths and stereotypes often held by rehabilitation staff, patients, and their partners. No current studies examine the effects of the drug Viagra on impotent CVA patients.

Frequently, the therapist will perceive elements interfering with speech therapy. The patient or the spouse may be unaware of them. A therapist who has sufficient rapport with the family may delicately suggest they seek further assistance to identify and resolve the problem in order to enhance speech therapy efforts.

We were treating a 48-year-old patient who had made significant and rapid progress in achieving limited communication but, after six months of speech therapy, had suddenly hit a plateaue. Through gentle probing, we learned that his wife had been distressed about their son, who had dropped out of high school during his senior year. They were eager to participate in family therapy, particularly once the son agreed, although grudgingly at first, to do so. Through several sessions, it was learned that the son had been concealing his depression concerning his father's stroke and feared that he, too, might suffer one at an early age. Once further information was provided about conditions that could lead to stroke and pent-up feelings among all parties ventilated, the son reenrolled in

school, the wife became calmer, and the patient's communicative abilities began to climb.

Certainly, not all cases follow such neat progression, but the watchful therapist may do much to at least help mollify a situation that perhaps does not have an easy solution or no solution at all, except to assist the family in adapting to a reality that does not portend an ideal outcome.

The decision to initiate family therapy will depend on the degree of cognitive, receptive, evaluative, and expressive function of the patient. This may be very difficult to ascertain when formal testing is of little value in determining the degree of true communicative competence. Holland (1977) has been critical of language tests that do not measure communicative competence, particularly in a natural environment. Her concerns led to the development of the CADL (communicative abilities in daily living) assessment inventory, which provides the therapist a dynamic and pragmatic tool to determine the nature of how the aphasic patient relates communicatively in a social or the family milieu (Holland, 1980). Her belief is that spouses may be more sensitive to the patient's verbal and nonverbal communicative attempts in the environment just described. We would concur and would use the initial family therapy session to decide continuation of the family therapy process. It may be argued that a severe Wernicke's or globally aphasic patient would be totally confused, bewildered, distracted, and oblivious to the communicative process in family therapy. We would counter that the patient may be receiving valuable but unmeasurable input from other family members and perhaps is deriving some satisfaction from the experience of being included in the family discussions.

Family therapy should not be considered a substitute for other speech-language therapy strategies. No research has yet determined the superiority of one approach over the other, although the importance of avoiding so-called cookbook approaches cannot be understated. It would appear, though, that family therapy can enhance traditional strategies by revealing communicative competencies and personal attitudes heretofore undetected or undetermined.

During the course of family therapy sessions with a severe apraxic patient and his spouse, the author learned of the patient's displeasure with the method his wife was using with him during home practice with visual and auditory materials. We originally had been consulted by the patient's speech-language pathologist, who informed us that the patient had been vocally abusive to his wife and that the therapist felt overwhelmed by the situation. What had not been revealed previously in therapy were the factors surrounding the abusive behavior. Providing both the patient and his wife an opportunity to inform me what was going on opened up a very emotional outpouring of sadness, loss, anger, and frustration related to the onset and aftermath of the stroke. We now took steps to educate his wife to a different approach and a more positive attitude in helping. While pretraumatic marital issues also emerged, discussion of these was helpful in resolving the immediate issues. Family therapy provided the atmosphere in which both parties were able to verbalize their discontent and pain and assuage their frustration after weeks of intense marital discord and inappropriate home therapy.

Guidelines for the Therapist

Once the determination to intervene with family therapy has been made, the therapist (either a speech-language pathologist trained in family therapy or a psychotherapist with knowledge of aphasia) can follow a series of guidelines that best meet the needs of the patient and family. Rollin (1984) developed such a plan, which is outlined here:

1. The therapist must determine how much information the patient or family needs about specific issues to be dealt with during therapy.
2. It must be recognized that the aphasic patient is not necessarily the only identified patient and that shifts to other family members may occur for underlying dysfunctional elements to be expressed.
3. Other family members must be aided in permitting the patient to function as a separate person during family therapy, communicating *with* the patient, too, rather than *about* the patient.
4. The therapist must be prepared to verbalize thoughts and feelings the patient may be struggling to express.

5. The therapist must be sensitive to what may be expressed nonverbally by all family members.
6. The therapist must gently facilitate the expression of feelings by all to uncover hidden angers, resentments, frustrations, or anguish.
7. The patient and other family members must be helped to confront self-destructive and self-defeating behavior and focus their energy on positive goals and the needs of other family members as well.
8. The therapist needs to help the patient and other family members discover or adjust to new roles for themselves, consistent with the reality of the changed family circumstances. Also important is the recognition that roles may return to their original place or perhaps to some modified alternative.
9. The therapist may struggle with his or her own role, avoiding the role of rescuer or presuming a role of one "who knows all."
10. Finally, the therapist should have resolved or continue to work with his or her own personal inner conflicts, doubts about therapeutic competence, misjudged perceptions of the family, and other personal insecurities.

Counseling the Patient

As noted, family therapy should not be considered a panacea for all the problems and difficulties confronting the patient or the family. Often, direct or indirect counseling with the patient alone may be effective or beneficial in promoting real progress, particularly during the first several months following the trauma. Ireland and Wotton (1996) offered 20 dysphasic patients, including several with severe language deficits, 20 sessions of individual counseling, using trained counseling speech-language pathologists and a teacher with personal experience with aphasia. While this was a qualitative study, the participants found considerable value in the experience based on posttherapy interviews. Also, in the United Kingdom, Cunningham (1998), using the principles of personal construct therapy in six sessions, demonstrated that a counseling approach with a severe aphasic patient was effective in improving comprehension. Cunningham used a repertory grid to facilitate patient communication as well. It is important to note that communication improvement may have been related to the greater confidence the patient experienced as a communicator in adapting to the clinical situation.

Initial Considerations

Davis (1983), in reviewing Tanner (1980), applied rules facilitating the grieving process with patients who have suffered a CVA. Suggestions are presented that the counseling therapist avoid certain behaviors that interrupt the grieving process and encourage behaviors that ease the process:

1. *Positive reinforcement of denial* should be avoided, and the reality of current and future circumstances discussed. Although a realistic prognosis may not always be determined, the patient must be given some degree of hope for recovery.
2. Recognizing and accepting rather than *punishing anger* will help to reduce and neutralize it. The patient must be helped to understand that what is felt is a natural consequence to what has been experienced.
3. *Bargaining with the patient* can be counterproductive, in that it may present false hopes to the patient while assuaging the therapist's own uncertainty and insecurity.
4. Care should be taken to avoid *providing secondary gains* to the patient that may reinforce or interrupt the grieving process. The therapist must be alert to the fostering of unrealistic dependency by the patient on the therapist and instead foster patient responsibility for decision making and ultimate progress.
5. The therapist should help the patient avoid *early distractions,* such as untimely suggestions that the patient get "his mind off things" or get immersed in other activities for which the patient may not be prepared.
6. The therapist must avoid *displaying anxiety about the patient's depression* and accept it as a natural consequence and a stage to be experienced before the patient can develop more constructive attitudes.
7. The therapist can *permit patient control* by encouraging specific decision making and taking responsibility in the therapy process.

8. The therapist must *provide the patient with perspective* so that a more realistic and rational understanding about reaction and attitudes that are quite normal for aphasia can be developed. Learning that what is being experienced is not unique will help remove the fright induced by personal reaction to the disabilities.
9. To *acknowledge the reality of the loss* of functions and to encourage the free expression of concerns the patient may have personally about the condition will strengthen the speech therapy program and further acceptance of the personal reality.
10. Therapists must *listen to the patient without defending or explaining their concerns* and not feel that they must have all the answers to the patient's problems. Unconditional positive regard and empathy without judgment are of utmost importance (pp. 916–928).

Indicators and Rationale for Continued Counseling

We now consider how counseling therapists can best respond to the ongoing emotional and language problems associated with aphasia, using appropriate counseling strategies while respecting their limitations but at the same time attempt to integrate with traditional symptomatic techniques.

Dealing with Continuing Denial   Patient denial manifests itself in several ways but may not be readily evident to the therapist. One such example is the patient's inability to accept the disability and the belief that full recovery is imminent. It is debatable whether or not this is similar to the "sleeping beauty syndrome" referred to elsewhere in the text, but it may be indicative of the patient's refusal to have therapy or comply with home practice. A similar example is the patient who perceives the disability as less than is objectively identified by formal or informal testing. Although this behavior, like the previous example, represents self-protection or defensiveness and may be highly resistant to change, the therapist at least can acknowledge verbally to the patient what he or she believes, even if not expressed verbally by the latter. This could provoke the patient to confront the contradiction between what is reality and what is not; but the patient must make the choice either to acknowledge the reality or continue to reject it.

As long as the patient is willing to continue in therapy, the likelihood is greater that the attitude will change. The therapist certainly will have to exercise considerable patience and understanding to enable the patient time to consider all the facts and ultimately make a personal decision either to continue or terminate therapy. Although the therapist may be tempted to enlist the aid of the spouse, we believe it may be counterproductive and could alienate the patient from therapy, the spouse, and the therapist. The therapist, however, might share with the patient professional judgment and ask permission to speak to the spouse about the issue, either alone or with both of them together. As long as the patient is aware of and alert to his or her immediate environment, no interpersonal transaction between the therapist and spouse should be concealed.

Dealing with Emotional Lability   Therapists frequently have difficulty in coping with their emotionally labile patients, who weep persistently at what seems the slightest provocation. The response may be prompted by such diverse comments as, "Your husband tells me you have eight grandchildren," "Are you aware how much more verbal you are today?" or " I understand you had some difficulty sleeping last night." Unlike the typical emotional response to depression or anxiety, it is best to neutralize it by either affirmation, reflecting the feeling, acknowledging the fact, by turning to a different subject, or if the therapeutic task has instigated the response, changing the task. We also find it helpful to say simply, "What you're experiencing now is natural for what you've been through," or "Because of your stroke, it's hard to control your feelings all the time," or "As you improve physically you'll have better control of crying when it doesn't seem appropriate."

One poignant example of emotional control regards a patient we had treated for several months for dysarthria. Throughout our sessions, George would begin weeping whenever I commended him for correct approximations of his articulation, from single word usage to 90% intelligibility in conversational speech. His lability had diminished considerably within six months. I hadn't seen him for

three years later when he walked into a stroke support group where I was to be the main speaker. When he first noticed me, he rapidly walked over, aided by no cane, and burst into tears. Throughout my presentation I noticed that he was frequently dabbing his eyes with his handkerchief. His reactions would be difficult to interpret but I believe that, while some emotional lability still may have been present, he just was delighted to see me and could not thank me enough for assisting in his communicative recovery.

In most situations or cases it is important for the therapist to help remove the affectual response to the weeping. If the labile response is only a momentary lapse of control, it is probably best ignored and the planned therapeutic task continued with. Emotional lability sometimes is fused with the overall emotional status of the patient. In such a case, it is important to verbalize as intuitively as possible, if necessary, that which is being experienced or felt.

Dealing with Guilt   We sometimes are confronted with patients whose guilt in having become ill is so pervasive as to interfere with the overall therapeutic process. These individuals apparently are bearing the full burden of their illness as well as the burdens of the spouse and other members of the family. Although depression may be an obvious expressed emotion, the underlying feelings are of remorse, self-pity, self-denigration, and resentment. They feel as if they should not have survived the stroke and, feeling unworthy, will frequently resist therapeutic assistance or even spousal support.

Guilt can be traced back to premorbid unresolved interpersonal relationships, but it is likely that the therapist would encounter either patient or spousal resistance to discussion of these issues. Therefore, the therapist will need to focus attention on alleviating or modifying the patient's current attitude by providing the maximum in encouragement, support, and empathic understanding. The patient is helped to realize that none of us is responsible for all the unfortunate events that befall us, and were such an event as a CVA to strike another member of the family instead, we would certainly do all in our power to help.

By encouraging the patient to allow the spouse or other family member to take on the burden or responsibility is to show respect and caring for that person. The therapist helps the patient understand that there indeed is enough burden for all to bear. Once more, the therapist attempts to neutralize the unrealistic or irrational concerns of the patient by directing him or her to assume positive and major responsibilities, such as trying to get better, following the rehabilitation regimen, and even helping others to cope.

Modifying Concrete Responses   Patients who are impaired in the "abstract attitude" manifest linguistic and emotional material concretely. Although the therapist may find it difficult to help the patient generalize more effectively because of the combined organic and emotional bases of the problem, some adjustments are possible. The patient who believes her spouse does not remain in the waiting room while she is having therapy because he does not care about her is perhaps a rare example of a concrete attitude tinged with premorbid attitudes of paranoia. For a situation such as this, the therapist can design a linguistic task that includes several possibilities for the spouse's absence. The patient is encouraged to contribute reasons for him not remaining in the waiting room. Together, the patient and therapist can identify other situations, particularly at home, in which he has helped her improve. It also is likely to take many therapeutic sessions to strengthen a more abstract or cognitive appreciation of reality and much will depend on the extent of premorbid attitudes as well as on the degree of organic involvement.

Care should be taken to avoid judging the patient's attitude as foolish or malicious but rather to acknowledge to the patient that such reactions are not unusual. If the patient's evaluative capabilities are impaired, the therapist's task will be considerably more difficult. In such a case, efforts will have to be directed at improving cognitive functioning first, if at all possible.

Enhancing Adjustment in the Extended Care Facility or Nursing Home   Speech-language pathologists have been seeing more and more aphasic individuals in settings that have become permanent "homes" for them.[2] Either because these persons no longer can care for themselves at home or because they have no families to which to turn, they must rely on the often impersonal assistance of nursing personnel. Those facilities with social workers on their staff certainly can help provide a richer support system for the patients who feel lonely, depressed, and withdrawn. Although the major objective of the therapist is to help the aphasic patient gain the communicative competence for functioning at least adequately in the facility, the daily emotional struggle cannot be ignored. The task, unfortunately, is made more difficult by understaffed nursing and nursing aide personnel, who no longer provide the extra attention that was more typical 10 years ago.

An ideal illustration of an assisted approach can be drawn from our experiences with aphasic patients in a particular convalescent hospital. A nursing aide is frustrated by her inability to determine what her patient is attempting to communicate. The patient in turn is frustrated because she cannot get through to the aide. Rather than dwell on airing only the patient's frustration, we bring them together and reenact the verbal interchange attempted previously. This satisfies the practical and emotional needs of both parties and acts as an impetus for both to practice such interchanges throughout their daily contact. It is not difficult to establish appropriate baseline responses and demonstrate behavioral changes objectively.

Patients who are sad because they cannot go home may need to be assisted in sharing their concerns because their fragile emotional state could interfere with further therapeutic intervention. This does not mean bombarding a person with judgmental reassurances or unrealistic pronouncements but rather helping the person to focus on improving the daily activities that prevent going home. These may consist of being able to use the telephone for emergency purposes or to shop for themselves. Ideally, a team approach, involving physical, occupational, and recreational therapy with a social worker, would be most effective.

---

[2]As of this writing, speech-language therapy services for patients in extended care facilities have been seriously curtailed by the U.S. Congress, and this should be considered in the context of the discussion.

Some patients resign themselves to the reality of the hospital existence and the realization that they will never go home. They present a considerable challenge to all caregivers who want to intervene in the patient's best interest. But, do we really know what that best interest is? Some time ago, we evaluated a patient who showed considerable promise for becoming a limited communicator. Following one month of traditional therapy along with a blending of communication-centered and rationale emotive therapy, it became clear she did not wish to continue therapy. She appeared very relieved, in fact, when informed her therapy would be terminated.

A short time later, the facility's social worker informed the author that, shortly after leaving, the patient had been hospitalized with pneumonia but had since returned to the convalescent facility. What had been a depressed, noncommunicative person was now one who attempted to communicate with others and was delighted when asked if she wanted therapy. Unfortunately, in this case, her physician refused to write orders because, as he put it, "She doesn't know what she wants."

This anecdote, although perhaps somewhat disturbing to most readers, raises serious moral, ethical, and professional issues that cannot be dismissed readily. While we prefer to believe that few physicians hold such an attitude, we nevertheless are challenged to determine objectively the efficacy of therapy when patient disengagement is a significant factor. Perhaps by providing this patient a therapeutic milieu in which she could air a particular desire consistently and by engaging periodically with the patient, she might have taken a more positive position from the beginning. Regardless, this therapist need not have been so definitive in his original termination of therapy report.

Dealing with Spontaneous Stress in the Midst of Speech-Language Therapy   The therapist should feel free to suspend symptomatic therapy when the patient is observed to be distracted, depressed, anxious, or uncooperative. Therapist sensitivity to subtle verbal or nonverbal clues is desirable, so that patient will not have to endure continuation of the session as planned. The therapist needs to share his or her own perception that "something seems to be bothering you" and give the patient an opportunity to ventilate concerns. In some instances, the patient may be hesitant in doing so, for fear of offending the therapist, who has a well-planned lesson. Or, the patient, unaccustomed to the expression of feeling, may feel uncomfortable in doing so.

Insensitive coaxing or cajoling could alienate the relationship and thereby interfere further with the therapeutic process. In such instances, the patient must be given the responsibility to make an independent choice as to how best to proceed, with the therapist accepting whatever choice the patient makes. If that means early termination of the session, so be it: The patient may be capable of working out the difficulty prior to the subsequent session or be more open to discuss the problem the following session. If the patient, though, welcomes the opportunity to talk about what is disturbing him or her, the therapist should listen and attempt to understand what the patient is experiencing. Providing instant solutions or making personal or professional value judgments not only will be counterproductive, because the therapist could be wrong, but may inhibit the patient from revealing further information. Also to be considered is the patient's choice to allow the spouse to enter into the discussion. If the difficulty experienced by the patient relates to the marital relationship, a rich opportunity presents itself toward resolution of the problem.

Dealing with Premorbid Psychological Problems
It may be difficult for the therapist to identify premorbid deep-rooted psychological problems when they have been exacerbated by the trauma of the CVA. The situation gets even more complex when the problems interweave with problems resulting from the initial trauma. Even if the therapist has been able to sort them out, based on information gathered from the case history or from spousal or family therapy, focus nonetheless can be directed to the patient's immediate affectual state. The mere opportunity for the patient to express feelings to a trusting and accepting confidant may be sufficient to reduce the stress associated with the problem, regardless of solutions for it, if any. Frantic referrals to psychiatrists or clinical psychologists may

not only be resisted by the patient or family but also be interpreted to mean rejection by the therapist or raise doubts regarding the therapist's competency. We do not suggest that the therapist bear the burden of the patient's deep-rooted conflicts and anxiety or assume the role of a professional psychotherapist. But, neither do we suggest that the therapist unwittingly apply superficial strategies to pacify the patient and in all likelihood submerge the problem further. The therapist who is willing to listen and to understand first what the patient is experiencing is in a better position to suggest gradually and gently further psychotherapeutic consultation.

Many therapists, however, have treated patients who do not necessarily fit the patterns just suggested. For example, premorbidly angry, selfish, abusive patients sometimes postonset transform into kind, gentle, cooperative patients to the considerable surprise and pleasure of the spouse. In other instances, premorbidly kind, loving, caring, gentle patients become tyrants, striking out either physically or verbally (even if only vocally) at their spouses or children. The dismay experienced by the family will have to be addressed by the therapist, if any further progress is to be forthcoming. We will not attempt to explore this likely bioneuropsychological change, but it is an area that certainly deserves further study.

Counseling the Depressed or Frustrated Nonverbal Patient   On occasion, we have heard psychiatrists, psychologists, social workers or family therapists refusing to see depressed nonverbal patients, with the apology that "I couldn't possibly help her because she doesn't speak, and anyway I don't really know anything about aphasia." Too often, in such cases, antidepressants or serotonergenic agents become the treatment of choice, typically prescribed by the family physician or neurologist. While such medications have been shown to positively alter the patient's mood, their negative side effects must be taken into consideration (Montgomery, 1998; Miyai and Reding, 1998; Gareri et al., 1998). Given such possible circumstances, the speech-language pathologist is placed in the awkward position of attempting to work around the presented behavior, particularly if medications are changed. Sometimes this is possible; other times, either the side effects interfere with therapy or, in some cases, enhance it. Regardless, the therapist need not feel the burden of any imposition as long as basic guidelines for counseling are followed and the therapist trusts his or her own skills for facilitating language. One of the most effective ways to do this is to verbalize for the patient in complete sentences whatever minimal verbal and nonverbal messages the patient is sending. If, for instance, the patient tilts her head downward and appears sad when asked, "How are you feeling this morning?" the therapist might say, "You look as if you're feeling down today." If the patient nods in agreement, the therapist could assist by having her say in unison, "I'm not feeling very well today," and then encourage her to say so independently or with some assistance.

Such an acknowledgment by the therapist of the patient's mood then can lead to further questions and responses, which not only would help relieve the patient of several personal concerns but also contribute to functional language usage. Unfortunately, we may not always be that adept in recognizing what the patient is feeling and in fact miss the point entirely. Although perhaps momentarily frustrating for both patient and therapist, it need not deter us from continuing the process until the patient's feelings are revealed more accurately. Surely, the aphasic patient recognizes that we too are human, that we are not always entirely accurate and can make mistakes. Even if the therapist cannot reach the heart of the matter by the end of the session, the patient might find some solace in the therapist's frustration so as to assuage the patient's own. It indeed might be appropriate for therapists to share their frustration in trying to understand the patient, commenting on their own limitations.

One further strategy the therapist could use to uncover hidden feelings is to share information surrounding an incident about which the patient may be concerned, thereby maintaining a constant flow of information. In doing so, the therapist should be alert to the patient's confirmation of that information and modify whatever is necessary to gain agreement. Such an approach also can shift the emphasis to other therapy matters. We recall an incident with one patient who was scheduled for the removal of a skin cancer on his hand. By acknowledging the circumstance, the therapist helped the patient explain that he had been told by his physician that it was not the kind that would metastasize. A productive session followed, in which the patient, with the verbal assistance of the therapist, expressed relief that things could be a lot worse, as in the case of a neighbor who was dying of lung cancer. Thus, the change of self-focus helped to reduce the patient's anxiety and depression.

Dealing with the Patient's Response to Linguistic Errors   One of the most typical behaviors therapists encounter during therapy is the patient's emotional response to errors made while attempting linguistic tasks. These responses may be characterized by evocations of self-depreciation, frustration, anger, or the desire to cease the task. The quality and intensity of the affect, of course, varies from patient to patient, depending on a combination of such elements as premorbid personality, postmorbid psychological attitudes, spousal or family support, and the degree of overall deficits. Therapists often observe that such responses may mentally block the patient, thereby triggering further inaccurate linguistic responses. For example, it is not uncommon for perseverative behavior to increase at such times and the wish to terminate the entire session.

It is appropriate, then, for the therapist to "take time out" to comfort the patient by acknowledging the difficulty and frustration being experienced and encourage further responses regardless of accuracy. All of us are familiar with our need to respond accurately in a problem-solving situation and are well aware of the blocks that arise when we try too hard. We find that, by being willing to risk error, we are more apt to arrive at the appropriate place. Similarly, for the aphasic patient, it is better to risk committing the error than to inhibit the attempt at all. Merely suggesting the patient relax may contribute to further tension and subsequent blocks to verbal communication. We suggest it is more productive to offer the person the notion that it is very natural and normal to want to be right and that if the correct response is not forthcoming, it might be so later on during the session or subsequent ones. What is most important is not just the correct response but the development of a more positive attitude toward oneself and the various verbal tasks confronted. These

considerations, we believe, will be most effective in reducing the patient's level of stress and enhancing continued retrieval of language competency.

Dealing with Patient Attitudes Toward Therapy and Options for Behavioral Change   The expectations of therapists are not always consistent with expectations of their patients. Regardless of a particular issue, it is important for the therapist to open up discussion or provide the patient opportunity to do so. Those therapists who restrict themselves to one particular therapeutic technique or routine when patient progress is at a standstill may not be aware that the patient's negative attitude about the strategy or exercise could be inhibiting progress. What may be appropriate in the mind of even the skilled clinician may not be necessarily appropriate for the patient who has a sense of "what works for me." The open, unthreatened, creative therapist can take advantage of this opportunity to explore with the patient what is not working, why it is not working, and what might work. The approach described could well lead to the use of a more fruitful approach and provide greater patient responsibility for personal recovery.

Frequently, the patient adheres to an unbending attitude, which may prove to be counterproductive. Self-effacement, expressions of futility, noncompliance with home practice (regardless of technique or strategy)—all these must be noted and brought out in the open. Once again, the therapist can listen, empathize, and clarify for the patient that such negative attitudes are not unusual, considering the trauma the patient has experienced. Still, the patient should be aided in realizing that the attitude can be self-defeating, delaying further progress. Here, counseling demands great patience by the therapist, who must now guide the patient with persistence yet not sacrifice the rapport already established.

Conceivably, a patient may want to terminate therapy, confronting the therapist with a difficult decision. Although not a life or death issue, it nevertheless presents the therapist with the choice either to acknowledge and accept the patient's resignation or to encourage the patient to continue therapy. This ethical issue of personal choice is one for which we have no simple answer, given the communicative difficulty the patient may have in expressing the wish. We also must be aware that the spouse may be the one who lost all hope, with the patient passively acquiescing. Nonetheless, it is incumbent on us to respect the patient's feelings and be sensitive to the persistence in the desire to terminate therapy. Whatever obstacles face the therapeutic relationship, the spouse or family members may be engaged to discuss the issue with the mutual consent of the patient.

Significance of Community Outreach Programs

The efficacy of community outreach programs, including group therapy and family support groups, has achieved greater prominence over the last 15 years with the emergence of outpatient day care centers, hospital auxiliaries, community agencies, and college and university programs. These have been particularly important developments in the light of managed health care, which, in its present form unfortunately, will continue to reduce delivery of rehabilitation services for the CVA patient. Therefore, therapists have been put in the position of providing more for less and determining how best to build the bridge to less costly, more socially based community programs. M. T. Sarno (1998) alludes to this dilemma in her discussion regarding follow-up care once individual therapeutic services have been terminated. The problem of social isolation in many cases of stroke patients with aphasia was exacerbated even one year following the stroke. As reported by Sarno and by anecdotal material supplied by clinicians, a large number of aphasic families think that people consciously avoid them.

Given the rationing of poststroke rehabilitation by the government and insurance companies, the efficacy of group therapy is receiving more attention in the literature, and such groups continue to emerge in hospitals, community agencies, clinics, and colleges throughout the United States. The formation of such organizations as the National Stroke Association[3] (NSA) has been a significant means to provide information to both stroke and nonstroke

families regarding prevention, treatment, stroke data reports, rehabilitation, survivor-caregiver support, and research. The NSA has also been instrumental in the formation of stroke support and peer group chapters throughout the country.

Purpose of Group Therapy

One of the chief objectives of group therapy for aphasic patients, it would seem, is to provide psychological support from participation in a group. A second objective would be to provide opportunities for patients to practice communicating with each other with the expectation that such experiences will enhance whatever the patient is trying to accomplish in individual therapy at home or other facility. A third, and perhaps the most far-reaching objective, is the peer interaction that may help to assuage the loneliness, depression, hopelessness, psychosocial isolation, and other effects experienced by the patient.

Value of Group Therapy

On first glance, it would appear that, despite the rapid growth of group therapy for aphasic patients, there has been only limited objective research to document its value in fostering language or recovery or psychosocial adjustment. Davis (1983) and Eisenson (1984), in their reviews of the literature, cite the studies of Wertz et al. (1981), Redinger et al. (1971), and Aten, Caligiuri, and Holland (1982), which reveal limited value at least in contributing to enhanced use of language, particularly in conjunction with individual therapy.

Brown and Abby (1999), following over 20 years of provocative group work with persons over 65 years of age, found that group sessions including exercises, discussion, and socializing were key elements in helping to restore motivation not only to manage the golden years more dynamically but to gain greater communicative skills. The authors describe how a wide variety of settings, including churches, adult day programs, and senior centers, can serve the population described, involving not only speech-language pathologists, but nurses, social workers, physical and occupational thera-

---

[3]National Stroke Association, 96 Inverness Drive E, Suite 1, Englewood, Colorado 80110.

pists, and students in training for all rehabilitation professions.

Still, research supporting group therapy as a means for improving psychosocial behavior has not been as definitive as desired. Albert et al. (1981) report the ineffectiveness of traditional group therapy techniques for aphasic patients but cite psychosocial benefits to be derived. Jenkins et al. (1975), in discussing the effect of group therapy in Veterans Administration hospitals, view its greatest value to be in helping the patient feel less isolated and encouraged by the progress other patients are making. We might note that one disquieting feature might be the depression that could result in patients who are *not* progressing, particularly when they observe other patients who *are*. Brumfitt and Sheeran (1997), in a short-term group therapy program, found significant improvements in communicative competence and a reduction in depression and enhancement of psychosocial well-being. Eisenson (1984) convincingly summarizes the value of group therapy for achieving the following social values:[4]

1. *Group training provides an opportunity for socialization* which would include the singing of popular and well-known songs, and the practicing of "social gesture" speech. Participation by all should be the objective but it could be encouraged gently.
2. *Group training provides an opportunity for "motivation from peers" rather than from the unimpaired therapist.* Patients are more likely to be motivated to attempt verbalizations when encouraged by other patients rather than by the linguistically proficient therapist.
3. *The group approach provides a situation where awareness of certain aphasic speech "habits" such as telegraphic and agrammatical language structure, becomes apparent;* patients would be able to better their self-monitoring skills through the corrective input of other patients as well as identifying with the incorrect "habits" of others.
4. *Group training provides an aphasic patient with an opportunity to observe the techniques of other aphasics for evoking speech and for getting speakers to make themselves understood.* The patient can learn either actively or vicariously without risking failures or detriment to his or her ego.

5. *. . . provides the aphasic with an opportunity in a learning situation to respond to more than one manner of speech and language usage.*
6. *. . . The group approach . . . provides for "ventilation of feelings" and "airing of grievances."* By identifying with the feelings of others in the group the patient is less likely to feel isolated and made a better adaptation to living with other members of his family.

Eisenson adds to his discussion of group therapy other admonitions:

1. *Withdrawn patients may find it difficult to attempt expression as members of a group.*
2. *Group pressure may provoke some patients into talking about personal problems before they are entirely ready for such revelations.*
3. *The rate of a group is usually slower than the best member can manage and somewhat faster than the weakest member can master.*

Eisenson concludes, as have other aphasiologists, by emphasizing that group therapy should be used only to supplement individual therapy. While group therapy may be inappropriate for some patients and the decision to use it must depend on the therapist's awareness of the principles of group dynamics and the individual patients' emotional needs and states, we believe it should be an option, particularly if nothing else is available. We need to bear in mind also that group therapy can be a realistic, even if not an ideal, substitute for families who can ill-afford the expense of individual therapy. All this may be moot in light of our discussion of cost containment in rehabilitation services as they presently worsen as of this writing. Elman and Ellis (1999) found statistically significantly positive effects of group treatment on linguistic and communicative performance in patients with chronic aphasia and make a strong case for its use, particularly in the light of our discussion.

Outcomes and Efficacy Research

This chapter has raised many issues regarding psychosocial correlates of aphasia and resultant implications. Many inferences were made based on the literature investigated as well as on anecdotal and clinical material. Consequently, we consider the directions research needs to take to validate several

---

[4]The two lists are reprinted with permission from J. Eisenson, Adult Aphasia, 2nd ed. (Englewood Cliffs, NJ: Prentice-Hall, 1984), pp. 236–238.

of the assumptions made and collaterally discuss design problems.

Personality Type

The study of personality type as a precipitating factor in the onset of a CVA has yet to be thoroughly investigated. The value of such research could add to other definitive factors already known. The nagging problem still appears to be the issues of tight experimental design, heterogeneity of population variance, difficulties with retrospective studies, and single-subject versus multisubject designs. Rabkin (1993) refers to the difficulties incurred by use of retrospective designs in terms of errors of recall by subjects, retrospective falsification to justify illness, and the differences between the evidence gathered by case study and results from prospective research. The problem, she indicates, is not so much the method as it is the misinterpretation of the results. Multisubject designs demand strict homogeneity and process delineation of personality patterns (oftentimes difficult to describe), psychosocial factors, and the complex interweaving of the two. Single-subject designs may be more precise, allowing for intensive clinical studies, but they hinder us in generalizing the results to other subjects. Probably the most sophisticated, but unfortunately most costly as well, approach would be the longitudinal study in which a randomly selected and tested population is followed over a period of time as in the Framingham studies.

Meta-analytical studies are being made more extensively during the present decade. While counseling treatment per se received minimal attention, Robey (1998), in an extensive search of aphasia treatment literature confirming an earlier meta-analysis, demonstrated that favorable outcomes of therapy depended on the amount of treatment, type of treatment, severity of aphasia, and type of aphasia. Only two types of treatment were reported as representative of most treatment strategies: one identified as "individualized multimodality stimulation" and the other "various linguistic and cognitive tasks." A considerable number of treatments were either too vague or absent and assigned a code of *not specified*. The use of family therapy was nei-

ther identified nor specified; nor were the issues of overall family adjustment addressed.

An unusual but valuable study by Warren (1999) stresses the need to incorporate a rehabilitation model in which client-centered interests are addressed in the light of the payer-driven environment we now all face. In essence, Warren suggests that outcome measurement will have to be determined by how patients cope with their handicap and take more individual responsibility for enhancing the quality of their lives. His findings are consistent with those of Clark and Smith (1998), who found that functional outcome could be measured by the stroke patient's satisfaction with progress manifested in a return to previous lifestyle activities, level of depression, cohesive family functioning, understanding of stroke, and clarity of expectations on admission to rehabilitation.

Family Communication and Caregiving

The efficacy of home health care services has received some support, as evidenced in the research by Ricauda et al. (1998), Dowswell et al. (1997), Dennis et al. (1998), and Stewart et al. (1998). Among several of the consistent conclusions reached by these investigators were that the emotional stability, sensitivity, and outlook of the caregiver (either spouse or hired person) were pertinent factors in patient outcome. Intermittent visits by nurses were found to be a rich support system for both patient and family. Peer visitor support was found to assist caregiver support needs, lessened caregiver demands, and aided the patient to feel part of the world again. It also was obvious that intermittent visits by therapists, regardless of discipline, almost equally enhanced both communicative and psychosocial recovery.

The development of a family functional communication scale for the measurement of pragmatic language competence as the result of varied therapeutic strategies yet needs to demand our attention. We have already alluded to the work of Holland and Code and Muller and their environmentally based testing and treatment strategies. We propose using the family therapy process as the model for determining how the family and nonfamily caregiver use language in relationship to the patient's disordered usage. We would attempt to measure the patient's functional usage over time, from onset, using a modification of the microanalysis method developed by Labov and Fanshel (1977). Such an approach certainly would not be free of obstacles. The complexity and uniqueness of "family communication" could defy standardization and predictability. It would appear that a precisely engineered linguistic discourse computer software program could facilitate the task. As a measure of the way an individual's disrupted language system may recover over a period of time, however, it presents us with challenging opportunities for constructive family participation in recovery and a method for complementing traditional strategies, not to ignore objective outcomes.

Conclusion

In this chapter, we document the most current literature and research associated with the many-faceted psychological ramifications of CVA and also identify and explore how eclectic individual and family systems therapy may be applied. We would be remiss, however, in not identifying certain aspects that require not only further inquiry but more extensive research regardless of their, perhaps, controversial aspects. We present these in the form of questions now, but they are alluded to in later chapters, too.

1. How do we modify counseling and family systems therapy to meet the needs of aphasic patients of various cultures, ethnicity, and race, without imposing traditional values that may be suitable only for white Americans?
2. How can we integrate either the introduction or examination of spiritual, mind, and body integrative values in a holistic approach that may defy objective analysis or validation? Or, should we ignore them?
3. Finally, although perhaps related to the preceding, how can we reconcile traditional with homeopathic medicine, particularly with respect to the use of acupressure and acupuncture, meditation or ayurveda practices, and use of natural food supplements and vitamins?

References

Adler R. Intense psychoperceptual disorientation during the acute stage post-stroke and brain trauma. Unpublished doctoral dissertation. Walden University, Naples, FL; 1980.

Affleck G, Tennen H, Pfeiffer C, Fifield J. Appraisals of control and predictability in adapting to a chronic disease. *J of Personality and Social Psychology.* 1987;53:273–279.

Albert MA, Goodglass H, Helm NA, Rubens AB, Alexander MP. *Clinical Aspects of Dysphasia.* New York: Springer-Verlag; 1981.

Artes MA, Hoops R. Problems of aphasia and non-aphasic stroke patients as identified and evaluated by patients' wives. In: Lebrun Y, Hoops R, eds. *Neurolinguistics: Recovery in Aphasics,* Vol 4. Amsterdam: Swets and Zeitlinger; 1976.

Aten JL, Caligiuri MP, Holland AL. The efficacy of functional communication therapy for chronic aphasic patients. *J of Speech and Hearing Disorders.* 1982;47:93–96.

Awata S, Ito H, Konno M, Ono S, Kawashima R, Fukuda H, Sato M. Regional cerebral blood flow abnormalities in late life depression; relation to refractoriness and chronification. *Psychiatry Clinical Neuroscience.* 1998; 52:1,97–105.

Baretz RM, Stephenson GR. Unrealistic patient. *New York State J of Medicine.* 1976;76:54–57.

Birkett PD. *The Psychiatry of Stroke.* Washington, DC: American Psychiatric Press; 1996.

Bjorntorp P. Stress and cardiovascular disease. *Acta Physiol Scand Suppl.* 1997;640:144–148.

Boone KB, Lesser IM, Miller BL, Wohl M, Berman N, Lee A, Palmer B, Back C. Cognitive functioning in older depressed patients: Relationship of presence and severity of depression to neuropsychological test scores. *Neuropsychology.* 1995;9:390–398.

Boswell S. ASHA submits comments to HHS on health objectives. *ASHA Leader.* 1999;4(1):1.

Bowlby J. *Separation and Loss.* New York: Basic Books; 1970.

Brand AN, Jolles J, Gipsen-de-Wied C. Recall and recognition memory deficits in depression. *J of Affective Disorders.* 1992;25:77–86.

Breslau LD, Haug MR, eds. *Depression and Aging: Causes and Consequences.* New York: Springer-Verlag; 1983.

Broderick J, Brott T, Kothari R, Miller R, Khoury J, Panciolia A, Gebel J, Mills D, Minneci L, Shukla R. The greater Cincinnati/northern Kentucky stroke study: preliminary first-ever and total incidence rates of stroke among blacks. *Stroke.* 1998;29:414–421.

Brookshire RH. *Introduction to Neurogenic Communication Disorders.* St. Louis: Mosby; 1997.

Brown W, Abby V. *Still Kicking: Restorative Groups for Frail Older Adults.* Baltimore: Health Professions Press; 1999.

Brunfitt SM, Sheeran P. An evaluation of short-term group therapy for people with aphasia. *Disability Rehabilitation.* 1997;6:221–230.

Burgess C, Morris T, Pettingale KW. Psychological response to cancer diagnosis—II. Evidence for coping styles. *J of Psychosomatic Research.* 1988;32:263–272.

Burns MS. Use of the family to facilitate communicative changes in adults with neurological impairments. In: Andrews JR, *New Directions in Speech-Language Pathology: Systems, Context, and Change.* Seminars in Speech and Language. New York: Thieme, 1996;17(2): 115–122.

Campbell TL, Patterson JM. The effectiveness of family interventions in the treatment of physical illnesses. *J of Marital and Family Therap.y* 1995;21(4):545–583.

Cannon WB. *The Wisdom of the Body.* New York: W. W. Norton, 1939.

Christenson JM, Anderson JD. Spouse adjustment to stroke: aphasic versus nonaphasic partners. *J of Communication Disorders.* 1989;4:225–231.

Clark MS, Smith DS. Factors contributing to patient satisfaction with rehabilitation following stroke. *Int J Rehabil Res.* 1998;2:43–154.

Code C, Muller DJ. *The Code-Muller Protocols.* Kilworth, United Kingdom: Far Communications; 1992.

Costa PT Jr, McCrae RR. Personality as a lifelong determinant of well-being. In: Malatesta C, Izards C, eds. *Affective Processes in Adult Development and Aging.* Beverly Hills, CA: Sage; 1984.

Costa PT Jr, McCrae RR, Locke BZ. Personality factors. In: Cornoni-Huntley J, Huntley R, Feldman JJ, eds. *Health Status and Well-Being of the Elderly: National Health and Nutrition Examination I—Epidemiologic Followup Study.* New York: Oxford University Press; 1990.

Crowe TA, ed. *Applications of Counseling in Speech-Language Pathology and Audiology.* Baltimore: Williams and Wilkins; 1997.

Cummings JL. Neuropsychiatric manifestations of right hemisphere lesions. *Brain and Language.* 1997;57: 1,22–37.

Cummings JL, Sultzer DL. Depression in multi-infarct dementia. In: Starkstein SE, Robinson RG, eds. *Depression in Neurologic Disease.* Baltimore: Johns Hopkins University Press, 1993:165–185.

Cunningham R. Counseling someone with severe aphasia: an explorative case study. *Disability Rehab.* 1998;20(9): 346–354.

Davis GA. *A Survey of Adult Aphasia.* Englewood Cliffs, NJ: Prentice-Hall; 1983.

————. Family adjustment to aphasia. *ASHA.* 1990;32(11): 63–64.

Denman A. Determining the needs of spouses caring for aphasic partners. *Disability Rehab.* November 1998; 20(11):411–423.

Dennis M, O'Rourke S, Lewis S, Sharpe M, Warlow C. A quantitative study of the emotional outcome of people caring for stroke survivors. *Stroke.* 1998;9:1867–1872.

Dohrenwend BP, Levay I, Shrout PE, et al. Life stress and psychopathology: progress on research begun with Barbara Snell Dohrenwend. *Am J of Community Psychology.* 1987;15:677–715.

Dowswell G, Lawler J, Young J, Forster A, Hearn J. A qualitative study of specialist nurse support for stroke patients and caregivers at home. *Clinical Rehab.* 1997;11(4):293–301.

Eckenrode J. The impact of chronic and acute stressors on daily reports of mood. *J of Personality and Social Psychology.* 1984;46:918–970.

Eisenson J. *Adult Aphasia,* 2nd ed. Englewood Cliffs, NJ: Prentice-Hall; 1984.

Elman RJ, Ellis EB. The efficacy of group communication treatment in adults with chronic aphasia. *J Speech Lang Hear Res.* 1999;42(2):411–419.

Engels GL. Grief and grieving. *Am J of Nursing.* 1964;64:93.

Evans RL, Griffith J, Haselkorn MD, Hendricks RD, Baldwin D, Bishop DS. Poststroke family function: an evaluation of the family's role in rehabilitation. *Rehab Nursing.* 1992;17:127–131.

Evans RL, Matlock AL, Bishop DS, Stranahan S, Pederson C. Family intervention after stroke:does counseling or education help? Stroke. 1988;19:1243–1249.

Eysenck H, Faulkner D. The components of type A behavior and its genetic determinants. *Act Nerv Super (Praha).* 1982; suppl 3, pt 1:111–125.

Felton BJ, Revenson TA, Hinrichsen GA. Coping and adjustment in chronically ill adults. *Social Science and Medicine.* 1984;18:889–898.

Ferrand C. *Introduction to Organic and Neurogenic Disorders of Communication: Current Scope of Practice.* Boston: Allyn and Bacon; 1997.

Finger WW. Prevention, assessment and treatment of sexual dysfunction following stroke. *Sexuality and Disability.* Spring 1993;11(1):39–56.

Friedman MH. On the nature of regression in aphasia. *Archives of General Psychiatry.* 1961;5:60–64.

Friedman MH, Rosenman RH. Association of specific overt behavior patterns with blood and cardiovascular findings. *JAMA.* 1959;169:1286–1296.

Gareri P, Stilo G, Bevacqua I, Mattace R, Ferreri G, De Saro G. Anti-depressant drugs in the elderly. *Gen Pharmacol.* 1998;30(4):465–475.

Geschwind N. The borderland of neurology and psychiatry: some common misconceptions. In: Devinski O, Schachter SC, eds. *Norman Geschwind: Selected Publications on Language, Epilepsy, and Behavior.* Boston: Butterworth–Heinemann; 1997:513–520.

Goldberg SA. The aphasic's need to understand his linguistic disability. Paper presented to: annual convention of California-Speech-Language-Hearing Assocation. Los Angeles, 1980.

Goldberger L, Breznitz S. Stress research at a crossroads. In: Goldberger L, Breznitz S. eds. *Handbook of Stress: Theoretical and Clinical Aspects,* 2nd ed. New York: The Free Press; 1993:3–6.

Goldstein K. *Aftereffects of Brain Injuries in War.* New York: Grune and Stratton; 1942.

———. *Language and Language Disturbances.* New York: Grune and Stratton, 1948.

———. The effect of brain damage on the personality. *Psychiatry.* 1952;15:245–260.

———. Functional disturbances in brain damage. In; Arieti S, ed. *American Handbook of Psychiatry.* New York: Basic Books, 1959.

Heilman KM. The neurobiology of amotional experience. *J of Neuropsychiatry and Clinical Neuroscience.* 1997; 9(3):438–439.

Herrmann N, Black SE, Lawrence J, Szekely C, Szalai JP. The Sunnybrook Stroke Study: a study of depressive symptoms and functional outcome. *Stroke.* 1998;29(3): 618–624.

Hemsley G, Code C. Interations between recovery in aphasia, emotional and psychosocial factors in subjects with aphasia, their significant others and speech pathologists. *Disability Rehab.* 1996;189(11):567–584.

Holland A. Comment on "Spouses' understanding of the communicative abilities of aphasic patients." *J of Speech and Hearing Disorders.* 1977;42:307–310.

———. *Communicative Abilities in Daily Living.* Baltimore: University Park Press; 1980.

Horenstein S. Effects of cerebrovascular disease in personality and emotionality. In: Benton AL, ed. *Behavioral Change in Cebrovascular Disease.* New York: Harper and Row; 1970.

House A, Dennis M, Mogridge L, Hawton K, Warlow C. Like events and difficulties preceding stroke. *J of Neurology, Neurosurgery, and Psychiatry.* 1990;53:1024–1028.

Ireland C, Wotton G. Time to talk: counseling for people with dysphasia. *Disability Rehab.* 1996;18(11):585–591.

Kannel S, Sorlie P, Gordon T., Labile hypertension: a faulty concept? The Framingham Study. *Circulation.* 1980(61):1183–1187.

Jenkins CD. Recent evidence supporting psychologic and social risk factors for coronary disease. *New England J of Medicine.* 1976;274:987–994,1033–1038.

Jenkins CD, Rosenman RH, Friedman M. Development of an objective psychological test for the determination of the coronary-prone behavior pattern in employed men. *J of Chronic Diseases.* 1967;20:371–379.

Jenkins JJ, Jimenez-Pabon E, Shaw RE, Defer JW. *Schuell's Aphasia in Adults,* 2nd ed. New York: Harper and Row; 1975.

Kim JS, Yoon SS, Lee SI, Yoo HJ, Kim CY, Choi KS, Lee BC. *European Neurology.* April 1998; 39(3):168–173.

Kinsella G, Duffy F. Psychosocial readjustment in the spouses of aphasic patients. *Scandinavian J of Rehab Medicine.* 1979;11:129–132.

Kirschner HS, ed. *Handbook of Neurological Speech and Language Disorders.* Neurological Disease and Therapy, Vol 33. New York: Marcel Dekker; 1995.

Krishnan K, Ranga R, Gadde KM. The pathophysiologic basis for late-life depression. Imaging studies of the

aging. *Am J of Geriatric Psychiatry.* 1996; 4(4, suppl 1): S22–S33.

Kubler-Ross E. *On Death and Dying.* New York: Macmillan; 1969.

———. *Death: The Final Stage of Growth.* Englewood Cliffs, NJ: Prentice-Hall; 1975.

Labov W, Fanshell D. *Therapeutic Discourse: Psychotherapy as Conversation.* New York: Academic Press; 1977.

Lamendella JT. The limbic system in human communication. In: Whitaker H, Whitaker HA, eds. *Studies in Neurolinguistics,* Vol 3. New York: Academic Press; 1977.

Lawlor BA, Anderson MC. The neurobiology of late-life depression: impact of silent cerebrovascular disease. *Human Psychopharmacology, Clinical and Experimental.* November 1995;10 (Suppl 4): S223–S227.

Lazarus R, Launier R. Stress-related transactions between persons and environment. In: Pervin L, Lewis M, eds. *Perspectives in Interactional Psychology.* New York: Plenum; 1978.

Letourneau PY. The psychological effects of aphasia. In Lafond D, DeGiovani R, Joanette J, Ponzio J, Taylor-Sarno M, eds. *Living with Aphasia.* San Diego, CA: Singular Publishing Group; 1993.

Linebaugh CW, Young-Charles HY. The counseling needs of the families of aphasic patients. In: Brookhaire RK, ed. *Clinical Aphasiology Conference Proceedings.* Minneapolis: BRK Publishers; 1978.

Lubinski R. Environmental language stimulation. In: Chapey R, ed. *Language Intervention and Strategies in Adult Aphasia.* Baltimore: Williams and Wilkins, 1981.

Luterman D. *Counseling Persons with Communication Disorders and Their Families.* Boston: Little, Brown and Company; 1996.

Malone RL. Expressed attitudes of families of aphasics. *J of Speech and Hearing Disorders.* 1969;34:146–151.

Manuel M. Doing it the family way. *Nursing Mirror.* 1979;149:28–34.

Matthews KA. CHD and type A behavior: Update on an alternative to the Booth-Kewley and Friendman quantitative review. *Psychological Bulletin.* 1988;104:373–380.

McEwen BS. Stress and hippocampal plasticity. *Annual Review of Neuroscience.* 1999;22:105.

McEwen BS, Mendelson S. Effects of stress on the neurochemistry and morphology of the brain: counterregulation versus damage. In: Goldberger L, Breznitz S, eds, *Handbook of Stress: Theoretical and Clinical Aspects,* 2nd ed. New York: The Free Press; 1993: 101–126.

Mega MS, Cummings JL, Salloway S, Malloy P. The limbic system: an anatomic, phylogenetic, and clinical perspective. *J of Neuropsychiatry and Clinical Neuroscience.* 1997;9(3):315–330.

Meichenbaum D, Turk D. Coping and disease: a cognitive-behavioral perspective. In: Neufell WJ, ed. *Psychological Stress and Psychopathology.* New York: McGraw-Hill; 1982.

Miyai I, Reding MJ. Effects of anti-depressants on functional recovery following stroke: a double blind study. *J of Neurologic Rehabilitation.* 1998;12(1):5–13.

Montgomery SA. Efficacy and safety of the elective serotonin reuptake inhibitors in treating depression in eldely patients. *Int Clin Psychopharmacol.* 1998;13 (suppl 5):49–54.

Moustakas CE. *Loneliness and Love.* Englewood Cliffs, NJ: Prentice-Hall; 1972.

Nagaratnam N, Pathama NN. Behavioral and psychiatric aspects of silent cerebral infarction. *British J of Clinical Practice.* 1997;51:160–163.

Orbrist PA. *Cardiovascular Psychophysiology: A Perspective.* New York: Plenum Press; 1981.

Ormel J, Kempen GI, Pennix BW, Brilman EL, Beekman AT, Van Sonderen E. Chronic medical conditions and mental health in older people; disability and psychosocial resources mediate specific mental health effects. *Psychol Med.* September 1997; 27(5):1065–1077.

Porter J, Dabul B. The application of transactional analysis to therapy with wives of aphasic patiends. *ASHA.* 1977;19:244–248.

Rabkin JG. Stress and psychiatric disorders. In Goldberger L, Breznitz S, eds. *Handbook of Stress,* 2nd ed. New York: The Free Press; 1993:477–495.

Redinger RA, Forster S, Dolphin MK, Goodduhn J, Weisinger J. Group therapy in the rehavilitation of the severely aphasic and hemiplegic in the late stages. *Scandinavian J of Rehabilitation Medicine.* 1971;3:89–91.

Ricauda NA, Pla FL, Marinello R, Molaschi M, Fabris F. Feasibility of an acute stroke home care service for elderly patients. *Arc Geron and Geriat.* 1998;(suppl 6):17–22.

Robey RR. A meta-analysis of clinical outcomes in the treatment of aphasia. *J Speech Lang Hear Res.* 1998;41(1): 172–187.

Robinson RG, Benson DF. Depression in aphasic patients: frequency, severity, and clinical-pathological correlations. *Brain and Language* 1981; 14:282-291.

Rollin WJ. Family therapy and the aphasic adult. In Eisenson J. *Adult Aphasia,* 2nd ed. Englewood Cliffs, NJ: Prentice-Hall, 1984.

———. Counseling spouses of the communicatively impaired. In: Curlee RF, ed. *Seminars in Speech and Language* 1988;9(3):269–281.

Roskies E, Lazarus R. Coping theory and the teaching of coping skills. In: Davidson P, ed. *Behavioral Medicine: Changing Health Lifestyles.* New York: Brunner/Mazel; 1979.

Sackeim HA, Greenberg MS, Weiman AL, Gur RC, Hungerbahler JP, Geschwind N. Hemispheric asymmetry in the expression of positive and negative emotion. Neurological evidence. *Archives of Neurology,* 1982;39:210–218.

Sackeim HA, Weber SL. Functional brain asymmetry in the regulation of emotion: Implications for bodily manifestations of stress. In: Goldberger L, Breznitz S, eds. *Handbook of Stress.* New York: Macmillan; 1982.

Salzman C, Shader RI. Depression in the elderly, part I. Relationship between depression, psychologic defense mechanism and physical illness. *J of the American Geriatric Society*; 1978(26):210–235.

Santos ME, Farrajota ML, Castro-Caldas A, De Sousa L. Problems of patients with chronic aphasia: different perspectives of husbands and wives. *Brain Injury.* 1999;13(1):23–29.

Sarno JE. Emotional aspects of aphasia. In Sarno MT (ed), *Acquired Aphasia.* New York: Academic Press, 1981.

Sarno JE, Gainotti G. The psychological and social sequelae of aphasia. In: Sarno MT, ed. *Acquired Aphasia,* 3rd ed. New York: Academic Press; 1998:569–594.

Sarno MT. Recovery and rehabilitation in aphasia. In: Sarno MT, ed. *Acquired Aphasia,* 3rd ed. New York: Academic Press; 1998:595–631.

———, ed. *Acquired Aphasia,* 2nd ed. New York: Academic Press; 1991.

Satir V. *Conjoint Family Therapy.* Palo Alto, CA: Science and Behavior Books; 1967.

Scheir MF, Weintraub JK, Carver CS. Coping with stress: divergent strategies of optimists and pessimists. *J of Personality and Social Psychology.* 1986;51: 1257–1264.

Selye H. *The Stress of Life,* rev. ed. New York: McGraw-Hill; 1976.

Shipley KG. *Interviewing and Counseling in Communicative Disorders: Principles and Procedures,* 2nd ed. Boston: Allyn and Bacon; 1996.

Shontz F. Reactions to crisis. *Volta Review.* 1965;65: 364–330.

Skelly M. Aphasic patients talk back. *American Journal of Hearing.* 1975;(7):1140–1142.

Skilbeck C. Psychological aspects of stroke. In: Woods RT, ed. *Handbook of the Clinical Psychology of Aging.* New York: John Wiley and Sons; 1996:283–301.

Spencer KA, Tompkins CA, Schulz R. Assessment of depression in patients with brain pathology: the case of stoke. *Psychological Bulletin,* 1997;122(22):132–152.

Stein PN, Gordon WA, Hibbard MR, Silwinski MJ. An examination of depression in the spouses of stroke patients. *Rehabilitation-Psychology.* Summer 1992; 37(2):122–130.

Stewart MJ, Doble S, Hart G, Langille L, MacPherson K. Peer support for family caregivers of seniors with stroke. *Can J Nurs Res.* 1998;30(2):87–117.

Sweet JJ, Newman P, Bell B. Significance of depression in clinical neuropsychological assessment. *Clinical Psychology Review.* 1992;(12):21–45.

Tanner DC. Loss and grief: implications for the speech-language pathologist and audiologist. *ASHA.* November 1980;22:916–928.

Ullman M. *Behavioral Changes in Patients Following Strokes.* Springfield, IL: Charles C Thomas; 1962.

Van Amburg S, Barber C, Zimmerman T. Aging and family therapy: prevalence of aging and later family life concerns in marital and family therapy literature (1986–1993). *J of Marital and Family Therapy.* 1996; 22(2):195–204.

Visch-Brink E, Bastiaanse R, eds. *Linguistic Levels in Aphasiology.* Neurogenic Communication Disorders Series. San Diego: Singular Publishers Group, 1998.

Warren RL. Creating value with measurement: moving toward the patient. *Topics in Stroke Rehab.* 1999;5(4): 17–37.

Webster EJ, Newhoff M. Intervention with families of communicately impaired adults. In Beasley DS, Davis GA, eds. *Aging: Communication Processes and Disorders.* New York: Grune and Stratton; 1981.

Weinstein E, Kahn R. *Denial of Illness.* Springfield, IL: Charles C Thomas; 1955.

Wenz C, Hermann M. Emotional reactions and illness perception in chronic aphasia. A comparison between patients and their relatives. *Psychotherapie-Psychosomatic-Medizinische-Psychologie.* 1990;40 (12):488–495.

Wertz RT, Collins MJ, Weiss D, Kurtzke JF, Friden T, Brookshire RH, Pierce J, Holzapple P, Hubbard DJ, Porch BE, West JA, Davis A, Matovitch V, Morley GK, Resurrecicion E. Veterans Administration cooperative study on aphasia: a comparison of individual and group treatment. *J of Speech and Hearing Research.* 1981;24: 580–594.

Williams RB, Haney TL, Lee KL, Kang Y, Blumenthal JA, Whalen RE. Type A behavior, hostility, and coronary arteriosclerosis. *Psychosomatic Medicine.* 1980;40: 538–549.

Xu S, Wang X, Liu Y, Zhang J, Yan X. The relationship between neuropsychological characteristics and therapeutic outcome as well as prediction of rehabilitation in non-aphasic stroke patients. *Psychological Science, China.* 1998;21(2):102–107.

3

Psychological Considerations
for the Traumatically
Brain-Injured and Their Families

The Nature of Traumatic Brain Injury

To understand the magnitude of TBI, we define it as a cognitive, intellectual, emotional, and physical impairment resulting from multiple or diffuse lesions in the brain due to sudden injury from an external source. Griffith (1983), adapting from Rosenthal (1979), presents an extensive list of the posttraumatic psychological sequelae in patients of severe TBI (see Table 3–1).

Although precise figures are unavailable, the two major types of TBI are closed head nonmissile injury, due to vehicular accidents and other blunt traumas to the head, and missile injury, such as gunshot wounds. As Levin, Benton, and Grossman (1982) state in the Preface of their book on TBI,

The personal, social, and economic consequences of head injuries, particularly those resulting from automobile accidents, assaults, and athletic mishaps, can scarcely be overestimated. Thanks to the remarkable life-saving capabilities of modern neurosurgical management of acute severe head injuries, the number of patients surviving such injuries mount steadily . . .

Today, however, we are becoming more cognizant of TBI occurring in children and women who are physically abused. The effects of TBI also are experienced by the individual's family, often resulting in profound psychological and social changes in the family constellation and within individual family members.

Comparison to Aphasia

TBI presents a very different picture from aphasia. Except for penetrating missile wounds, TBI generally results in diffuse lesions of the cerebral cortex rather than the characteristic focal ones in aphasia. In TBI, cognitive deficits, in conjunction with emotional and behavioral changes, are more pronounced. Although these persons may also be aphasic, as in the case of those who suffer a penetration wound, their prognosis for recovery appears more favorable than that of aphasia victims (Levin, 1981).

A further distinguishing characteristic is that aphasia, which generally results from a CVA, is related to the overall aging process, whereas TBI usually occurs in a much younger population. And, as we explain later, the psychosocial ramifications are much different. Finally, there is a greater likelihood of direct subcortical lesions and severance or shearings of the hemispheres at the corpus callosum in TBI patients. These may have significantly greater consequences than in CVA. Levin and Chapman (1998) provide an extensive literature review and discussion, indicating that the brain-language paradigm established by classic theory in aphasia has contributed to our understanding of language deficits in TBI.

Incidence and Prevalence—Statistical Data

From the results of a major project conducted by the Santa Clara Valley Medical Center (SCVMC), a major regional TBI rehabilitation center in San Jose, California, it was estimated that nearly 500,000 cases of TBI occur in the United States annually (1982). It also was determined that, between 1970 and 1974, more than 900,000 TBI individuals were still suffering from the effects of their injuries. Thus, at any one time in the United States, 1 out of approximately 220 individuals is suffering the effects of TBI and requires medical, restorative, maintenance, or rehabilitative care. The figures cited, however, do not include those with permanent disabilities who are not using nor have access to the health care system. It is important to note that the data collected in the SCVMC study also do not include those individuals who, because of minor brain injuries, were not admitted for hospital care despite significant cognitive impairment from transient loss of consciousness or severe concussion.

The data reported by the SCVMC may be somewhat misleading in that a more recent study, conducted by the National Center for Injury Prevention and Control (Thurman, Branche, and Sniezek, 1998), reported approximately 300,000 people, generally young, incur sports-related TBIs per year. The study identifies exactly what is meant by *sports related*, but does not identify acts of "drag racing," or other "road games." They also report that, in 1995, the rate of TBI-associated deaths due to all external causes was 19.2 per 100,000 population (50,000 deaths; unpublished data obtained from multiple cause-of-death public use data tapes, Atlanta, Georgia, 1997).

Other investigators such as Naugle (1990) and Sorenson and Kraus (1991) put the incidence of TBI in the general population at approximately 200 per 100,000 people. For young adult males, the incidence is approximately 400 per 100,000. Winslade (1998) states that, of the 2 million Americans who suffer from TBI each year (most from car and motorcycle accidents), nearly 100,000 will die prematurely. More than 90,000 of these individuals will require nearly 10 years of extensive rehabilitation, at a cost of $4 million each.

According to one of the Morbidity, Monthly, Weekly Reports of the National Center for Injury Prevention and Control, motor vehicle crashes still are the leading cause of injury-related deaths in the United States, accounting for 31% of all such deaths in 1996 (U.S. Department of Health and Human Services, 1999; Center for Disease Control, unpublished data, 1949). Further reported is that motor-vehicle crashes resulted in 41,967 deaths (16 per 100,000 population), 3.4 million nonfatal injuries (1,270 per 100,000 population), and 23.9 million vehicles in crashes at a cost estimate of $200 billion. While exact figures related to TBI are inexact, the outcome of such accidents cannot be ignored.

Regardless of exact figures, TBI has been characterized by many as the "silent epidemic," a term suggesting that the actual number of TBIs is much higher because physicians often fail to recognize head injuries when other injuries are more apparent. Recovery is impeded, and the head injured often do not receive needed treatment because of the absence of easily observable symptoms. These may be people who generally look well and seemingly act appropriately, are in denial perhaps, but who indeed may be suffering emotionally.

Fortunately, more and more physicians are recognizing the real damage that may be brought about by supposedly minor brain injuries. Because of the development and refinement of sophisticated diagnostic instruments—computerized axial tomography scanners (CAT), positron emitted tomography (PET), nuclear magnetic resonance (NMR), brain electrical activity mapping (BEAM), regional cerebral blood flow (rCBF), magnetoencephalogram (MEG), single photon emission computer tomography (SPECT)—brain injury that escaped detection earlier is now revealed. Our increased knowledge of cranial physiology has further contributed to our understanding.

Profile of the Patient

According to Jennett and MacMillan (1981), the incidence of TBI is highest among men between the ages of 15 and 35. Similar findings have been verified by Kraus (1980) and Miller and Pentland (1989). Research by Kerr, Kay, and Lassman (1971) has shown the ratio of male to female patients admitted to hospitals is approximately 4:1, with an incidence rate peaking in the 15–24 age range.

Kerr et al. (1971) were able to establish a relationship between hospital admissions for TBI and a lower socioeconomic class in their Newcastle, Eng-

Table 3-1. Psychologic Disabilities

A. Cognitive-intellectual
1. Disorders of consciousness
2. Disorientation
3. Memory deficits
4. Decreased abstraction
5. Decreased learning abilities
6. Language-communication deficits
7. General intellectual deficits
8. Deficits in processing-sequencing information
9. Illogical thoughts
10. Poor judgment
11. Poor quality control
12. Inability to make decisions
13. Poor initiative
14. Verbal, motor perseveration
15. Confabulation
16. Difficulty in generalization
17. Short attention span
18. Distractibility
19. Fatigability
20. Perplexity
21. Dyscalculia

B. Perceptual-perceptual motor
1. Reduced motor speed
2. Reduced eye-hand coordination
3. Poor depth perception
4. Spatial disorientation
5. Poor figure-ground perception
6. Auditory perceptual deficits
7. Anosognosia
8. Autotopagnosia
9. Tactile, auditory, visual neglect
10. Apraxias

C. Emotional
1. Apathy
2. Impulsivity
3. Irritability
4. Aggressiveness
5. Anxiety
6. Depression
7. Emotional lability
8. Silliness

C. Behavioral-personality
1. Lack of goal-directed behavior
2. Lack of initiation
3. Poor self-image, reduced self-worth
4. Denial of disability or its consequences
5. Aggressive behavior
6. Childlike behavior
7. Bizarre, psychotic ideation and behavior
8. Loss of sensitivity and concern for others: selfishness
9. Dependency, passivity
10. Indecision
11. Indifference
12. Slovenliness
13. Sexual disturbances
14. Drug, alcohol abuse

Adapted from M.Rosenthal, Psychological deficits in the brain-injured adult and family. Paper presented at the Conference on Rehabilitation of the Traumatic Brain-Injured Adult, June 1979, Williamsburg, VA. (As cited in Griffith, 1983.)

land, study of 386 patients. They also noted a tendency toward a relationship between assault as a cause of injury and the lowest socioeconomic class, whereas sports-related injuries were common to upper socioeconomic groups. The findings in Great Britain and the United States have been supported by those in Australia, where Selecki, Hoy, and Ness (1968) found TBI admissions to predominate for laborers and craftsworkers, with incidence among business people, clerical workers, and women who work only at home being significantly lower.

Jennett (1983) reports, in a study in the United States, that 72% of TBI patients had had alcohol in their bloodstreams on hospital admission and 52% were intoxicated by legal definition. Kerr et al. (1971) had earlier found alcohol to be a predisposing cause for brain injury, particularly in motor vehicle accidents and in domestic accidents and assaults. Levin et al. (1982) indicate that, based on previous studies, one fourth to one half of all severe head injuries are among chronic alcoholics. Even though annual motor-vehicle crash-related fatalities involving alcohol has decreased 39% since 1982 (according to the Center for Disease Control, CDC) to approximately 16,000, these deaths account for 38.6% of all traffic deaths with alcohol being the chief instigator. In 1997, the death rate among young (ages 16–20 years) motor-vehicle occupants was 28.3 % per 100,000 population—more than twice that of the U.S. population of 13.3 per 100,000. "Teenaged drivers are more likely than older drivers to speed, run red lights, make illegal turns, ride with an intoxicated driver, and drive after drinking alcohol or using drugs" (U.S. Department of Health and Human Services, 1999, pp. 369–374).

Despite the suppositions we might make regarding the data thus reported, from a psychosocial perspective, the literature establishing a precise relationships between specific psychiatric disorders and incidence of TBI is inconclusive. Yet, we cannot ignore the evidence of psychological factors appearing to be a contributing risk factor in the occurrence of TBI (Thurman et al., 1998, and in a personal conversation with this author). An early study by Fahy, Irving, and Millac (1967) in Great Britain revealed that 46% of the patients with TBI

admitted to hospitals presented evidence of social maladjustment. And, in their study, Kerr et al. (1971) found the incidence of TBI among the divorced to be four times that expected in the general population. One inference from such a connection is that some persons who have not recovered psychologically from their divorce might be more prone to serious accidents. Hibbard et al. (1998) found definitively that a significant percentage of subjects were found to have had substance abuse disorders prior to TBI.

There appears to be some evidence also that individuals who have sustained one TBI are three times more likely to be brain injured a second time and eight times as likely to have subsequent injuries, according to Annegers et al. (1980). They conclude that alcohol abuse is the predominant behavioral pattern contributing to repeated brain injury in adults. These latter results must be viewed cautiously, however, considering the profound characterological changes that may occur following the first TBI.

Although the research thus far has only begun to explain the epidemiological aspects of the incidence of TBI, it is apparent that socioeconomic and psychosocial factors play a major contributing role. We must contend with these factors if we are to cope successfully with the posttraumatic patient. Also, less is known about the premorbid personality of the characteristics of the person with TBI, but it would be presumptuous to assume a pre-accident-prone personality type, particularly when we consider the incidence of TBI among presumably innocent victims. Nonetheless, we cannot ignore the cited evidence that suggests a prevalence of self-destructive individuals, who have sustained TBI and who are being treated in hospitals and rehabilitation centers.

We view with considerable interest another major cause of injury, with two groupings: under age 15 and over age 70 (Rimel and Jane, 1983). Cartlidge and Shaw (1981) found that more than one third of the over-70 group of patients had recently taken alcohol and that the group also is more vulnerable to such hazards as unlit stairs, uneven pavement, and icy patches on the road, as well as confusion and unsteadiness.

The younger group is prone to injuries from falling for different reasons. In fact, Oddy (1984) stated that accidents in the home are the more common cause of TBI in children under 3 years of age, with "baby battering" responsible for an unknown proportion. Falls occur so frequently that they often are used to cover up child abuse. Sadder is the fact that child abuse is common enough that medical personnel have found skull fractures with particular features to be indicative of child abuse (Hobbs, 1984). Hobbs acknowledges, though, "that more 'gently battered babies' might be indistinguishable from those having minor falls" (p. 251). An even subtler TBI event is the "shaken baby syndrome," well documented by Spicknell (1998). Some authorities have advised consideration of TBI wherever abuse is suspected. The battered too frequently are assigned the more socially acceptable label of "nonaccidentally injured" (Cartlidge and Shaw, 1981). The Committee on Child Abuse and Neglect, 1993–1994, report that the "data regarding the nature and frequency of head trauma support a medical presumption of child abuse, when a child younger than one year of age has intracranial injury" (1997, p. 365). Shaken baby syndrome was the most serious form of infant abuse particularly under 6 months of age. Occurring frequently and often overlooked in its subtle form, it is easily underdiagnosed because of an absence of externally visible injury. Some parents may not even have any knowledge of the cause.

It is worth noting, unfortunately, that injury caused by abuse is not necessarily unique to the younger population; the media continue to bring to the public's attention the increased numbers of elderly who are physically abused by their adult children or by disturbed personnel in some nursing homes. A review of these events has been noted by Kingston and Reay (1996) but report of actual evidence is somewhat tentative and unsubstantiated in the literature.

Rehabilitative Needs

During the last 30 years, we have seen not only a dramatic increase of those individuals who suffer TBI but also, as noted earlier, the advent of almost miraculous medical procedures that save their lives. The modern efficiency of paramedic emergency teams and hospital trauma centers has played a part, along with the medical knowledge gained in the battleground surgical theaters of the Vietnam War. Consequently, the need for acute and long-term care and rehabilitation has been accompanied by a demand for new procedures and techniques to cope with the personal, social, educational, vocational, and economic needs of the patient.

The Nature and Extent of the Injury

Throughout the United States and abroad, rehabilitation programs, often part of major medical centers, have been established to assist survivors of TBI and their families. Because these programs vary in magnitude, breadth, and kind, the patient may not always receive the individualized attention necessary for multidimensional recovery. Worse yet, escalating medical costs limit the amount of time the patient may reside in rehabilitation centers. What happens, then, becomes of serious concern to the patient and the families who must take on the burden of care.

Levin et al. (1982), citing reports by Najenson et al. (1974, 1978) and Rosenbaum et al. (1978), describe one of the foremost rehabilitation programs established. Responding to the casualties suffered by Israel in the Israeli-Arabic conflicts, the Lowenstein Rehabilitation Hospital in Raanana, Israel, was established to provide the most comprehensive treatment facility for TBI patients.

Throughout the United States, either regional rehabilitation centers or rehabilitation centers are directly connected to hospitals. While the TBI patient typically obtains immediate assistance related to restoration of disturbed ventilation, treatment of large lesions of vital organs, attention to swallowing problems (if required), cognitive and communicative assistance, control of inappropriate psychosocial behavior, and mobility training, among other interventions, the actual facility stay seldom goes beyond six months, if that.

Administration of the Glasgow Coma Scale (GCS), The Rancho Los Amigos Levels of

Cognitive Functioning Scale (LCFS), and cognitive and motor components of the Functional Independence Measure (FIM(SM)-COG and FIM(SM)-M) have been used to predict morbidity, mortality, and efficacy in prediction of functional outcomes (Zafonte et al., 1996; Wilson, Pettigrew, and Teasdale, 1998; and Satz et al., 1998b). While these scales have been found to be of limited value regarding functional outcome measures, they can be of assistance in measuring status of recovery, as we discuss later.

Active management of TBI patients begins with physical therapy for comatose patients, and during the transition from coma to normal orientation, the patient is encouraged to participate more actively. With wakefulness also emerges behavioral disturbances, which to an extreme may consist of transient psychoses. The patient's family always is included and encouraged to participate in providing a supportive and calm environment to facilitate a sense of security and orientation for the patient. The recovery program also includes a comprehensive cognitive, intellectual, and communication assessment based on formal testing (if possible), family interviews, and informal behavioral observation. These procedures, unfortunately, do not always fit the reality of a possibly dysfunctional family situation, mediocre rehabilitative care, degree and quality of patient injury, or the sometimes negative circumstances of a rural environment.[1]

Nevertheless, among the goals of treatment are helping the patient develop skills indirectly or directly related to assistance with independent living activities and acquiring adaptive behaviors to deal with personal problems, including the vast array of emotional changes, and to enhance cognitive and communicative skills, particularly when the patient is released from the environs of the rehabilitation facility. The psychotherapist or neuropsychologist, if one is consistently available, ideally should be primarily responsible for the patient's cognitive and psychodynamic treatment in conjunction with the speech-language pathologist, physical therapist, and occupational therapist.

It is not unusual, though, for the responsibility to fall on the expertise of the speech-language pathologist, who must guide the patient-therapist-family relationship in encouraging the widest range of skills and activities.

A Team Approach

We believe the elements that should characterize the best of rehabilitation centers is a team approach. Because of the wide range of problems encountered with TBI and the different types of injuries that vary along differing stages, many disciplines need to be involved in patient care. Among these we would include medical-surgical, nursing, neuropsychology, speech-language pathology, audiology, teaching, physical, occupational, and vocational therapy, and social work. Although each area has its own distinctive goals to pursue with the patient, no one of them can be totally effective without interacting with the others.

It appears to us that the convergence of all of these disciplines must occur at the loci of the cognitive-behavioral changes. In this chapter, we focus on the psychosocial components, recognizing the difficulty in separating these from purely cognitive-linguistic elements. Several books, including Brooks (1984), Rosenthal and Miller (1999), and Krych et al. (1999), present comprehensive databases and conceptual frameworks for understanding the psychological, social, and family consequences of TBI. With contributions from experts in the field, the most recent evidence is discussed relative to the psychiatry of closed head injury, attentional deficits, the psychological implications of TBI during childhood, and the psychological management of behavior disorders following severe TBI, among other related topics.

Psychosocial and Neuropsychological Factors and Adjustment Problems for the Family

Changes in Affectual State

The quality and the degree of changes in the affectual state following TBI may vary from acute psy-

---

[1]Having lived in a rural area for over 10 years and treating TBI patients during that length of time, we can personally attest to some of the factors just alluded to.

chosis through character disorders to specific and generalized dysfunction.

Levin et al. (1982) describe the psychiatric consequences in terms of four states:

1. *Acute posttraumatic psychosis,* in which the patient may exhibit such behaviors as depressive psychosis, manic-depressive psychosis, paranoid psychosis, or reactive psychosis. These may be observed in patients who are not comatose but confused and stuporous.
2. *Acute confusional state,* which includes acute agitation, traumatic delirium, disorientation, increased psychomotor activity, incoherent talkativeness, and indiscriminate movements, with perhaps transient periods of coma. "Agitation in these patients was manifested by thrashing of extremities, truncal rocking, dislodging intravenous tubes and catheters, yelling, combativeness, and attempts to get out of bed" (p. 175).
3. *Affective psychosis* in the subacute phase of recovery, which may include euphoria, depression, and prolonged disinhibitory behavior.
4. *Postconcussional syndrome,* which includes combined psychological and somatic symptoms characterized by "headache, anxiety, insomnia, hypochondriacal concern, hypersensitivity to noise, and photophobia" (p. 175).

Levin et al. note, however, that differentiation between neurological and psychological changes is not clear, as is reflected in the current literature on the subject (Manchester, Hodgkinson, and Casey, 1997; Suhr et al., 1997; and Satz et al., 1998a, among others).

Neuropsychological Changes

Gronwall and Wrightson (1980) support the view that, after even minor brain injury, there is pathological evidence of microscopic lesions and that concussion is related to both a breakdown in information processing and characteristic behavioral symptoms. Bukay and Glasauer (1980) view postconcussion syndrome in minor head injury as a constellation of headache, irritability-restlessness, depression, insomnia, defective memory, fatigue, impaired concentration, dizziness-vertigo, and alco-

hol intolerance. Kushner (1998), in fact, declares that the term *minor brain injury* (MBI) may be misleading, in that it may include a wide array of symptoms from mild to disabling. Its manifestations and treatment need to be recognized by even general medical practitioners, according to Kushner. Harvey and Bryant (1998), in their study of determinants of acute stress disorder (ASD) following MBI, found that, of 48 patients who had sustained MBI following a motor vehicle accident, nearly half had difficulty coping and experienced ASD. In a somewhat later study, Bryant and Harvey (1998), using a larger sample of victims of motor vehicle accidents found 82% of their sample to still be suffering from ASD six months following their diagnoses.

Major brain injuries typically provide a more definitive picture of the profound changes that occur following either minor or major accidents. Blumer and Benson (1975) report on the now-famous case of Phineas Gage, who in 1868 was brain injured as a result of an explosion that sent a crowbar through his frontal lobe, penetrating his corpus collosum. Although he was thought to be a premorbidly psychologically healthy person, the injury was responsible for profound personality changes and intellectual regression. His behavior was characterized by fitful moods of mania with associated childlike tantrums, inability to respond to advice from his friends, and marked impatience. He lived for 12 more years, never returning to his premorbid state, and meandered directionless until his death. They considered the destruction of the prefrontal convexity, basal ganglia, and thalamus to result in antisocial, childish, and euphoric behavioral patterns somewhat akin to a "pseudopsychopathic" personality.

Rosenthal and Miller (1999) consider the behavioral effects of closed TBI frequently related to the frontal lobes. Among the behavioral consequences are a diminution of drive, apathy, insufficient goal-directed behavior, lethargy, childishness, lack of judgment, social disinhibition, inappropriate sexual behavior, aggressiveness, and emotional dullness and flatness. Because the frontal lobes are known to fulfill an "executive function," it is understandable why frontal-lobe-injured persons are unable to regulate or integrate their behavior and characteristically wander aimlessly with little sense of identity and lack of self-esteem. Leon-Carrion et al. (1998), in their study of impairment of executive function, found that neurosurgical intervention, even two years following the initial injury, did not improve problem solving and executive functioning.

Most crucial to our understanding of the relationship of focal neurological evidence of destructive lesions with the presence of behavioral dysfunction is Rosenthal's (1984) admonition:

> Problems such as fluctuating depression, irritability, poor frustration tolerance, inability to deal with stress, and sexual dysfunction are often seen in head injured persons, irrespective of the neuropathology of their injury. These behavioral changes may be attributable to the diffuse and widespread organic damage, the presence of pre-existing emotional and behavioral problems, or perhaps the response of the environment to the newly head injured person. (p. 200)

We now address the response of the environment, in conjunction with the secondary psychological manifestations.

Environment and Psychological Changes

Regardless of focal or diffuse TBI, the individual is thrust into a strange, frightening, and unfamiliar world, with the body and the brain struggling to regain a grip on reality. The perception of actual reality by the patient may be colored by the unique features that characterize the person's premorbid state and previous environment and certainly by the injury itself.

Bond's categorization of the five major effects on personality and behavior are still relevant. (1983). These are summarized, interspersed with our observations.

1. *Capacity for social perceptiveness.* The patient loses the ability to be empathic with others, generally is self-centered, and does not appear capable of self-criticism.
2. *Capacity for self-control.* The patient is impatient, randomly restless, and impulsive.
3. *Learned social behavior.* The patient is impaired in the ability to organize, plan, and make judgments with concomitant loss of initiative.
4. *Ability to learn.* Learning capacity is reduced, the patient demonstrating a slowing down and rigidity of mental processing abilities.

5. *Emotion.* The patient becomes labile, apathetic, often silly, and irritable, with reduced or increased sexual drive. Depression, obsessiveness, bizarre ideation, panic disorder, bipolar disorder, or anxiety may dominate much daily behavior.

Indicating the apparent overlap of these categories and the apparent relationship with other cognitive-behavioral-social changes, Bond also cautions that there is significant variation in the defects among TBI individuals. Furthermore, the pretraumatic personality characteristics certainly must be considered. More recent writers, like Hickling et al. (1998), investigated the effect of TBI on the development of posttraumatic stress disorder (PTSD) in motor vehicle accidents. Subjects who suffered TBI were found to have developed PTSD as frequently as those who had not reported TBI. There are interesting implications here relative to pretrauma personality characteristics.

The reader may recall the discussion of premorbid profiles of TBI patients, in which we noted that specific factors and certain personality characteristics appear to predispose many of them to injury. Therefore, such premorbid features as aggressiveness, anxiety, and anger are likely to be exacerbated. It is obvious, also, that, depending on premorbid personality, patients will respond to their immediate hospital, skilled nursing facility, rehabilitation center, and family environment in a unique manner. We need to be mindful, though, that the nature of the physical injury itself may cause devastating psychological changes regardless of premorbid tendencies and postmorbid reactions.

We recently worked with a 28-year-old TBI patient who was sent home to his mother and father following eight weeks of intensive therapies in a rehabilitation center. Although ambulatory and linguistically and vocally unimpaired, among his major deficits were impairment of judgment, inappropriateness of behavior, cognitive confusion, and inconsistent intermediate and short-term memory loss. His delusional behavior, in which he refused to believe that his main caregiver was his mother, and his total rejection of her, including physical attacks, needed to be managed before meaningful cognitive, occupational, and physical therapy could be of value.

There is no available evidence to suggest how neural reorganization occurs in individual patients and how these same patients establish their own organic homeostasis. Perhaps many of the behavioral changes occur relative to the way in which each patient adjusts or responds to the trauma experienced. In the case just discussed, the young patient had been very loving to his mother premorbidly and had a very close relationship with her. Interestingly, while in his comatose state following his auto accident, only she remained by his side, constantly verbalizing, encouraging him to "hang in there" while all attending physicians were encouraging her to "let him go; he'll likely be in a vegetative state anyway." His remarkable recovery of most modalities was a shock to all except his mother, who was devastated by his total rejection and his denial that she indeed was his mother.

While such anecdotal reports are not unusual, one could speculate that his rejection reflected an organic desire to die rather than to bear the aftermath of a life in which he likely would be unable to live independently. What we have discussed previously and presently as pathological behavior in part may be described as a quite normal reaction to an extraordinary shock to the brain, psyche, and body. Certainly, even less is known about the overall recovery process following brain injury in individual patients. Nevertheless, we are left with the task of understanding as much as we can about the personality and behavior changes in order to assist all TBI patients toward recovery.

Specific Personality and Behavioral Changes

In discussing personality and behavioral changes, it is necessary that we consider them in the light of the various levels of change each patient undergoes. Further, because the severity and loci of injury in part determine the extent of the various disabling characteristics, we discuss personality and behavior changes regardless of injury type.

Impairment of Judgment

Luria (1980) first described deficits in judgment in patients with damage to the prefrontal area. More recent authors, McDowell, Whyte, and D'Esposito

(1998), using a D2 dopamine receptor agonist on such patients, found some improvement in their executive function and cognitive processes in general. Such patients may not be aware of all that is occurring in their immediate environment and often appear to act impulsively and hyperactively, without regard for others. They do not appear to process all the information available to them. Ben-Yishay and Diller (1983) describe impaired judgment in terms of the cognitive function, too. These patients are unable to use good judgment in self-care activities such as dressing, eating, and elimination needs. Verbal and nonverbal expressions or gestures often are inappropriate to the occasion, and such patients will invade the privacy of others. They seem unable "to maintain 'friendliness' or 'chumminess' within proper bounds" (p. 175).

Denial

According to Rosenthal (1983) and Rosenthal and Miller (1999), patients in a later stage of recovery (three to six months post morbid) tend to deny the extent of their disability, particularly when they have made substantial progress in ambulation and performance of daily activities. Disturbed by restrictions placed on their behavior, they become confused and upset. It is not so much the physical disability that is being denied but the cognitive and other mental concomitants to the brain insult. Although cooperating with members of the rehabilitation team in assessment and treatment procedures structured to deal with cognitive and other mental difficulties, the patient continues to deny overtly their presence and significance. The degree and quality of denial may range from an extreme euphoric, "all is well" reaction to an opposite one of depression; that is, one of self-denigration and disavowal of abilities still intact. As we discuss presently, the degree to which patients manifest may depend on the family's own response to the patient and the injury.

Denial may be viewed as an adaptive mechanism that may fend off major emotionally disturbed behavior. Further, it should not be confused with the patient's disordered thinking, which interferes with the awareness of his or her actual deficits. Because patients are not reacting emotionally in a manner we think appropriate does not necessarily mean they are in denial but, rather, that they are coping.

Finally, we need to be cautious in not equating real memory loss with denial, particularly when patients cannot recall unpleasant events such as the initial trauma or accident itself.

Impaired Capacity for Control and Regulation

Under this rubric, patients demonstrate impatience, impulsiveness, and random restlessness, according to Lezak (1978b). In the extreme state, patients are confused and agitated, detached from the present, and unable to process information. Less extreme is the tendency for patients to respond prematurely or inappropriately to requests or input from others. As Ben-Yishay and Diller (1983) describe it, patients demonstrate an inability to attend and concentrate. They are abnormally "stimulus bound" (distractable), disinhibited, and unable to modulate their responses.

Apathy and Withdrawal

Under the heading of initiative, activity level, and emotional "tone," Ben-Yishay and Diller (1983) describe several subclasses: (1) the inability to initiate simple behaviors, verbal or nonverbal, without assistance from others; (2) the abnormal slowing down of responses, manifested by motor behavior with a fragmented rhythm; (3) the abnormal reduction in the way activities are carried out, which includes passivity and displays of "lack of stamina"; and (4) manifestations of an inability to relate emotionally to others as characterized by "flatness" of affect or "remoteness."

These patients also appear to be self-involved; that is, they are preoccupied with themselves or with extraneous stimuli from their immediate environment. Their inability to remain tuned in may give others the impression of severe intellectual impairment when it actually may represent a defense coping mechanism. Withdrawal from and apathy to activities structured by caregivers should not be interpreted as necessarily indicating stubbornness, rigidity of thought, or uncooperativeness but may be the manifestation of complex primary or secondary effects of the injury.

Irritability, Paranoia, and Hostility

The degree to which TBI patients demonstrate any one or combination of these traits depends on the interrelationship of many factors, including the premorbid personality and behavior, neurological effects, and family dynamics. Caregivers can significantly help to modify or extinguish such behaviors as long as they do not personalize them when bearing the brunt of attacks from the patient. To do otherwise is to reinforce the patient's negative attitude, causing greater frustration for all. Certainly, it may be very difficult to determine what triggers irritable, paranoic, and hostile responses and how much is based on reality. Sometimes nothing more than uncaring handling by a rude aide may unleash a torrent of rage, out of proportion to the provocation. Such may be evident in the formal rehabilitation setting or, as described earlier, even in the most caring of home situations.

Depression

The onset of depression may be viewed from either a primary perspective or as a secondary manifestation. Rosenthal, Christensen, and Ross (1998) conducted one of the most exhaustive studies to date, employing virtually all of the computerized database searches of the English-language literature on TBI. While few studies appeared, depression was found to predominate among the consequences of TBI. They see depression as a major impediment to the achievement of optimal functional outcome in both the acute and chronic stages of recovery. They found that a combination of neurochemical and neuroanatomic factors was chiefly responsible for its persistence. It appears that psychopharmacologic treatment, particularly the use of nontricylic antidepressants, achieves the most effective results. They conclude that confirmation of the underlying causes would have to consist of demographic, biologic, and psychosocial investigations. Our own search of both the American and foreign literature found similar results in the investigations of Gomez-Hernandez (1997), who focused on the effects of depression on interpersonal relationships and concern over job loss. Busch and Alpern (1998) found a prevalence of 35% of their patients with mild brain injury as having left frontal damage. In a study conducted in the United Kingdom, Deb et al. (1999) found depression to be pervasive and supported by the Glasgow Outcome Scale (GOS), informal testing, and the Mini-Mental State examination. Ownsworth and Oei (1998), in Australia, found pretraumatic psychiatric illness to have been present in their patients, which supports the findings of other investigators. Satz et al. (1998b), in their investigation, while finding no association between depression status and neuropsychological measures did find a relationship with overall recovery, including feelings of personal competency and employability.

Whether a primary or secondary manifestation of TBI, the patient experiences a profound feeling of loss. The patient, less able to function physically and feeling impotent and more dependent socially, in a sense, finds safety in the depressed state. According to Rosenthal (1984), during the rehabilitative phase of recovery, such depression may be viewed as a compensatory means to reduce denial and may reflect the patient's further understanding and insight into the recognition of the reality and degree of the disability.

Although depression may not interfere profoundly with the patient's rehabilitation program as long as physical recovery continues and even with careful monitoring of antidepressant medication, the prospect of new adjustments socially, vocationally, and educationally may yet sustain depression. Once physical recovery reaches a plateau, the likelihood of anxiety, frustration, sadness, and anger could increase. In some cases suicide is contemplated.

In a very real sense, the patient experiences a partial death and, while not mourning in the way the family may (as we discuss later), nevertheless passes through the stages of mourning, as discussed earlier. The TBI patient feels overwhelmed, finds the problem insurmountable, and realizes that life may never return to quite the way it once was. The extent to which TBI patients come to the latter realization cannot be determined, however, given the paucity, still, of scientific investigations in the subject.

Regression to Childlike Behavior and Dependency

It is not unusual to see a regression to childhood behavior in TBI adults. Their behavior is characterized by a desire to have needs satisfied immediately, unusual affectionateness, and demands for attention. They often defer from taking responsibility, relying on others to do things for them. They also might ignore the needs of others and seem unconcerned with the expression of others' needs or problems. Family members frequently feel as if they are talking to a stone wall. Interestingly, some young

TBI adults will acknowledge to family members or caregivers that they realize what they are doing but add they find it difficult to control their behavior. The degree to which these are primary or secondary effects of the TBI cannot be ascertained due to our present state of knowledge.

Other Personality and Behavioral Changes

Varying degrees of anxiety, hypochondria, hypersensitivity, and poor self-esteem are noted in some cases of TBI, but as with other behavioral changes, these may subside following the subacute stage. According to Levin et al. (1982), cerebral dysfunction may be partly reversible, but in cases of psychoses, residual behavioral disturbance is more than likely.

In the last few years, several investigators have seen a frequent manifestation of posttraumatic stress disorder in TBI patients. PTSD may best be described briefly as involving intense fear, helplessness, and the persistence of the experience of the event. Schnyder and Buddeberg (1996), in their own Medline search (1985–1995), found among the scarcity of references to psychosocial effects some incidence of PTSD, along with the effects noted earlier. Ohry, Rattok, and Solomon (1996) found 33% of their sample of 24 TBI outpatients to have met their criteria of PTSD, distinguishing it from other traumatic events. Hibbard et al. (1998), in their investigation of 100 TBI adults, found, along with prior substance abuse disorders, select anxiety disorders such as PTSD, obsessive-compulsive disorder (OCD), and panic disorder. Childers et al. (1998) also illustrate the importance of treating obsessional symptoms if other behaviors are to be better managed.

Regardless of the degree and quality of the initial brain insult, the premorbid personality and psychosocial environment, along with premorbid factors such as family attitudes, personal problems, and poorly conceived rehabilitation attempts, may exacerbate and extend the symptom complex.

Adjustment Problems for the Family

The psychological and social upheaval to the family brought about by TBI to one of its members is well known and documented (O'Neill and Carter, 1998; Pittman and Fowler, 1998; DePompei and Zarski,

1989). In terms of family systems theory (discussed in Chapter 2), the equilibrium of the family has been traumatically disrupted, creating not only profound changes in other members but also altering the interpersonal relationships of all members, including the patient. Regardless of the extent of the initial insult, the family shares with the victim the long and tedious process of recovery. Barry (1984) describes the early period of the medical crisis as a time when everyone's energy is geared toward surviving the initial crisis. As the patient proceeds through the recovery period, family members also experience varying stages of recovery. The way in which each family member copes with the recovery process and the reality of the life and home situation affects all family members, including the patient and the family as an entity. Because family members differ from each other, no two will respond similarly, so the adjustment process and its time line vary for each.

The Grieving Process

Not unlike the grieving process experienced by family members in response to the physical death of another family member is the response to brain injury when actual death does not occur. Grief is both a natural response to loss and an important aspect of the recovery process. While the entire process appears similar to family reaction to a member who has had a CVA, the dynamics are different because the injured person typically is younger, with different predisposing factors and vocational status, the presence of family members who are young children, and so forth. As described by Kubler-Ross (1969), the family goes through various stages to reach a point where the loss finally can be accepted. (In many cases, though, this may not occur.) Because the "death" is within the personal system and incomplete, it has been characterized by Muir (1978) as "mobile mourning." Unlike the finality of death, the process appears to be more diffuse, involving the various stages through which the family passes. Nonetheless, these stages can be determined.

The first stage is shock caused by what has happened and the denial of its occurrence. Denial may assume the form of optimism that the patient has

survived a life-threatening injury and thus has taken on aspects of immortality (Lezak, 1978a, 1978b; Bond, 1983). Unrealistic pressure may be put on the patient in efforts to deny the reality of the condition. For example, the patient's limitations may be criticized as "laziness." This tends to overshadow the fact that the patient actually has survived due to the most modern lifesaving technology possible. So, overjoyed by this, family members fail to recognize the real consequences of the injury. The need to reject any negative outcome immediately post onset can be strong and appropriate, at least for the time being.

Within this is anxiety or panic, where family members feel helpless in coping with the disruption in their lives. According to Bond (1983, 1984), the family transforms the anxiety or panic into anger and may express this to members of the hospital staff when staff members refuse to confirm the family's false hopes and to the victim, when becoming irritable and egocentric or when spontaneous recovery reaches a plateau. The anger toward others transforms into anger at oneself, culminating in feelings of guilt, particularly when family members contrast their good health with the precarious health of the patient (Lezak, 1978a; Barry, 1984). Resnick (1993) found that families expressed anger because of limited information given them about TBI and little support. This would exacerbate the anger already felt as part of the grieving process. Bargaining, according to Lezak (1978b), is evidenced as the family exhausts itself in providing excess care in hope and expectation for a rapid recovery. This may have a negative effect on the patient, who may make unrealistic demands on the family, when in fact the person should be initiating self-care

Eventually, depression becomes part of the grieving process. Overwhelmed by all that has happened, the reality of loss finally is realized. The still bewildered family may gradually accept what has happened, attaining a realistic understanding of the patient's assets and limitations. The patient may be accepted and dealt with in his or her present reality. According to Barry (1984), the family recognizes the actual limits dictated by the disability.

In a study of 13 TBI patients over a four-year period, Romano (1974) found negligible movements through the grief stages described previously. She found denial to be the prominent stage, evidenced in the common fantasy (the "sleeping beauty" syndrome) that the person would awaken from the present condition in his or her premorbid state. Families also fantasized improvement when, in fact, none had occurred. Once the patient emerged from the coma, denial would persist that the patient had changed in any way. Romano maintains that anger—at the hospital staff, doctor, and patient—still was a denial of the patient's condition. Denial was further manifested in isolation from social activities, as the family defensively protected the patient's "normalcy." As the patient began the recovery process, the family members would deny to the patient personal limitations and thus would do the patient (and themselves) irreparable harm. Romano suggests that persistence of this denial stage indicated rejection of the mourning process because, although the body was still alive, the family could not accept that the person known premorbidly essentially was dead.

Our own experience over 35 years with families of TBI patients, as well as anecdotal reports from fellow workers, confirms the extent of the denial process. We remind the reader, however, that it may be important for the family to deny, to an extent, in order to reestablish family equilibrium. Denial helps families come to terms with their life change, but if it persists, social isolation may result and life might then center around the impaired individual only. Virtually no published data indicate how long a family can remain stuck in the denial stage without it being characterized as abnormal. Perhaps, as with other stages of grief, each family responds uniquely with its own adjustment process, so that any absolute criteria may be impossible to establish. Although the concept of denial may be interpreted in various ways, as described, the key is to examine each distinct family and honor and support the system each may need to employ. Only if the means, in our clinical estimation, appears to be destroying the family, may we need to intervene more directly.

Earlier, Fahy et al. (1967) surveyed 26 families six years posttrauma and concluded that, where family support was lacking, patients became socially withdrawn. Romano (1974) also appears to support these findings, suggesting that social deprivation may lead to depression in the patient.

Thomsen (1974) did a follow-up study of 50 young TBI patients and reported that most patients continued to suffer from lack of family contact and nearly all relatives complained of the patient's change in personality and behavior. Thomsen stresses the need for long-term treatment and support of the patient as well as the family.

There is little doubt that family support is critical to satisfy progress in TBI patients. Fortunately, more writers, such as Resnick (1993), DePompei and Zarski (1989), Nagle (1989), DePompei and Williams (1994), O'Neill and Carter (1998), and Holland and Shigaki (1998), among others, have written about how families can be integrated within the rehabilitative process to help the TBI patient.

The Plight of the Spouse

In Chapter 2, we discuss the profound effects a CVA has on the family and in particular on the wife. We believe the effect is even greater for the spouse (usually the wife) of a person with TBI, because the patient typically is much younger than the CVA patient, and further, because the use of excessive alcohol shortly before injury is the most firmly established correlate. As noted by Levin et al. (1982) and Thurman (1998), as well as a history of impulse-control and antisocial behavior problems, the significance of the premorbid marital relationship cannot be underestimated.

The Premorbid Relationship

Little research, prospective or retrospective, has been done to isolate a characteristic dysfunctional premorbid relationship or environmental difficulties that may have been present and their effect on rehabilitation efforts with TBI individuals or their families. Gillen et al. (1998), from findings in their retrospective study of depression among caregivers, including spouses, found a suggestion of premorbid depression in the marital relationship. They acknowledge that much more research needs to be conducted to identify dysfunctional marital factors. As Lishman (1973) found, premorbid traits of instability and inadequacy contribute to the form that postmorbid dysfunction takes, so must the nature of the premorbid marital relationship.

The Postmorbid Relationship

Romano (1974), Lezak (1978b), Bond (1983), De Pompei and Zarski (1989), Gillen et al. (1998), and others report the wife to be particularly victimized by the plight of the TBI patient, as she agonizes over the loss of a partner whom she cannot mourn in the typical sense. Her attempts to mourn are unsuccessful because the "body" (that is, the patient) is still functioning. The wife's despair is intensified by a society that neither truly acknowledges her grief nor provides support and comfort as would benefit a bona fide widow.

Rosenbaum and Najenson (1976) discuss how the wife's role changes abruptly from equal partner to mother surrogate or nurse. Emotions ranging from desolation to hostility accompany such role changes as she copes with the social isolation, after initial support by friends and extended family. Increased responsibility for household affairs, child rearing, medical costs, economic catastrophe, as well as having to deal with often critical and overprotective in-laws, may also result in a conflict between hostility toward the patient and guilt at having such feelings. According to Pittman and Fowler (1998), it is not unusual for the spouse to respond with anxiety and cognitive disassociation, classified as acute stress disorder. The latter has been further substantiated by the experimental research of Leathem, Heath, and Wooley (1996), Kreuter et al. (1998), and Marsh et al. (1998). Depression was found to be prevalent in all these investigations.

According to studies by Oddy, Humphrey, and Uttley (1978b), Thomsen (1974), and Painting and Merry (1972), the primary cause of depression in the spouse is related to the personality changes of the injured person. Bond (1983) sees the wife enjoying little in her life now that she no longer feels she has a husband as confidant. Because she receives little positive reinforcement from others in caring for her husband and children, she easily becomes vulnerable to depression. In the Rosenbaum and Najenson study (1976), the wives of TBI servicemen were considered to be more depressed and socially isolated than those of physically disabled servicemen, because the former had lost their cognitive capabilities, which more profoundly limited their function in society. Similar results were found by Smith and Schwirian (1998), who reviewed previous studies and affirmed that functional ability and cognition both negatively affected and burdened the caregiving spouse.

Further stress is brought to bear on the spouse when the patient becomes emotionally dependent and demands constant attention. As described by Rosenthal (1984) and Rosenthal and Miller (1999), the spouse may reinforce this behavior to avoid further distress in the patient, herself, or the family. Often this encourages a negative situation, as "pampering will foster dependency, resentment and behavioral stagnation" (Lezak, 1978b, p. 594). Other significant causes of stress to the spouse might be the patient's poorly controlled behavior, such as pathological laughter or emotional lability, fear of epilepsy, coping with associated physical disabilities, concern for the patient's prognosis, and fear of another accident (Oddy et al., 1978b).

The incidence and prevalence of sexual dysfunction have been reported in several studies. Lezak (1978b) describes how the spouse's sexual and affectional needs are frustrated by the injured husband's inability to empathize and be sensitive to those needs. Childlike and dependent, the patient may be self-involved, unintentionally inconsiderate, or demanding of purely physical sexual relief. In research by Rosenbaum and Najenson (1976) concerning wives of TBI survivors one year after the Yom Kippur War, there was drastic reduction in sexual relations. Although Oddy, Humphrey, and Uttley (1978a) claim that sexual dysfunction was not indicated in their six-month posttrauma study, a decrease as well as an increase in intercourse was evidenced. We would question, however, what the authors mean by their use of the term *dysfunction*.

Mauss-Clum and Ryan (1981), citing their own research and that of others, indicate that approximately 47% of the spouses reported either sexual disinterest or preoccupation in their TBI husbands. The most comprehensive investigation and reporting is in the work of Griffith and Lemberg (1992), who provide extensive information concerning sexuality and the diversity of sexual dysfunction in TBI patients and their spouses. While written for a lay audience, it is technically complete for the professional to use in rehabilitative efforts. The text dispels many of the myths surrounding sexual issues in the population under discussion. More recently, Elliot and Biever (1996), in an extensive review of the literature, describe specific sequelae such as impulsiveness or inappropriateness and changes in libido and sexual frequency; and they discuss the limited treatment models available to the clinician. In a most recent study, Medlar (1998) does not separate the sexual dysfunction in the patient from diminished social skills, intimacy, the need for closeness and affection, consideration, and empathy. Medlar describes the implementation of the Massachusetts Statewide Head Injury Program to respond effectively to these behavioral concerns as they relate to staff, client, and family education.

Prospects for the Future Relationship

Many factors will determine the outcome of the marital relationship, among which are (1) degree of personality and behavioral change in the patient, (2) premorbid marital relationship, (3) the spouse's attitude and level of support, (4) level of support for both patient and spouse from members of the extended family, and (5) the degree and quality of formal rehabilitation efforts, with particular emphasis on family counseling integrated with traditional therapies.

Oddy and Humphrey (1980), in their study of 54 TBI patients, found that, after one year, of the 7 patients who were married, three spouses were rated as feeling less affectionate toward their partners. After two years, one spouse and two patients reported their marital relationship to be worse than before the trauma. Thomsen (1974), in her follow-up study of 50 patients, found that the relationship between single patients and their mothers essentially was better than between married patients and their spouses. In six families where car accidents had been involved, persistent feelings of spousal guilt continued to affect the relationships.

Bond (1983), summarizing earlier studies, concludes that the mental problems persist longer than the physical ones and have a more profound effect on the marital relationship. In time, as the reality of the new circumstances is acknowledged, the recovery reaches a plateau, and the marital couple no longer receive the support given by outside sources, a new family homeostasis is formed. Although Painting and Merry (1972) report a divorce rate of 40%, there is no definitive evidence that describes how the couple relate to one another within the context of their changed lives. Moreover, given the generally high divorce rate in this country, the results could be skewed. Perhaps many of these relationships would be characterized more by toleration than by mutual understanding and acceptance. Certainly the couples who premorbidly were functioning well would be more likely to resume their lives, albeit differently and with considerable difficulty.

In general, patients with less severe injuries in time would be more likely to settle into acceptable relationships with their spouses, other factors notwithstanding. Those with more severe injuries, who are likely to be more dependent, may have less satisfactory relationships, unless adequate counseling and support have been given the spouse and the family to help them with the adjustment. People with unsatisfactory premorbid relationships are likely to find such adjustment very difficult to cope with, particularly if alcoholism had been a factor. These may be families where separation and divorce could be inevitable.

It would seem from Oddy and Humphrey's findings that the period when the family, and the spouse in particular, need the most support usually is when services are being withdrawn and the patient is returning home to face a very uncertain future. This needs to be recognized by the rehabilitation team and provision made for home health and counseling services to be available even when the patient is no longer receiving the intensive services previously provided. This very significant issue is addressed in a later section of this chapter.

Specific Effects on the Family

Having discussed the possible effects of head injury on the spouse, it is necessary to consider what effects there may be on other members of the family as well. Although to a degree some similarities exist, the intrinsic nature of the patient, spouse, and children relationships will determine different outcomes. Of considerable interest are the effects on the children and the familial ramifications when children are brain injured.

The Children

When the father has been injured, it is not unusual for the children to suffer silently as attention is drawn to the victim and the plight of the spouse. The unbalancing of the family system may bring about temporary or permanent changes in family interrelationships, depending on the nature of the premorbid family system, the various premorbid roles of each member, and how each copes with the distress caused by the trauma.

Lezak (1978a, 1987b) describes the children as being confused, fearful, and desperate. The young child tends to rely more on the uninjured parent for stability and comfort, thus increasing his or her burdens further. The uninjured wife finds herself caught in a web of conflicting loyalties that she may resolve by either abandoning her mate or passively abandoning her child. The uninjured husband might do likewise. The situation is further aggravated by the TBI parent, who may deliberately tease or upset the child by immaturely competing for the spouse's attention. The patient is likely to react abnormally to noise, making house play impossible. Large family gatherings during the holidays may have to be discontinued as the patient becomes withdrawn or irritable. Pathological laughter and outbreaks of verbal abuse or crying may make the home and home life intolerable for all.

Frequently, the child's personal agony is reflected in truancy, delinquency, failure at school, or psychosomatic illness. Oddy et al. (1978b) indicate that 25% of the relatives of TBI patients reported an illness at intervals of six months post morbidly. Older children may attempt to cope with their own feelings or the family feelings by leaving home prematurely.

Rosenthal and Muir (1983) found that the social isolation of the family is felt most keenly by the adolescent and young adult, because they tend to lose the peer contacts so vital to them. They also found that the child who sustains TBI has a marked effect on siblings. Poor performance in school

accompanied by guilt is not unusual, particularly when there have been unresolved premorbid sibling issues. There also may be a role reversal for the children, whereby the big brother becomes the younger child.

Sander and Kreutzer (1999) also found guilt in the siblings of TBI patients. In addition, they found that the patient who played a significant positive role in their sib's life but who no longer is available for a meaningful and supportive reationship will profoundly affect the uninjured siblings. In a comprehensive study of parental TBI on parenting and child behavior, Uysal et al. (1998) found spouses of individuals with TBI reported less feelings of warmth, love, and acceptance toward their children. Children from families in which a parent had TBI perceived both parents as more lax in their discipline, with the parent without TBI perceived as less actively involved in parenting roles. While no differences were found in the frequency of behavior problems between children of parents with TBI and children of parents without TBI, parents with TBI and their children were significantly more depressed. The necessity for proactive interventions to maximize family adjustment and minimize affective distress were definitively indicated.

The Parents

Lezak (1978b) found that families of children with TBI often have unrealistically high expectations regarding how much their children will recover. The inability to understand and appreciate fully the profound changes that have occurred is related to natural family optimism, fostered by their conception of the event. Bond (1983) noted that families may develop overly high expectations for two reasons. First, in the beginning, children tend to recover rapidly; second, the hospital staff may be reluctant to be specific about long-term outcome. In this case, the family may push the child too hard. For many parents, the concept of irreversible disease is alien to their past experiences. After all, children, when they do get sick, usually recover. Lezak also believes that overly low expectations may be related to the family's need to protect the child. This, however, can lead to the child's dependency, resentment, and behavioral stagnation.

Regardless of the reasons, parents of TBI children often have unrealistic expectations. Whether too high or too low, such expectations may interfere with recovery.

Intertwined with the unrealistic expectations of the parents is their denial of the severity or long-range effects of the injury. Romano (1974) found that, in families of TBI children, denial did not give way to anger, bargaining, and grief, as usually is the case in loss of a loved one. Instead, it persisted for months, even years. She found that denial manifested itself in many ways—first, in fantasies, families would actually state that "He is only sleeping"; second, in verbal refusals, "He always did have a temper." Often the family can recognize and even accept the physical but not the mental limitations of the child. Third, family members responded inappropriately by overprotecting the patient.

Several more recent investigators, in the United States as well as abroad, have substantiated and added to our previous discussion and with greater experimental scrutiny. Andrews, Rose, and Johnson (1998), in their study of 27 TBI children with matched non-TBI controls, demonstrated significantly lower levels of self-esteem and adaptive behavior, higher levels of loneliness, and aggressive-antisocial behavior. Sokal et al. (1996) found parental stress to be related to perceived and actual thought disorders and attention problems. Over time, though, parents perceived their children as less behaviorally impaired. Max et al. (1998a), in one of several experimental studies, found oppositional defiant disorder/conduct disorder (ODD/CD) to be significantly related to impaired family functioning in TBI children and adolescents; also shown was a trend toward a greater family history of alcohol dependence or abuse.

In determining predictive factors of psychiatric outcome of TBI children six months post onset, Max et al (1998b) found that unique psychiatric disorders could be predicted based on a premorbid family history of family dysfunction, behavior-adaptive function, and class-intellectual function. Their study suggests that some children, identifiable through clinical assessment, are at increased risk for psychiatric disorders following TBI. Further substantiation of these findings was made, again by Max et al. (1998c), that severe TBI is a profound

risk factor for the development of a psychiatric disorder. In a later investigation, Max et al. (1999) concluded that postinjury negative outcome added significantly to family dysfunction and that a premorbid family history added significantly to lower socioeconomic status in explaining diminished cognitive functioning.

While family adaptation might be viewed as the stage when emotional homeostasis is developing, it usually is the last stage and most difficult to achieve according to Martin (1990). Many factors, such as type and severity of injury, extrinsic social support, and the family's coping mechanism, all of which are touched on in the discussion of adult TBI, play a role in recovery.

The Abused Child as Brain-Injured Patient

Earlier we documented the extensive epidemiological evidence suggesting the high incidence of TBI in children, with physical abuse as a determining factor. The implication of such evidence will significantly influence the child's recovery, particularly if the child is to live with the abusing parent or parents once again. Parker (1994) discusses the difficulty in establishing an effective prognosis for these children, since it is not until the child matures that definitive findings are made. These include cognitive, personality, and adaptive dysfunctions that easily could have been missed because of the lack of early rigorous investigation. Ewing-Cobbs et al. (1998) examined 40 children hospitalized for TBI who had no documented history of previous brain injury in a prospective longitudinal study. For the 20 subjects whose TBI had been inflicted in later outcome measures 1.3 months following TBI, those with inflicted TBI were found to have greater mental deficiency and significantly impaired cognitive dysfunction along with evidence of preexisting TBI.

Unfortunately, because of the legal-medical complications and ramifications surrounding child abuse in general, the difficulties in providing a safe, healthy, and encouraging environment conducive to recovery are obvious. Only with a close-working, congruent relationship between the professional team and legal authorities can the child at least have the opportunity for even a modest outcome.

Counseling Intervention

The need to intervene psychotherapeutically with TBI children and adults and their families is justified not only by the marked behavioral and personality changes that occur but also by the neuropsychological changes. Although our attention will be directed mainly to procedures focusing on psychosocial changes, we cannot ignore the influence of cognitive deficiencies on such adaptation. While not focusing on specific cognitive workbook tasks, the rehabilitation effort, as we see it, is both educational and psychotherapeutic, in that each contains elements of the other. For this reason, we do not believe any one provider or caregiver can lay claim to any one strategy. It does imply, however, that all those involved with the patient work in an integrated fashion and have some understanding of all the procedures that constitute the rehabilitation process.

Educating the Family and the Patient

We already infer from earlier discussions that the family must play a significant role in the overall and specific aspects of the rehabilitation program. Diehl (1983) believes that the program should be flexible and varied enough to adapt to the specific needs of the patient and the family, with input from all members of the rehabilitation team. Of utmost importance is the establishment of "careful environmental control" in both the home and treatment facility, as both the victim and the family will have distinctive time lines for adjustment and adaptation to the injury.

Providing Information

In Chapter 2, we discussed the value and importance of providing information about CVA to aphasic patients and their families. Although we believe it is as valuable to provide information about TBI to these victims and their families, qualitative differences between the two types of brain insult dictate a somewhat different approach. To begin with, denial of the brain injury and its concomitant sequelae appear to be more intense and of longer duration. It is doubtful that the patient or family

members could process and assimilate any substantial amount of information during the initial stages of the grief process. Yet, it is crucially important to provide basic data concerning the initial impact of the injury to all members of the family, particularly when the patient emerges from coma.

Also, because the course of recovery in the TBI patient is much less predictable than in cases of CVA, prognostic indications by the informant by necessity must be deferred or given with great caution. The profound behavioral and personality changes that occur in TBI, either immediately post onset or later, are unlikely to be understood, by either the patient or the family, even when discussed by the most sensitive expert. Furthermore, the younger age of the TBI person would oblige us to direct attention to the far-reaching implications on both patient and family and cautions us to withhold our opinions until such time as some stabilization has occurred.

Of considerable importance during the early and later periods post onset is that opportunities for continued communication between the professionals and family caregiver must be maintained. Nothing is more frustrating and insulting than for family members to be uninformed of what is occurring during the rehabilitation program. Naturally, it is self-evident that the family be completely involved in the program so that changes in their own feelings and attitudes are recognized and managed. Obviously, they will then have a clearer sense of what is in store for them when the patient comes home.

Probably the greatest challenge to the information provider, however, is the often unstated ambiguities and the incongruent messages family members give regarding their desire for information. We need to understand that such behaviors are not necessarily psychopathological or naive but rather natural defenses related to coping with the tragedy. It entails great patience in attempting to determine exactly how much and what kind of information family members may indeed wish. We also assume that the information providers understand their own uncertainties about the patient and will not allow their own egos to distort the reality of the patient's condition and thereby exacerbate ambiguities and misinformation. For complete professional honesty, all that is required is the statement "I really don't know," which is nothing to be ashamed about.

Given the reality of rationed health care in rehabilitation facilities and home health care, Holland and Shigaki (1998) provide a three phase family and caregiver educational model that can be used in a rehabilitation setting that satisfies the family's acute education needs as they arise and a standardized delivery of information meeting certain knowledge criteria.

We next discuss how, from a somewhat different perspective, this problem can be dealt with during the counseling process.

Major Areas of Information

In addressing the needs of the family, Millard (1983), the mother of a 24-year-old TBI man, provides us several summarized guidelines that we believe are particularly useful:

1. Encourage the family to make use of its own knowledge of the patient to ascertain even minimal return of awareness.
2. Inform the family of the function of the acute care and rehabilitation facility and particularly the extended care facility (ECF), if that will be an interim requirement.
3. Prepare the family for the necessary financial requirements so that the transfer process between facilities will be facilitated and the family given enough time to make whatever arrangements are necessary.
4. Help the family understand that it is dealing with an adult (if such is the case) and an intelligent person regardless of the current behavior and encourage it to treat the patient appropriately.
5. Inform the family that the uniqueness of individuals, different types of injuries, and different recovery factors will determine the possible outcome, and all of what it now observes may not necessarily be permanent.
6. Explain exactly what constitutes the various therapies to be employed and what values they serve. We would add, explain how the family may assist in the various therapeutic processes (without overwhelming them).

7. Encourage limited home visits by the patient, when appropriate, with the understanding that such visits would not necessarily be under the best circumstances. These visits will give the family members a better understanding of what may be in store for them, but they should also be made aware that the permanent reality may be experienced only after the patient is discharged.
8. Discharge planning must include continuous open communication with the family. We would add that families must have access to advice long after discharge.

Specific Areas of Information

Lezak (1978b) consolidates the specific problem areas we need to cover with the family:

1. Anger, frustration and sorrow are natural emotions for close relatives of TBI individuals;
2. Caregiving persons must take care of themselves first if they are going to be able to continue giving the patient good care;
3. The caregiver must ultimately rely on their own conscience and judgment in conflicts with the patient or other family members;
4. The role changes that inevitably take place when an adult becomes dependent or irresponsible can be emotionally distressing for all concerned;
5. The family members can probably do little to change the patient and thus need not feel guilty or wanting when the care does not result in improvement;
6. When it appears that the welfare of dependent children may be at stake, families must explore the issue of divided loyalties and weigh their responsibilities. (pp. 595–596)

It already was noted that many TBI families, in the beginning, have difficulty assimilating the information provided. Nevertheless, it is important to give information on some topics that the family could process. Among these are several we have found significant for the family to know:

1. A basic description of the physical trauma with reference to which part of the injured brain may affect which behavior.
2. An explanation of incontinence and how the patient may respond to it. Emphasis must be placed on the fact that such physiological behavior could correct itself in time.

3. An explanation of any one or combination of typical behaviors, such as patient self-centeredness, depression, paranoia, hostility, and inability to respond to family members as they would wish. Here, we would include patient apathy, withdrawal, confusion, agitation, disorientation, and clinging to family members.
4. A clarification of the nature of the patient's memory problems and how these interfere with personal day-to-day functioning.
5. An explanation of the cognitive-linguistic changes and how these influence, or are influenced by, other behaviors, particularly psychological in nature.

We presently discuss how providing information about TBI to the family becomes a vital aspect of the entire counseling process for the entire family as well as for the patient.

A Framework for Psychotherapeutic Counseling

The rationale and justification for intervening psychotherapeutically when a brain insult has occurred are quite different than that for the typical emotionally disturbed individual. Also, with TBI, we feel that its effects on the patient and the family system generally are more profound than in case of CVA. Rosenthal and Muir (1983) believe that the patient's "emotional regression," "inappropriate social behaviors," and in the case of frontal lobe syndrome, maladaptive behaviors such as lethargy, reduced drive, flat affect, irritability, lack of spontaneity, and inappropriate goal-directed behavior are the most devastating to the family system.

The spouse, family, and patient can be seen to react to the initial event and ensuing circumstances in a discernable pattern. Recognition of the effects on the individual, the family, and their lifestyle by the rehabilitation team is vital for the patient's progress. It would appear that the team's support of the family and the patient and the adjustments they make are an important factor in successful rehabilitation. It also is clear that information and support for the patient and the family need to continue well after the patient has completed a rehabilitation program and returned home. The need for individual counseling and family education and counseling or

therapy is clear; by this, we mean the family and patient will receive emotional support and assistance in understanding and coping with the disability and its potential long-term consequences. Most important will be the attempt at reorganizing a different but functional family system. Resnick (1993), in her retrospective survey of how family and marital relationships are altered, emphasizes the importance of a continued interaction with a case management representative to monitor long-term outcomes.

Guidelines for Intervention

1. The degree and quality of counseling intervention will depend on the way in which the family is mourning. The therapist must be sensitive to the need of some families to cope independently and of others who want help but have difficulty requesting it.
2. Counseling must be conducted within the context of understanding the pretraumatic family system and the behavioral and personality characteristics of individual family members and the patient in particular. Rosenthal and Muir (1983) note: "The 'diagnosis' of the family and 'prescription' for treatment will aid in preventing secondary disability produced by maladaptive interactions between patient and family" (p. 410). (We would add particularly when maladaptive patterns were there previously.)
3. The quantity and complexity of information to be provided the patient and family depend not only on the need to know but also on how necessary it is for them to have the information to assist in the rehabilitation process. For example, the spouse who gets upset with her TBA husband over his childish behavior should be informed of its meaning so that she can not only assist perhaps in modifying that behavior but at least understand it.
4. Determining the degree to which the patient should be counseled or be involved with the family in the counseling process is based in part on the feedback from members of the rehabilitation team and family members. Many speech-language pathologists find that counseling is an intrinsic aspect of cognitive retraining, and occu-

pational therapists find counseling to be helpful in encouraging self-help skills. It is important that counseling, no matter to what degree utilized, be coordinated by one professional sufficiently trained in counseling psychotherapy and in the area of TBI.

5. The choice of family intervention techniques, which include patient-family education, family counseling, and family therapy, is based on the appraisal of the unique TBI family by the various rehabilitation personnel. De Pompei and Zarski (1989) outline three different family intervention techniques: educational counseling to inform the family about any cognitive-communicative disorder and promote adaptive skills, family counseling to deal with the emotional aspects of the TBI event, and family therapy to examine and explore the conflicts, attitudes, nature of the family system. In their preliminary investigation of changes in levels of distress and marital adjustment following TBI, Perlesz and O'Loughlin (1998) found that, while anger had increased over a period of two years of therapy, family conflict, family distress, and feelings of burden and strain had diminished in the families they investigated. We believe that, while no approach should be considered a panacea for significant family recovery, the use of family therapy for TBI, as employed for CVA families, is a more comprehensive approach (Rollin, 1984).

6. The role of nonprofessional support groups for families of TBI patients should not be underestimated, because they play a major role in providing the emotional support and practical assistance such families need, not only in the initial stages post onset of TBI but continuously when all other services have been withdrawn. For the TBI family, it is probably the least threatening method psychologically and financially. We do not suggest that it replace professional assistance, if available, but that it be a complementary activity.

Family Counseling

Initially, family counseling should be convened to provide whatever information is deemed necessary for the family to have and whatever information it requests immediately following the brain injury. We would not expect the process to be particularly dynamic at that time because the family may be resistant to counseling intervention. Nonetheless, as long as the family is aware that such services are available and is aided in the understanding that such therapy will be of value to their injured member (should that person be able to participate in the process), it is more likely to be amenable.

Mauss-Clum and Ryan (1981), based on their experiences with families of TBI patients in the rehabilitation unit at a Veterans Administration hospital in California, found that families unanimously "ranked their need for a clear and kind explanation of the patient's condition as first priority" (p. 166). Most important, however, is the need to include families in the planning of acute and long-term care of their injured member. We believe this to be fundamental to family counseling, in that it can help reduce the guilt-ridden, self-pitying, and defeatist attitudes aroused in the grieving process by reinforcing all of the positive possibilities. Excluding families from the rehabilitation process not only will induce negative consequences for the patient but also distance family members from the patient, thereby alienating them from one another.

Family Therapy

In family therapy, a far more dynamic and complex process than family counseling, the focus is away from individual family members and directed toward the entire family system. De Pompei and Williams (1994) provide guidelines for engaging the family in what they describe as a family-centered approach. Rollin (1984) and Webster and Newhoff (1981) also provide the rationale, justification, and guidelines to follow with TBI families.

Because the evidence identifies clearly defined premorbid psychosocial patterns that may be present—social maladjustment, alcoholism, marital-family instability, and so on—the therapist would have to give careful consideration to these factors in the quest for family harmony. Long established individual and family patterns are not readily modified regardless of the premorbid reality and, in fact, may become more firmly entrenched. Of course, it also is possible that the trauma may produce such a dramatic change in the realignment of family members that some positive changes may ensue. For example, alcoholism, drug abuse, or run-ins with the law, as in the case of some families known to us, may cease. The opposite may occur as well; in which case, the advent of the injury may bring to the surface premorbid issues that had been concealed and not only exacerbate the present situation but tear the family apart.

A second major consideration with regard to family therapy is the younger age of those with TBI. Unlike the CVA patient, the TBI patient is likely to have many more years of life ahead; and therefore, educational, vocational, and social factors become more crucial to the overall family therapy process. In the case of older or elderly parents of the victim, the issue of future independent living must be recognized and acknowledged by all and dealt with appropriately. Younger marital couples in TBI cases further dictate consideration of role and social adjustments, as well as realistic vocational possibilities.

A third consideration is the quality, nature, and degree of the cognitive, emotional, and communication deficit. Rosenthal and Miller (1999) edited a comprehensive and up-to-date rehabilitation approach in their text to assist clinicians and related professionals. The often profound changes in behavior certainly will challenge the family therapist to establish and maintain interpersonal family communication conducive to family homeostasis. Although the temptation might be to exclude a patient who exhibits inappropriate language, affect, and behavior from family therapy, we believe it is unwise to do so, because all will need somehow to cope with the reality of living together. Should participation by the patient in family therapy interfere with the process, we would advise that the therapist allow the person to guide the direction of the session, if at all possible, and then carefully allow other family members to take part.

A final consideration is the recognition that certain high-risk families may not be amenable to any form of counseling intervention. Although Rosenthal and Muir (1983) do not preclude such families from counseling assistance, we believe that the severe "maladaptive behavior patterns," "prolonged use of denial," and "severe chronic physical and/or mental deficits" that they describe would resist well-intentioned psychotherapeutic efforts.

As a concluding note, we agree with Rosenthal and Muir that, regardless of postmorbid problems, not all families require extensive counseling intervention and would add that we must trust such families to determine their own livable reality apart from our presumably objective professional judgment.

Individual Counseling

In treating the individual patient, it is apparent that psychological dimensions are involved in every aspect of the rehabilitation process and that the chief provider of services (very likely the speech-language pathologist) must take on the task of integrating the cognitive, communicative, and emotional behaviors psychotherapeutically.

Makmus et al. (1980) of the Adult Head Trauma Team of Rancho Los Amigos Hospital in California, one of the foremost and earliest rehabilitation teams to work with TBI patients on the West Coast, states the responsibilities precisely:

> All personnel, regardless of their specific disciplines, are psychotherapists in that they possess human qualities of warmth, understanding, empathy, genuineness, caring and respect and as such, set the therapeutic environment. It is most important to view the patient as a person, to understand and respect his confused and fractured state of identity and his struggle and frustration to regain his previous identity and place in life. One does not have to be a psychologist to be facilitative. Often because of failure to understand behavior, one becomes fearful and uncomfortable and the tendency is to refer such problems to a psychologist to diagnose and "cure." Psychotherapy, more often than not, is a lengthy process in that a person must be allowed time to progress and reassess ways of being in light of his consequences and life dynamics. The psychologist does not possess any magical power or potent words that will somehow transform a situation and miraculously cause the patient to perform and "behave." (p. 51)

We would concur and add that, not only is it possible to continue to combine cognitive treatment strategies with psychotherapeutic ones, it is of utmost necessity to do so. To act otherwise is to neglect the very needs presented by the patient. Of course, how much emphasis is to be given to cognitive retrieval and how much to psychological adjustment is not easy to determine. The speech-language pathologist typically uses traditional methods including workbooks, computerized software programs, and structured discourse to enhance cognitive skills and indirectly to deal with emotional issues. Or, is it possible to rely more on counseling procedures to do the same thing, providing the clinician is trained in these methods?

While not addressing psychotherapeutic intervention directly, McGann and Werven (1995) propose the utilization of the patients' insight into their own social communication problems to enable them to be primary managers of their activities, rather than allow therapist directed tasks to guide the patient. What they describe as "principle-centered therapy," an attitude rather than a methodology, challenges the clinician to relinquish his or her authoritative and paternalistic role. Essentially, a communicative interaction is fostered whereby the clinician acts as a resource for the patient and together they engage in activities that focus more on principles of communication than specific skills per se. McGann and Werven believe that the pressure to use only quantifiable, outcome-based programs obscures what our therapeutic goals are—to be sensitive to the patient and how the individual best can enhance his or her social skills.

We already described how the behavior problems presented by the patient are made more complex by the variables of premorbid psychosocial factors and the presence of postmorbid neurobiolgical variables, including cognitive deficits. The Rancho Los Amigos team also describes the necessity for long-term psychotherapeutic treatment, often impossible to sustain if hospitalization is short term. The team believes the focus should be on using psychotherapy to prepare the patient for discharge and reentering the family and community and on helping the person determine a redefinition of his or her life. We believe these expectations, while commendable, might be somewhat unrealistic for most moderate and severe TBI patients and their families. Nevertheless, a bridge needs to be established as the patient is shifted to the subsequent environment.

Many of the psychotherapeutic guidelines described earlier for the CVA patient are applicable with the TBI patient but with some major differences. These differences are highlighted by the fact that emotional responses in the TBI patient are frequently mediated by their disordered thought processing. To assign diagnostic labels "or even psychopathological explanations" can be misleading and counterproductive. Still, the following are psychodynamic factors to consider:

1. *Marked egocentricity and inappropriateness of behavior.* The patient is aided in becoming aware of exactly what constitutes such behavior. Although told that these behaviors are natural consequences of the injury, they can be altered by recognizing that they occur, acknowledging their effects on others, and modifying them to produce more acceptable behaviors. Use of feedback through videocassettes has been found to be an effective means to achieve this end with many patients and can be utilized readily during the course of cognitive retraining procedures.

2. *Concrete thinking and impaired judgment.* An approach similar to the preceding one is used. Modeling by the therapist can help the patient more clearly recognize individual behavior and how it interferes with communication and interrelating with others. To be sure, the patient may not always have the ability to modify the behavior accordingly, but any positive change should be rewarded and reinforced.

3. *Confusion, disorientation, and restlessness.* Work being done on orienting the patient to reality should be carried over during counseling. We refer to not only the identification of such concepts as time, events, and places but also to the concentration on clarity of communication between the patient and therapist. For the patient to be confused by the psychotherapeutic process will add to the personal confusion surrounding other aspects of reality, particularly if feelings about being confused and disoriented are discussed.

4. *Anxiety and insecurity.* The therapist will need to distinguish between anxiety and insecurity based on actual reality from anxiety and insecurity that are reflections of the patient's personality pattern. For example, it is certainly understandable if the patient becomes anxious when not informed of schedule changes of various therapies, and it is incumbent on the counseling therapist to help correct the situation. If, on the other

hand, the patient is unable to risk expanding the range of experiences, say, going to the dentist or getting a haircut, then such fears need to be scrutinized and analyzed by both patient and therapist. Especially important is that the therapist also be aware of any developing transference or countertransference relationship. It is not unusual for TBI persons to cling to the professional caregiver who is most "there" for them or appears to understand them best. Weaning the patient away from the dependency, yet maintaining the therapeutic relationship, is a challenge to even the most experienced counselor.

5. *Denial and unrealistic expectations.* It is not uncommon for the patient, because of disordered thinking, to believe that a return to the premorbid state is imminent and life will continue as it had left off. We need to be cautious not to assign such a belief to a maladjusted emotional state, because it could well be the organism's attempt to reestablish homeostasis. Similarly, when we believe that the patient is not reacting in an appropriate emotional manner, we cannot assume that the problems are being denied. The therapist can attempt to help the patient identify the disparity between thought and feeling with the understanding that such reconciliation indeed can be very difficult to achieve.

6. *Memory problems.* Long- or short-term memory difficulties can hinder the psychotherapeutic relationship in that anything processed, understood, or presumably learned in one therapy session may be readily forgotten in another. There is no simple solution to this problem, except to help the person be aware that it is a natural consequence of the injury and, by maintaining a daily log of learned insights and practicing new behaviors, some retention is possible. Maintenance of a stable environment and schedules also will be helpful to the patient.

7. *Depression.* It is important to reinforce any slight gain the individual makes in order to minimize the effects of primary or secondary depression. The therapist sometimes must cope with the patient who becomes depressed about feeling depressed. Such a state of mind is very complex, and the patient should be helped to understand that which is being experienced is also a natural consequence of the injury and in fact may be a positive sign of progress. To be oblivious to it even may be counterproductive.

8. *Disinhibition.* Because of the injury, the inhibitory function of the cerebrum is reduced. Violent outbursts of temper and temper tantrums typically occur, and the therapist will have to be acutely sensitive in distinguishing these from secondary acting-out behaviors and behavioral manifestations of frustration and anger. As with depression, the patient must learn to reconcile the primary and secondary behaviors and, in doing so, gain some degree of control over them. Although many factors, such as resistance, avoidance, denial, or even euphoria, might mitigate against recognition, awareness, and control of disinhibitory behavior, the therapist may find confrontive cognitive-emotional techniques, used judiciously, helpful.

The neuropsychodynamic processes and psychotherapeutic strategies just described cannot be viewed discretely in every case, and therefore the therapist is urged to use his or her best professional judgment in intervening accordingly.

Furthermore, the therapist will have to determine judiciously how much the family must or should know of the patient's inner struggles as they emerge in counseling. Counseling or family therapy is used to complement individual counseling. Regardless, the patient's individual rights should be honored and respected while directed toward independent living. With those cases where independent living or reentering family life is contraindicated because of the extent of the disability, the therapist, as well as other caregivers, will be challenged to assist the patient adapt cognitively and emotionally to whatever living environment is deemed appropriate It would be useful, particularly in this regard, for readers to familiarize themselves further with the work of McGann and Werven, discussed earlier.

A Case Study

Brian K. was 26 years old when he ran off a remote country road into a culvert, following a long night of imbibing. Although the friend he was with was uninjured, Brian suffered a brain concussion and scattered and diffuse damage to the cortex. Comatose for several weeks, he emerged with spastic hemiparesis, severe cognitive dysfunction, infantile behavior, and impulsivity. After a year and a half of rehabilitation efforts, he rapidly progressed to the point where he was fully ambulatory, albeit with spastic movement of the right-side extremities. His cognitive-intellectual behavior was characterized by distractibility, poor judgment, and difficulty processing and sequencing information. Emotionally, he often acted foolishly, inappropriately, and generally insensitively to others while also overly friendly and often ingratiating. His speech was mild to moderately dysarthric, and his voice breathy and aprosodic.

Prior to the injury, Brian had lived at home with his father and stepmother and had been employed as a cook in a local coffee shop. Postmorbidly, he still lived at home. Clinical reports revealed some family counseling during the course of rehabilitation but no individual counseling per se for Brian except for some tangential work connected to cognitive retraining. Brian was referred to us by a social worker, who believed Brian needed more help in adjusting to his changed circumstances and acknowledging his deficits. Apparently, the family, his father in particular, was still caught up in the so-called sleeping beauty syndrome and believed that soon all would be normal again. The family had refused further family counseling or family therapy but agreed to individual counseling for Brian.

The following clinical protocol is intended as an example of the psychotherapeutic process that may be used in such cases as this one. It illustrates the complexity of dealing with the psychodynamics posed by some TBI individuals and represents an excerpt from the fifth session:

BRIAN: You know what my father told me yesterday?
THERAPIST: What was that?
BRIAN: As soon as I'm able to drive again, he's getting me a new Trans Am.
THERAPIST: You sound very pleased about that.
BRIAN: You bet!
THERAPIST: Do you remember last week when we talked about realistic expectations for yourself? Have you thought much about that?

BRIAN: And you know another thing, it's going to have all the equipment on it.
THERAPIST: What was it I just asked you, Brian?
BRIAN: If I know what to expect.
THERAPIST: Yes, if you thought about things you could realistically achieve with respect to your difficulties.
BRIAN: I know I'm getting better.
THERAPIST: Up to now you've come a long way and have worked very hard at getting better.
BRIAN: I know. And you want to know another thing, Walter?[2]
THERAPIST: Yes?
BRIAN: I like you.
THERAPIST: Oh?
BRIAN: Yeah. You're really gonna get me on my feet again.
THERAPIST: Do you know what you're doing now, Brian?
BRIAN: Yeah, I'm getting off the subject.
THERAPIST: Yes, it's really hard for you to stay on the subject, but it's important that you stay focused on what we need to talk about—like realistic expectations.
BRIAN: I get distracted.
THERAPIST: Yes you do, but it's good that you recognize that as you do now. I know you work very hard at doing that. Keep it up.
BRIAN: Do you think I'm going to get better?
THERAPIST: You've made a lot of progress already and I know you'll make more. How much, we don't know. You have to take one day at a time.
BRIAN: You bet! Like, I'd like to meet a nice girl.
THERAPIST: You have strong feelings about that.
BRIAN: I keep thinking about it all the time.
THERAPIST: And that's very natural for you to do.
BRIAN: Maybe when I get my TransAm.
THERAPIST: What do you mean?
BRIAN: I'll be able to impress her. (He laughs boastingly.)

---

[2]Note: Typically, at the start of the initial counseling session, I introduce myself with my full name, sans title, allowing the client to chose whatever form of salutation he or she might find comfortable. In Brian's case, I felt his choice was characteristic of his need to be liked and to establish a "buddy" relationship with me. The latter explanation has not necessarily applied with other clients.

THERAPIST: A relationship with a girl means more, much more, Brian, and I think you know that.

BRIAN: I do, but I need something to get it going.

THERAPIST: Like you feel that you personally won't attract her—that you need some kind of artificial object to begin the relationship?

BRIAN: I guess so. It's easier that way.

THERAPIST: Is that how you want it?

BRIAN: I don't care which way.

THERAPIST: I have trouble understanding that.

BRIAN: What do you mean?

THERAPIST: Because I think you want to be accepted for who you are, in spite of your disability.

BRIAN: And I'm better off now than I used to be, aren't I?

This therapeutic interaction identifies several aspects of cognitive-intellectual-emotional behavior sometimes characteristic of TBI. To what degree such behaviors relate to premorbid attitudes is not readily determined. Brian had graduated from high school and was generally an affable young man but prone to immature outbursts of anger. The latter behavior virtually disappeared following his injury, but other premorbid characteristics still were evident. Brian was counseled for eight months, during which time he gradually but slowly began to respond more appropriately to others and became more willing to look realistically toward his future. It should be noted that, during the course of counseling, I had the persistent feeling that he was making a greater effort at pleasing me and acquiescing in fulfilling contract goals while not really modifying his inappropriate behavior. How much of this was due to my own counseling competence or the persistent nature of primary and secondary neuropsychological factors cannot be ascertained.

Certainly, we do not wish to infer that all such counseling interrelationships in the case of TBI can be predicted. We, in fact, have seen many definitively successful outcomes. We merely suggest that the reader be fully cognizant of the manipulative behaviors that frequently characterize the TBI person's quest for survival in a differently perceived world.

Family Caregiver Support and Group Therapy

Because of the mutual frustration, dissatisfaction, helplessness, and financial strain often experienced by families in their search for appropriate facilities and support in returning TBI members to their realistic potential, many family survival programs have sprung up across the United States. Among the goals of the National Head Injury Foundation, a nonprofit corporation formed to advocate for TBI persons and their families, has been the development of a support group network to assist families in organizing local support groups in all states.

Levy (1979) describes the function of a support group in which a trained facilitator is used. He defines such groups as

> composed of members who share a common status or predicament that entails some degree of stress, and the aim of these groups is generally the amelioration of this stress through mutual support and the sharing of coping strategies and advice. There is no attempt to change their member; that is taken as more or less fixed, and the problem for members of these groups is how to carry on in spite of this. (p. 242)

Employing a health model, the support group focuses on current problem situations, not on the dynamics that created the situation or the interpersonal relationship among members. The approach essentially is nonconfrontational, supportive, and nonjudgmental, in which the members take responsibility for their own actions. Networking and socializing among members are encouraged for them to learn how to cope from each other, particularly when grief still is being experienced. In their study of distress, depressive symptoms, and depressive disorder among family caregivers, Gillen et al. (1998) found that depression persisted beyond six months following TBI.

The role of the facilitator is to[3]

---

[3]This text on the role of the facilitator and how emotional difficulties of caregiving are handled has been adapted, in part, from M.L. Boering and L. McKinney-Adler, "Facilitating Support Groups—An Instructional Guide," NIMH Training Grant 15718, Group Facilitation Skills for Health Professionals, made to Pacific Medical Center, 1981.

1. *Foster cognitive and emotional communication* by encouraging members to talk to each other and focus on feelings about specific situations. These feelings are verified by one another.
2. *Encourage mutual respect among group members* by modifying and emphasizing special aspects of each situation in order to decrease competitiveness, advice giving, or teaching.
3. *Encourage exploration of problems* through practical problem solving, alternative choices, brainstorming, and similar activities. All aspects of each individual member's problems are explored and interrelated to obtain a complete picture.
4. *Encourage the sharing and trying out of coping strategies and support efforts to change* by moving from exploring problems to making change, often very difficult. The facilitator uses as models those members who have made changes in their situation and asks how they accomplished it. The main focus is on flexibility and individual ways of achieving the desired goal.
5. *Focus on improvement* by giving mutual respect and supporting efforts to change, grow, adapt, and fight the system if necessary, to care for oneself.
6. *Maintain the group duties* by encouraging members to define and maintain ground rules. Include a structuring process—helping members develop appropriate norms, goals, roles, and values by providing structure and allowing structure to emerge.
7. *Maintain balanced participation of members* by keeping group discussion on topics pertinent to the focused group concerns.
8. *Mediate* (also done by members) when an inappropriate level of friction is observed.
9. *Coordinate* by handling arrangements, overseeing the newsletter, arranging the room, and so on.

How members of the group are helped to deal with the emotional difficulties of caregiving includes

1. *Coping with depression by decreasing the feeling of helplessness and hopelessness* through taking action to control parts of the situation when possible.
2. Reducing feelings of being overwhelmed by having a place to ventilate feelings with others, putting them into perspective, and helping *provide a structure for dealing with the problem.*
3. *Guilt* can be decreased by sharing common themes and seeing them as natural by-products of caregiving: "I want my husband to die," "How can I *place* my husband?" or taking time for *oneself.*
4. *Decreasing anger and frustration* by provision of a place to ventilate and receive validation for the reality of many frustrating situations, such as dealing with bureaucracies—difficult for all of us and not our fault. It may not decrease the frustration but can help provide a better perspective on it, and the frustration may decrease if a better understanding of how the system works is achieved.
5. *Anger and resentment* can be decreased through education gained in the group; for example, being angry at a spouse because he cannot perform a certain task. The group member may learn this is a common symptom of the injury and, by an increase in understanding, feel less angry and helpless.
6. Members have a place to express *grief* and work through it with others and view it as natural.

It is obvious that support groups cannot change the basic situation of caregiving, but members of different families can learn to cope more effectively by gaining increased control over time. We also must recognize that these groups are not a panacea and individuals may require individual psychotherapy or therapy within the context of family therapy. Further note that some individuals may resist all forms of counseling. Ideally, what Prigatano and Altman (1990) and Prigatano (1999) refers to as the *milieu* or *holistic approach*, in which the patient is aided to participate with others including other TBI patients and the professional personnel in real-life situations incorporating cognitive, psychotherapeutic, and social practices, we find to be a most practical and realistic approach in rehabilitation. More significant, it involves the patients participating with staff members in making the day-to-day decisions typical of a rehabilitation center. It resembles somewhat the social competence concept, discussed earlier, drawn by McGann and Werven (1995) and McGann, Werven, and Douglas (1997), in which TBI patients move toward becoming their own managers, taking control of their own lives, as the clinician serves as a resource person, not someone with all the answers.

Group Therapy

Given the reality of the increase of rationing of health care in the United States, those responsible for maximizing the potential of TBI patients have had to make the "most out of the little." One means has been the establishment of group therapy for TBI patients, focusing on the treatment of substance abuse and frustration management through education, social support, and developmental skills. Delmonico, Hanley-Peterson, and Englander (1998) describe such a service provided at Santa Clara Rehabilitation Center in San Jose, California. Johnson and Davis (1998) attempted group therapy, integrating TBI patients with matched non-TBI individuals from the community, and found that social integration can be enhanced with limited staff intervention.

Outcomes and Conclusion

During the past decade, considerable focus has been on follow-up outcomes of children and adults with TBI, beyond termination of formal rehabilitation. Rivera et al. (1996) determined that preinjury functioning was the best predictor of three-year outcomes. They concluded that families at risk for poorer outcomes can be prospectively identified and should be aided and encouraged in their attempt to develop new coping resources. Max et al. (1998b), in their study of predictors of family functioning following TBI in children and adolescents, found that the greatest influences on family functioning following TBI are preinjury family functioning, negative family events, and stressors.

It is clear that TBI presents counseling therapists with the most formidable challenge to their expertise in coping with the intricate issues manifest in the patient and family. It demands not only the highest degree of competence in both individual and family psychodynamics but a sound knowledge of all the related physical, cognitive, perceptual motor, intellectual, and communication concomitants. The reentry of the adult with TBI into family, social, perhaps educational, and vocational life and guiding the child with TBI in a direction approximating his or her premorbid life will demand many interdisciplinary resources. The major question and concern confronting us is that, once the TBI patient comes home, after all forms of health insurances are exhausted, how does the typical TBI family reintegrate without the professional resources?

References

Andrews TK, Rose FD, Johnson DA. Social and behavioral effects of traumatic brain injury in children. *Brain Inj.* February 1998; 12(2):133–138.

Annegers JF, Grabow JD, Kurland LF, Laws ER. The incidence, causes, and secular trends of head traumas in Olmstead County, Minnesota. *Neurology.* 1980:912–919.

Barry P. *Family Adjustment to Head Injury.* Framingham MA: National Head Injury Foundation; 1984.

Ben-Yishay Y, Diller L. Cognitive deficits. In: Rosenthal M, Griffith ER, Bond MR, Millers JD, eds. *Rehabilitation of the Head Injured Adult.* Philadelphia: F. A. Davis; 1983.

Blumer D, Benson DF. Personality changes with frontal and temporal lobe lesions. In: *Psychiatric Aspects of Neurological Disease.* New York: Grune and Stratton; 1975.

Bond MR. Effects on the family system. In: Rosenthal M, Griffith ER, Bond MR, Dougles JM, eds. *Rehabilitation of the Head Injured Adult.* Philadelphia: F. A. Davis; 1983.

———. The psychiatry of closed head injury. In: Brooks N, ed. *Closed Head Injury: Psychological, Social, and Family Consequences.* Oxford, England: Oxford University Press; 1984.

Brooks N, ed. *Closed Head Injury: Psychological, Social, and Family Consequences.* Oxford, England: Oxford University Press; 1984.

Bryant RA, Harvey AG. Relationship between acute stress disorder and posttraumatic stress disorder following mild traumatic brain injury. *Am J Psychiatry.* May 1998; 155(5):625–629.

Bukay L, Glasuer F. *Head Injury.* Boston: Little, Brown and Co.; 1980.

Busch CR, Alpern HP. Depression after mild traumatic brain injury: a review of current research. *Neuropsychol Rev.* June 1998; 8(2):95–108.

Cartlidge NEF, Shaw DA. *Major Problems in Neurology,* Vol. 10 *Head Injury.* London: W. B. Saunders; 1981.

Childers MK, Holland D, Ryan MG, Rupright J. Obsessional disorders during recovery from severe head injury: report of four cases. *Brain Inj.* July 1998; 12(7): 613–616.

Committee on Child Abuse and Neglect 1993–1994. Shaken baby syndrome: inflicted cerebral trauma. *Del Med J.* July 1997; 69(7):365–370.

Deb S, Lyons I, Koutzoukis C, Ali I, McCarthy G. Rate of psychiatric illness one year after traumatic brain injury. *Am J Psychiatry.* March 1999;56(3):374–378.

Delmonico RL, Hanley-Peterson P, Englander J. Group psychotherapy for persons with traumatic brain injury: management of frustration and substance abuse. *J Head Trauma Rehabil.* December1998; 13(6):10–22.

DePompei R, Williams J. Working with families after TBI: A family-centered approach. *Topics in Language Disorders.* November 1994;15(1):68-81.

DePompei R, Zarski JJ. Families, head injury, and cognitive-communicative impairments: Issues for family counseling. *Topics in Language Disorders.* March 1989; 9(2):78–89.

Diehl LN. Patient-family education. In: Rosenthal M, Griffith ER, Bond MR, Miller JD, eds.

Dougles JM. *Rehabilitation of the Head Injured Adult.* Philadelphia: F. A. Davis; 1983.

Elliott ML, Biever LS. Head injury and sexual dysfunction. *Brain Inj.* October 1996;10(10):703– 717.

Ewing-Cobbs L, Kramer L, Prasad M, Canales DN, Louis Pt, Fletcher JM, Vollero H, Landry SH, Cheung K. Neuroimaging, physical, and developmental findings after inflicted and noninflicted traumatic brain injury in young children. *Pediatrics.* August 1998; 102(2, pt 1): 300–307.

Fahy TJ, Irving MH, Millac P. Severe head injuries: A six year follow-up. *Lancet.* 1967;2:475–479.

Gillen R, Tennen H, Affleck G, Steinpreis R. Distress, depressive symptoms, and depressive disorder among caregivers of patients with brain injury. *J Head Trauma Rehabil.* June 1998;13(3):31–43.

Gomez-Hernandez R, Max JE, Kosier T, Paradiso S, Robinson RG. Social impairment and depression after traumatic brain injury. *Arch Phys Med Rehabil.* December 1997; 78(12):1321–1326.

Griffith ER. Types of disability. In: Rosenthal M, Griffith ER, Bond MR, Miller JD, eds. *Rehabilitation of the Head Injured Adult.* Philadelphia: F. A. Davis; 1983.

Griffith ER, Lemberg S. *Sexuality and the Person with Traumatic Brain Injury: A Guide for Families.* Philadelphia: F. A. Davis; 1992.

Gronwall D, Wrightson P. Duration of post-traumatic amnesia after mild head injury. *J of Clinical Neuropsychol-ogy.* 1980;2:51–50.

Harvey AG, Bryant RA. Predictors of acute stress following mild traumatic brain injury. *Brain Inj.* February 1998; 12(2):147–154.

Hibbard MR, Uysal S, Kepler K, Bogdany J, Silver J. Axis I psychopathology in individuals with traumatic brain injury. *J Head Trauma Rehabil.* August 1998;13(4): 24–39.

Hickling EJ, Gillen R, Blanchard EB, Buckley T, Taylor A. Traumatic brain injury and posttraumatic stress disorder: a preliminary investigation of neuropsychological test results in PTSD secondary to motor vehicle accidents. *Brain Inj.* April 1998; 12(4):265–274.

Hobbs CJ. Skull fracture and the diagnosis of abuse. *Archives of Disease in Childhood.* 1984;(59):246–252.

Holland D, Shigaki CL. Educating families and caretakers of traumatically brain injured patients in the new health care environment: a three phase model and bibliography. *Brain Inj* 1998; Dec v12(12): 993–1009.

Jennett B. Scale and scope of the problem. In: Rosenthal M, Griffth ER, Bond MR, Miller JD (eds), *Rehabilitation of the Head Injured Adult.* Philadelphia: F. A. Davis, 1983.

———, Macmillan R. Epidemiology of head injury. *British Med J.* 1981;(282):101.

Johnson K, Davis PK. A supported relationships intervention to increase the social integration of persons with traumatic brain injuries. *Behav Modif (9L5)* 1998; Oct v22(4): 502-528.

Kerr TA, Kay DWK, Lassman LP. Characteristics of patients, type of accident, and mortality in a consecutive series of head injury admitted to a neurosurgical unit. *British J of Preventive and Social Medicine* 197; 25: 1799-185.

Kingston P, Reay A. Elder abuse and neglect. In: Woods RT, ed. *Handbook of the Clinical Psychology of Aging.* New York: Wiley and Sons; 1996:423–438.

Kraus JF. Injury to the head and spinal cord: the epidemiological relevance of the medical literature published from 1900 to 1978. *J of Neurosurgery* (suppl). 1980; 53:3–10.

Kreuter M, Sullivan M, Dahll of AG, Si osteen A. Partner relationships, functioning, mood and global quality of life in persons with spinal cord injury and traumatic brain injury. *Spinal Cord.* April 1998; 36(4):252–261.

Krych D, Ashley MJ, Persel CH, Persel CS. *Working with Behavior Disorder: Strategies for Traumatic Brain Injury Rehabilitation.* San Antonio, TX: Psychological Corp.; 1999.

Kushner D. Mild traumatic brain injury: toward understanding manifestations and treatment. *Arch Intern Med.* August 10–24, 1998;158(15):1617–1624.

Kubler-Ross E. *On Death and Dying.* New York: Macmillan; 1969.

Leathem J, Heath E, Woolley C. Relatives' perceptions of role change, social support and stress after traumatic brain injury. *Brain Inj.* January 1996;10(1):27–38.

Leon-Carrion J, Alarcon JC, Revuelta M, Murillo-Cabezas F, Dominguez-Roldan JM, Dominguez-Morales MR, Machuca-Murga F, Forastero P. Executive functioning as outcome in patients after traumatic brain injury. *Int J Neurosci.* May 1998;94(1–2):75–83.

Levin H. Aphasia in closed head injury. In: Sarno MT, *Acquired Aphasia.* New York: Academic Press; 1981.

Levin HS, Benton AL, Grossman RG. *Neurobehavioral Consequences of Closed Head Injury.* New York: Oxford University Press; 1982.

Levin HS, Chapman SB. Aphasia after Traumatic Brain Injury. In: Sarno MT, *Acquired Aphasia,* 3rd ed. New York: Academic Press; 1998.

Levy LH. Processes and activities in groups. In: Lieberman MA, Borman LD, eds. *Self-Help Groups for Coping with Crisis.* San Francisco: Jossey-Bass; 1979.

Lezak MD. Subtle sequelae of brain damage: perplexity, distractibility and fatigue. *Am J of Physical Medicine.* 1978a;57:9–15.

———, Living with the characterologically altered brain injured patient. *J of Clinical Psychiatry.* 1978b;39:592–598.

Lishman WA. The psychiatric sequelae of head injury: a review. *Psych Med.* 1973;(3):304–318.

Luria AR. *Higher Cortical Functions in Man.* New York: Basic Books; 1980.

Makmus D, Booth BJ, Kadimer C. *Rehabilitation of the Head Injured Adult: Comprehensive Cognitive Management.* Downey, CA: The Professional Staff Association of Rancho Los Amigos; 1980.

Manchester D, Hodgkinson A, Casey T. Prolonged, severe behavioral disturbance following traumatic brain injury: what can be done? *Brain Inj.* August 1997;2(8):605–617.

Marsh NV, Kersel DA, Havill JH, Sleigh JW. Caregiver burden at six months following severe traumatic brain injury. *Brain Inj.* March 1998;12(3):225–238.

Martin D. Family issues in traumatic brain injury. In: Bigler ED, ed. *Traumatic Brain Injury.* Austin, TX: Pro-Ed; 1990.

Mauss-Clum N, Ryan M. Brain injury and the family. *J of Neurological Nursing.* 1981;13:165–169.

Max JE, Castillo CS, Robin DA, Lingren SD, Smith WL Jr, Sato Y, Mattheis PJ, Stierwalt JA. Predictors of family functioning after traumatic brain injury in children and adolescents. *J Am Acad Child Adolesc Psychiatry.* January 1998a;37(1):83–90.

Max JE, Koele, SL, Smith WL Jr, Sato Y, Lingren SD, Robin DA, Arndt S. Psychiatric disorders in children and adolescents after severe traumatic brain injury: a controlled study. *J Am Acad Child Adolesc Psychiatry.* August 1998b;37(8):832–840.

Max JE, Lingren SD, Knutson C, Pearson CS, Ihrig D, Welborn A. Child and adolescent traumatic brain injury: correlates of disruptive behavior disorders. *Brain Inj.* January 1998c;12(1):41–52.

Max JE, Robin DA, Lindgren SD, Smith WL Jr,, Sato Y,

Mattheis PJ, Stierwalt JA, Castillo CS. Traumatic brain injury in children and adolescents: psychiatric disorders at one year. *J Neuropsychiatry Clin Neurosci.* Summer 1998d;10(3):290–297.

Max JE, Roberts MA, Koele SL, Lindgren SD, Robin DA, Arndt S, Smith WL Jr, Sato Y. Cognitive outcome in children and adolescents following severe traumatic brain injury: influence of psychosocial, psychiatric, and injury-related variables. *J Int Neuropsychol Soc.* January 1999;5(1):58–68.

McDowell S, Whyte J, D'Esposito M. Differential effect of a dopaminergic agonist on prefrontal function in traumatic brain injury patients. *Brain.* June 1998;121(6):1155–1164.

McGann W, Werven G. New management concept. Social competence and head injury: a new emphasis. *Brain Inj.* 1995;9(1):93–102.

McGann W, Werver G, Douglas MM. Social competence and head injury: a practical approach. *Brain Injury.* September 1997;11(9):621–628.

Medlar T. The sexuality education program of the Massachusetts statewide head injury program. *Sexuality and Dis.* 1998;16(1):11–19.

Millard A. The family and communication: a letter from the mother of a head trauma victim. *The Coordinator.* June 1983:6–11.

Miller JD, Pentland B. The factors of age, alcohol, and multiple injury in patients with mild and moderate head injury. In: Hoff JT, Anderson TE, Cole TM, eds. *Mild to Moderate Head Injury.* Boston: Blackwell Scientific; 1989:125–133.

Muir CA. Mobile mourning: Psychodynamics of family and patient in brain trauma. Paper presented at: Western Psychological Association; April 1978; San Francisco.

Nagle TK. Effects on families of children with a traumatic brain injury to be studied. *Naric Quarterly.* Spring 1989;2(1).

Najenson T, Mendelson L, Schechter I, Daviv C, Mintz N, Grosswasser Z. Rehabilitaion after severe brain injury. *Scandinanvian J of Rehab Med.* 1974;6:5–14.

Najenson T, Sazbon L, Fiselzon J, Becker E, Schechter I. Recovery of communicative functions after prolonged traumatic coma. *Scandinavian J of Rehab Med.* 1978;10:15–21.

Naugle RI. Epidemiology of traumatic brain injury in adults. In Bigler ED, ed. *Traumatic Brain Injury.* Austin, TX: Pro-Ed; 1990:69–103.

Nikas DL. Commentary on cerebral perfusion pressure: management protocol and clinical results. *AACN Nursing Scan in Critical Care.* July–September 1996;6(3):13.

Oddy M. Head injury during childhood: The psychological implications. In: Brooks N, ed. *Closed Head Injury: Psychological, Social and Family Consequences.* Oxford, England: Oxford University Press; 1984.

Oddy M, Humphrey M. Social recovery during the year following severe head injury. *J of Neurology, Neurosurgery and Psychiatry.* 1980;43:798–802.

Oddy M, Humphrey M, Uttley D. Subjective impairment and social recovery after closed head injury. *J of Neurology, Neurosurgery and Psychiatry.* 1978a;41:611–616.

———. Stresses upon the relatives of head-injured patients. *British J of Psychiatry.* 1978b;133:507–513.

Ohry A, Rattok J, Solomon Z. Post traumatic stress disorder in brain injury patients. *Brain Inj.* September 1996; 10(9):687–695.

O'Neill LJ, Carter DE. The implications of head injury for family relationships *Br J Nurs.* July 1998.

Ownsworth TL, Oei TP. Depression after traumatic brain injury: conceptualization and treatment considerations. *Brain Inj.* September 1998;12(9):735–751.

Painting A, Merry P. The long-term rehabilitation of severe head injuries with particular reference to the need for social and medical support for the patient's family. *Rehabilitation.* 1972;38:33–37.

Parker RS. Neurobehavior outcome of children's mild traumatic brain injury. *Semin-Neurol.* March 1994;14(1): 67–73.

Perlesz A, O'Loughlan M. Changes in stress and burden in families seeking therapy following traumatic brain injury: a follow-up study. *Int J Rehabil Res.* December 1998;21(4):339–354.

Pittman D, Fowler S. Acute stress disorder: application to families of head-injured patients. *J of Neuroscience Nursing.* August 1998;30(4):253–256.

Prigatatano GP. *Principles of Neuropsychological Rehabilitation.* Oxford: Oxford University Press; 1999.

Prigatatano GP, Altman IM. Impaired awareness of behavioral limitations after traumatic brain injury. *Archives Phys Med Rehabil.* Decemeber 1990;71(13): 1058–1064.

Resnick C. The effect of head injury on family and marital stability. *Social Work in Health Care.* Binghamton, NY: The Haworth Press; 1993:18(2).

Rimel RW, Jane JA. Characteristics of the head injured patient. In: Rosenthal M, Griffith ER, Bond MR, Miller JD, eds. *Rehabilitation of the Head Injured Adult.* Philadelphia: F. A. Davis; 1983.

Rivera JM, Jaffe KM, Polissar NL, Fay GC, Liao S, Martin KM. Predictors of family functioning and change 3 years after traumatic brain injury in children. *Arch Phys Med Rehabil.* August 1996;77(8):754–764.

Rollin WJ. Family therapy and the aphasic adult. In: Eisenson J, *Adult Aphasia.* Englewood Cliffs, NJ: Prentice-Hall; 1984.

Romano MD. Family response to traumatic head injury. *Scandinavian J of Rehab Med.* 1974;6:1–4.

Rosenbaum M, Lipsitz N, Abraham J, Najenson T. A description of an intensive treatment project for the rehabilitation of severely brain-injured soldiers. *Scandinavian J of Rehab Med.* 1978;10:1–6.

Rosenbaum M, Najenson T. Changes in life patterns and symptoms of low mood as reported by wives of severely brain-injured soldiers *J of Consulting and Clinical Psychology.* 1976;44:881–888.

Rosenthal M. Psychological deficits in the brain-injured adult and family. Paper presented at Conference on Rehabilitation of the Traumatic Brain-Injured Adult; June 1979; Williamsburg, VA.

———. Strategies for intervention with families of brain-injured patients. In: Edelstein BA, Couture ET, eds. *Behavioral Assessment and Rehabilitation of the Traumatically Brain Damaged.* New York: Plenum; 1984.

Rosenthal M, Christensen BK, Ross TP. Depression following traumatic brain injury. *Arch Phys Med Rehabil.* January 1998;79(1):90–103.

Rosenthal M, Miller JD, eds. *Rehabilitation of the Adult and Child with Traumatic Brain Injury.* Philadelphia: F. A. Davis; 1999.

Rosenthal M, Muir CA. Methods of family intervention. In: Rosenthal M, Griffith ER, Bond MR, Miller JD, eds. *Rehabilitation of the Head Injured Adult.* Philadelphia: F. A. Davis; 1983.

Sander A, Kreutzer JS. A holistic approach to family assessment after brain injury. In: Rosenthal M, Miller JD, eds. *Rehabilitation of the Adult and Child with Traumatic Head Injury.* Philadephia: F. A. Davis; 1999.

Santa Clara Valley Medical Center. Head Injury Rehabilitation Project. Final Report; 1982; San Jose, CA.

Satz P, Forney DL, Zaucha K, Asarnow RR, Light R, McCleary C, Levin H, Kelly D, Bergsneider M, Hovda D, Martin N, Namerow N, Becker D. Depression, cognition, and functional correlates of recovery outcome after traumatic brain injury. *Brain Inj.* July 1998;12(7): 537–553.

Satz P, Zaucha K, Forney DL, McCleary C, Asarnow RF, Light R, Levin H, Kelly D, Bergsneider M, Havda D, Martin N, Caron MJ, Namerow N, Becker D. Neuropsychological, psychosocial, and vocational correlates of the Glasgow Outcome Scale at six months post-injury: a study of moderate to severe traumatic brain injury patients. *Brain Inj.* July 1998;12(7): 555–567.

Schnyder U, Buddeberg C. Psychological aspects of accidental injuries—an overview. *Langenbecks Arch Chir.* 1996;381(3):125–131.

Selecki BR, Hoy RJ, Ness P. Neurotraumatic admissions to a teaching hospital: a retrospective survey, part 2. *Head Injuries Medical Journal of Australia.* 1968;2:113–117.

Smith AM, Schwirian PM. The relationship between caregiver burden and TBI survivors' cognition and functional ability after discharge. *Rehabil Nurs.* September–October 1998;23(5):252–257.

Sokol DK, Ferguson CF, Pitcher GA, Huster GA, Fitzhugh-Bell K, Luerssen TG. Behavioral adjustment and parental stress associated with closed head injury in children. *Brain Inj.* June 1996;10(6):439–451.

Sorenson SB, Kraus JF. Occurrence, severity, and outcomes of brain injury. *J of Head Trauma Rehabilitation.* 1991; 6:1–10.

Spicknell K. Shaking babies . . . shaken baby syndrome. *Nursing Times.* March 25–31, 1998;94(12):34–35.

Suhr J, Tranel D, Wefel J, Barrash J. Memory performance after head injury: contributions of malingering, litigation status, psychological factors, and medication use. *J Clin Exp Neuropsychol.* August 1997;19(4): 500–514.

Thomsen IV. The patient with severe head injury and his family. *Scandinavian J of Rehab Med.* 1974;6:180–183.

Thurman DJ, Branche CM, Sniezek JE. The epidemiology of sports-related traumatic brain injuries in the United States: recent developments. *J Head Trauma Rehabil.* 1998;13(2):1–8.

U.S. Department of Health and Human Services. Injuries and deaths associated with use of snowmobiles, Maine 1991–1996. *Morbidity and Mortality Weekly Report.* January 10, 1997;46(1).

———. Achievements in public health, 1900–1999. Motor-vehicle safety: a 20th century public health achievement. *Morbidity and Mortality Weekly Report.* May 14, 1999;48(18):369–374.

Uysal S, Hibbard MR, Robillad D, Pappadopulos E, Jaffe M. The effect of parental traumatic brain injury on parenting and child behavior. *J Head Trauma Rehabil.* December 1998;13(6):57–71.

Webster EJ, Newhoff M. Intervention with families of communicatively impaired adults. In: Beasley DS and Davis GA, eds. *Aging: Communication Processes and Disorders.* New York: Grune and Stratton; 1981.

Wilson JT, Pettigrew LE, Teasdale GM. Structured interviews for the Glasgow Outcome Scale and the extended Glasgow Outcome Scale: guidelines for their use. *J Neurotrauma.* August 1998;15(8):573–585.

Winsdale WJ. *Confronting Traumatic Brain Injury: Devastation, Hope, and Healing.* Boston: Yale University Press; 1998.

Zafonte RD, Hammond FM, Mann NR, Wood DL, Black KL, Millis SR. Relationship between Glasgow Coma Scale and functional outcome. *Am J Phys Med Rehabil.* September–October 1996;75(5):364–369.

4

Psychological Considerations for Individuals Who Stutter and Their Families

Introduction

Over the last 60 years, at least, the quest by speech-language pathologists for answers to the mystery and dilemma of stuttering has not been unlike Jason's search for the Golden Fleece. The discussion in this chapter is no exception to that adventure, except that it will attempt to trace one further route to the source and explore some familiar and some unfamiliar paths toward further explanation of the stuttering phenomenon.

A hypothesis that will underscore our discussion is the assumption that people are not *stutterers* and that, if we are to understand the stuttering process, we must focus on what people *do*. To assume otherwise is to pigeonhole people categorically and, in a real sense, deny them the prerogative to represent something more than only their stuttering. To define people as "stutterers" not only defeats our own professional purposes but could forever guarantee the perpetuation of their stuttering behavior.

We do not claim to have discovered the ultimate solution to the problem of stuttering. We merely suggest that we shift our thinking and give more attention to an alternate aspect of the process itself. We would not deny that the stuttering process has received considerable emphasis over the last several decades, except that the value of such research has been undermined by our persistence in labeling. We view, with great irony in fact, Wendell Johnson's own consistent use of the term *stutterer* in his land-

mark work, *People in Quandries* (1946), yet elsewhere in his text he discusses *evaluative labeling* as follows:

> This term is designed to emphasize our common tendency to evaluate individuals and situations according to the names we apply to them. After all, this is a way of saying that the way we classify something determines in large measure the way in which we react to it. We classify largely by naming. Having named something, we tend to evaluate it and so react to it in terms of the name we have given it. We learn in our culture to evaluate names or labels, or words, quite independently of the actualities to which they might be applied. (p. 261)

We agree with Johnson, who further suggests that, by naming the individual who stutters and who is evaluated by others in the environment as a stutterer, the problem is apt to become self-perpetuating. Later, influenced by one of his former students, Dean E. Williams (1957, 1971), Johnson extended his semantic orientation to therapy. He challenged the stuttering person's view of self as a *stutterer* and described how that view set the person apart from others merely on the basis of the stuttering behavior. Dare we consider the possibility that, as speech-language pathologists, we have contributed as well to the self-perpetuation of stuttering?

Fortunately, in 1993, the American Speech and Hearing Association (ASHA), as a result of the influence of consumer and self-help groups, adopted a policy in which person-first language was to be used rather than direct labels. Authors now are required to use the term *person who stutters* instead of *stutterer* (ASHA, 1999).

Morgan (1980) and others, including Faden (1998), have written extensively on the iatrogenic factor that frequently occurs in doctor-patient relationships. Iatrogeny is the production or inducement of a harmful change in the somatic or psychological condition of a patient or client, by means of the words or actions of the doctor or therapist. Aronson (1985) describes how iatrogenic voice disorders may be caused as the result of injudicious medical advice regarding voice rest following laryngeal surgery. Conceivably, in our attempts to treat the stuttering person, we may be focusing too much on the negative features (dysfluencies) that these persons produce rather than on the positive elements (fluencies). Therefore, these individuals could be inclined to perceive themselves as more different than similar to those who do not stutter.

We prefer to leave the solution to this problem for consideration by individual practitioners and focus more positively on how they may approach their clients from a cognitive-emotional perspective. Before doing so, however, we will look briefly at several etiological perspectives to establish a rationale for a course of treatment to follow.

The Enigma of Etiology

Over the years, many writers have devoted considerable energy to documenting the plethora of theories on stuttering that evolved over the centuries and, in particular, during the latter half of the 20th century (Hahn, 1956; Eisenson, 1975; Rieber et al., 1976; Van Riper, 1971; Bloodstein, 1981, 1993, 1995; Silverman, 1996; Curlee, 1999). Today, most theorists would categorize the major factors as genetic, neurophysiological, neuropsychological, and behavioral-psychogenic.

We briefly review these, integrating several components of each, and family systems theory as a contributory explanation for the stuttering process.

The Neurophysiological Hypothesis

Modern-day investigators who support a neurophysiological hypothesis tend to consider constitu-

tional factors as major components. That is, they believe stuttering individuals to have had a predisposition to its occurrence or to a *breakdown* in speech. Although these theorists differ with regard to the exact predisposing factor, they all agree that stuttering is an inner organic condition that may be precipitated by any one of a combination of environmental circumstances. Research has yet to confirm how the breakdown may occur, and investigators continue to search for the definitive factor that would explain all stuttering behaviors.

Among the various explanations put forward today, many still are based on the early explanations of Orton (1927) and Travis (1931), who espouse a lack of cerebral dominance as the major factor. West (1958) and Kopp (1934) believe that a biochemical aberration is responsible. Later, Tomatis (1963) espoused the conflict of lateral auditory dominance and Schwartz (1976) saw stuttering as essentially laryngeal dysfunction. Representing a still intriguing neurofunctional theory, Blum (1984) postulates that stuttering individuals have an intermittently dysfunctional auditory monitoring system that interferes with the ballistic function of articulation, resulting in a breakdown of speech fluency. According to Blum, the integrity of the auditory feedback process depends on external environmental influences or stressors or internal ones. That is, the stuttering individual's auditory monitoring does not operate continuously but is invoked when vocalization and articulation begin and then is altered by their perception of a change in the external or internal environment. The difficulty the stuttering individual has is in modulating personal speech to varying moments of silence and external and internal stimuli, which in turn contributes to the disruption of the phonemic process. Leung and Robson (1990), in their review of theories of etiology, suggest that a major predisposing factor may be difficulty in learning the precise temporal patterns required for speech, suggesting a neurophysiological dysfunction.

More recently, Fox et al. (1996) employed PET (positron emission tomography), finding stuttering behavior to cause extensive overactivation of the motor system in both the cerebrum and cerebellum, with right cerebral dominance. They found inactivity of the auditory system during stuttered reading and a deactivation of the frontal-temporal system necessary for speech production. With fluency, overactivity was reduced in most motor areas and considerably reversed the underactive auditory and speech production system. While their conclusions do not necessarily point to a definitive etiology, they provide one more piece of the puzzle, suggesting multiple variations in neural systems involved in fluency and dysfluency. Kroll and DeNil (1998) also used PET in their ongoing studies of speech fluency in both stuttering and nonstuttering populations, and while suggesting a definitive neural basis to explain the phenomena, no conclusions have yet been reached.

In their EEG examination of stuttering preschool children, Ivanova et al. (1991), when comparing subjects with brain pathology and no stuttering with subjects who stuttered, found the presence of marked polymorphic activity in the parietal-temporal zone of the right hemisphere of those who stuttered. These findings suggest a disturbance of interhemispheric relationships not unlike the mixed dominance theory referred to earlier.

Despite these neural findings, we are left with the dilemma of a chicken or egg phenomenon and unable to distinguish a definitive cause-effect relationship relative to etiology.

Genetic Factors

While in no way rejecting outright neural dysfunction, we also choose to identify genetic factors as necessary components toward a fuller appreciation of the stuttering phenomenon—but only in the context of the preceding discussion and other significant factors to be discussed later.

Ludlow and Cooper (1983), in their survey of the genetic literature, contend that stuttering as a genetic disorder has gained in popularity. They caution that methodological problems prevent us from drawing significant conclusions about etiology. Nonetheless, they note that studies of familial incidence, spontaneous recovery, parental dysfluencies, and twinning suggest a connection between stuttering and a family history of stuttering. Ludlow and Cooper (1983) cite several studies that suggest the risk of stuttering is almost four times higher for individuals whose relatives stutter than those in nonstuttering families. They further note that, if one

parent stutters, the risk is even greater that one of the children will stutter. Confirmation of significant sex differences is cited in their review of the literature, with males four times more likely to stutter than females.

Based on a series of genetic studies, Kidd (1977) found that a genetic factor in stuttering represented by a "single major locus" is highly likely. In their retrospective study of family history of stuttering in 169 adults and adolescents who stuttered, Poulas and Webster (1991) determined that 112 individuals reported a family history of stuttering. Their data indicate that there appear to be two subgroups within the clinical population of those who develop stuttering. One group is characterized as having a genetically inherited predisposition for stuttering, while the other group appears to have sustained some form of brain insult.

More recent investigations also appear to support a genetic component to stuttering. Yairi, Ambrose, and Cox (1996) evaluated a substantial number of research tools used in familial studies of stuttering. They found that, while epidemiologic factors had likely contaminated earlier results related to the genetics of stuttering, there appears to be evidence, based on incidence and twinning factors, that spontaneous recovery and chronicity are influenced by genetic factors. They also claim that environmental factors cannot be ignored and that an interaction most likely exists.

In a later study Ambrose, Cox, and Yairi (1996) studied 66 children to determine the number of cases of persistent and recovered stuttering when comparing boys with girls. Among their results, they found recovery among girls to be more frequent than among boys. They further determined that, while the persistence and recovery from stuttering was transmitted, recovery did not seem to be a genetically milder form of stuttering nor were the two types genetically independent. They concluded that persistence appears related to additional genetic factors.

While the reader would not be surprised at the confirmation of a male to female ratio of 4:1 or 5:1 in adulthood, the open question remains of what role family environment, cultural factors, and learning processes play in stuttering behavior. Halpern (1997) attempts to address that question in his review of multiple studies, which suggest that males tend to dominate in areas of stuttering, delayed speech, and poorer fine motor skills but also admits to the evidence of a psychobiosocial model based on intelligence and environmental events.

Individual Adaptability to Stress

It is obvious that we have not yet reached that level of understanding that would allow us to determine which specific genetic precursors account for stuttering behavior. Having a genetic blueprint will not be enough, as we will need to determine how environment can activate or inhibit the blueprint to bring about specific behaviors. Farber (1982) cautions us in our use of the term *heritability,* which "refers to the proportion of variance in a group that can be associated with genetic variance." She notes that heritability is a population statistic and tells us nothing about individuals. Therefore, even if we were able to determine that a certain percentage of those who stutter do so because of a genetic predisposition, it still would not mean that, among that population, environmental factors would not be as significant. She notes, "heritability statistics are based on a cross-sectional, nondevelopmental approach and frequently are interpreted as though the actions or genes (or environment) were static and indeed immutable from the moment of conception" (p. 124). We believe that the work of Yairi, Ambrose, and Cox, discussed earlier, attempt to address these very issues raised by Farber.

We are led now to consider, how, given a genetic component, psychogenic and cognitive stress may play a part in activating the stuttering process. Hamilton (1982) defines *cognitive stressors* as "those cognitive events, processes, or operations that exceed a subjective and individualized level of average processing capacity" (p. 109). Using an information processing model, he suggests that we vary in our abilities to process the content to which we are exposed, as well as in the degree to which we utilize, extend, or overload our processing system. As an example, he explains how the ego-threatening content of the word *failure* may be received through the process of hearing and how the individual identifies the auditory features to understand the word. He further notes that short-term memory is the most vulnerable to overload.

Hamilton defines *psychogenic stressors* as "internal stimuli deriving from internal sources of information that is unpleasant, aversive, threatening, or dangerous for the person" (p. 112). He views psychogenic stressors as related to distinctive thought processes a person has about self in relationship to the action of others or to objects, situations, and events in the immediate life space of the individual. Thus, the person described is one who will be most sensitive to attacks on self-esteem, failing to achieve goals, or vulnerable "to situations in which performance may be adversely evaluated, or to any situations that are ambiguous with respect to meaning or personal implications that therefore signal unstable or uncertain events" (p. 113).

Hamilton reasons that psychogenic and cognitive stressors must be considered jointly because anxiety contributes to the information processing system. Similarly, with stuttering behavior, we would infer from Hamilton's research and the research of other cognitive psychologists whom he cites that the child learning language makes interpretations and assigns meaning not only in terms of a developing lexicon but to the environment to which the child is exposed. Adaptability to whatever stressors are present depends on unique constitutional factors, be they biophysiological, a specific diathetic factor, or constitutional predisposition, as originally put forth by Travis (1931).

Related to Hamilton's conceptualizations, Andrews et al. (1983) hypothesize that a central processing inadequacy is inherited. They believe that the development of stuttering depends on a special relationship between sensory-to-motor and motor-to-sensory transformations and on the capacity with which the individual copes with the speech act itself.

A considerable earlier body of research by speech scientists has strongly hinted at a possible relationship between language acquisition and the development of dysfluency in children (Murray and Reed, 1977; Westby, 1979; Stocker and Parker, 1977; Andrews et al., 1983). Among the evidence found have been delay in language development, greater risk of articulation disorders, and poor performance on some language tests. While Halpern's (1997) investigation appears to support this, definitive conclusions are far from being made. What is of interest, however, is that researchers from different disciplines appear to be drawing similar inferences about some relationship between cognitive development and stuttering. How individual adaptability to the stresses placed on the child during early development certainly demands our attention, particularly in our further discussion.

Repressed Needs Models

Most repressed needs models suggest that neurotic behavior is the basis of all stuttering. If we define *neurosis* lexically, it generally means a functional disorder of the mind or emotions involving anxiety, depression, phobia, conflict, or other behavioral symptoms that interfere with the individual's functioning in daily life. Such definition hardly provides any definitive explanation regarding the differentiation of behaviors manifest at varying times in most of us, the stuttering individual, notwithstanding. Moreover, we would have to define what we mean by *abnormal behavior*.

The classic repressed needs model is represented most clearly by the psychoanalytical explanation of Glauber (1958), who sees stuttering as essentially a neurosis in which a basic conflict emerges between satisfaction of the ego and the superego. Stuttering is viewed as a symptom manifestation, represented by anxiety, in which the ego has become fixated in its early childhood state. Representing a neoanalytic viewpoint, Barbara (1954) believes that stuttering resides in the child's inability to resolve inadequate interpersonal relationships. Anxiety is produced by parental pressures and inconsistent rearing practices, creating inappropriate means of coping. Stuttering essentially is a neurosis in which aberrant personality patterns develop as a means of reducing anxiety.

In their survey of the literature exploring the relationship between anxiety and stuttering, Menzies, Onslow, and Packman (1999) conclude that the research has yet to determine that anxiety is systematically related to stuttering. A major difficulty is that our methodological tools are not refined enough to draw a definitive relationship, yet many clinicians more frequently than not assume that anxiety must be addressed with their stuttering clients.

Tkaczenko (1990) sees stuttering as multifaceted and focuses on "organ inferiority" as espoused by the Adlerian school of neo-Freudian psychotherapy. In Adler's view, individuals may use their stuttering as a means of "preserving in fantasy their inflated longings for prestige against wounding encounters with reality, in the sense of what they might have become, if they had not stuttered" (p. 299). Stuttering is seen as a manifestation of a parent-child relationship in which there is conflict brought about in the separation-individuation process related to parenting.

Treon (1995) hypothesizes a bipolar theory that encompasses

> a psychosocial-emotional traumatic deprivation-distortion-conflict-disruption-dysfunction (disorder) emerging from early developmental environmental experiences interacting with innate (genetically determined) emotional temperament-reactivity predisposing tendencies. The other is innate predisposing neurolinguistically based psycholinguistic-prosodic sensorimotor speech dysynergy-dysynchrony possibly interacting with environmentally experienced-induced physical lesion/maldevelopment impairing sensorimotor speech synergy-synchrony emergence. (pp. 35–36)

It appears that Treon has left few stones unturned in reaching for etiologies that would cover virtually all instances of the development of stuttering, and perhaps further research will bear him out.

Given the scarcity of sound empirical investigation, there is little reason to support the contention that stuttering per se is a neurosis, particularly when we reconsider the definition of *neurosis* noted earlier. We prefer to support the contention made by many learning and nonpsychoanalytic theorists that stuttering is a maladaptive behavior brought about, in part at least, by interactional elements occurring in the individual's early childhood. We, of course, would not rule out the possibility that stuttering for some is associated with unresolved deep emotional conflicts and that stuttering itself, again for others, may bring about severe emotional hardship, which in turn could exacerbate the stuttering behavior. We, therefore, need to examine other explanations for its occurrence and development.

Anticipatory Struggle Models

Historically, one of the most popular explanations for the onset of stuttering has been the belief that individuals who stutter interrupt the manner in which they are attempting to speak because they believe they will have difficulty speaking. As a somewhat self-fulfilling prophecy, the anticipation of stuttering creates the stuttering.

This viewpoint is best illustrated by the diagnosogenic theory put forth by Johnson and elaborated by his associates (1959). According to the theory, stuttering is not brought about by what comes from the child's mouth but what is interpreted by the parents' ear. In essence, parents identify their child's normal dysfluencies as stuttering. Evaluated as such, the child tries to speak in a way to satisfy the parents' expectations for more fluent speech. The child responds to parental criticism and anxiety by beginning to speak differently in order to be relieved of the pressures. Bear in mind that the child's perception and response should not be considered conscious behavior but as an attempt by the organism to maintain homeostasis. Support for Johnson's theory has come from years of research, which tends to identify parents of those who stutter as perfectionistic, demanding, or overanxious.

A major criticism with such a generalization is that not all children of such parents develop stuttering. Moreover, self-reports by others who stutter have not always identified such parents nor even such significant others in their early environment. The question also may be asked, Why do most children or adults who have been exposed to the type of parenting just described not stutter?

Bloodstein (1981), in summarizing his own earlier research involving stuttering children, expands the anticipatory struggle hypothesis. He goes beyond mere labeling and believes stuttering to be activated by the child's perception of communicative failure. He suggests that anticipatory struggle reactions develop regardless of either a diagnosis of stuttering or normal dysfluencies in the child's speech. He notes,

> what is first identified as stuttering usually begins as a response of tension and fragmentation in speech, not sharply different from certain types of normal dysfluencies and is brought about largely by the provocation of continued or severe communicative failure in the presence of communicative pressure. (p. 56)

Adams (1990) appears to extend Bloodstein's work with his basic premise that fluency breaks down when environmental or self-imposed demands go beyond the speaker's emotional, cognitive, motoric, or linguistic capacities for responding fluently. Adams clearly indicates, through his model, how a wide variation of stuttering individuals may occur.

Going beyond only communicative pressure, we would suggest that other, often indirect, stressors within the child's environment could well contribute to the onset of stuttering or other maladaptive behaviors. But these we discuss later.

Learning Theory Models

Learning theory models cover a broad range of hypotheses that include formulations based on operant and classical conditioning and approach-avoidance conflict. Although these various theories give little attention to etiology per se, they relate in part to the models discussed earlier. Because thorough descriptions of these models have already been given in depth by others, we take only a cursory view of them here.

Sheehan's Double Approach-Avoidance Theory

Based on Miller's work with rats, in which approach-avoidance conflict was first demonstrated, Sheehan (1953, 1975) applied a similar paradigm to stuttering behavior. In essence, during any specific moment, the individual has a desire to speak and not to speak. Each desire has both negative and positive components that contribute to the conflict. The resulting vacillation is represented in the stuttering phenomenon. Although Sheehan's theory essentially is an attempt to describe the behavioral event of stuttering, it appears to fit the anticipatory struggle theory and repressed needs theory etiologies.

Sheehan views the conflict as occurring on various levels: *the word level*—sounds or words that have unpleasant meanings or are feared; *the situation level*—fear reactions to threatening speech situations; *the emotional level*—conflicts that include guilt, anger, and anxiety about speaking; *the interpersonal level*—anxiety with others, particularly with authority figures; and the *ego-protective level*—avoidance of competitive behaviors, which are viewed as threatening in terms of success or failure.

Two-Factor Theory

Brutten and Shoemaker (1967) represent a more classic conditioning viewpoint in believing that the disruption of speech is precipitated by stresses in particular situations in which the negative emotions aroused are linked to neutral stimuli. Thus, generalization of word and situational fears occurs through a complex series of stimulus-response conditions. As the child is penalized, reminded, or admonished for abnormal speech behavior, the communicative act produces conditioned negative reactions. In time, the child learns to associate words and people with communicative failure.

This theory is described as "two factor" in nature because the means by which the child attempts to cope are instrumentally conditioned. That is, the child attempts to avoid or escape fluency failures and thereby secondary stuttering features are developed. Although these avoidance reactions may lessen the anxiety about speaking, they also are reinforced and therefore maintained. Such operant behaviors, when combined with classical conditioning behaviors, define the process through which stuttering develops and is perpetuated.

Although two-factor theory does not identify any one etiology, it seems to come close to a breakdown hypothesis and it would not necessarily negate neurobiological factors. As Bloodstein (1981) notes, "The development of stuttering is ascribed, not to speech anxiety, but to stress in essentially any form, and constitutional predisposition, in the form of innate conditionability and autonomic reactivity, is considered to play a part" (p. 65).

A Family Systems Theory

The likelihood for stuttering to have a neurobiological or genetic base in conjunction with familial incidence already was noted. Nonetheless, the relationship becomes somewhat obscure when we consider the influence of the family environment. That is, neither a nature nor nurture hypothesis can stand alone, given the present evidence.

Bloodstein (1981), in surveying the literature through 1976, finds support for stuttering to be linked to environmental pressure for conformity and achievement. The exact nature of that relationship is not yet clear, particularly when we try to determine if we are dealing only with parental demands for precision in verbal communication, parental pressure for a standard of behavior beyond the capabilities of the child, or both. In later writings, Bloodstein (1993) describes the widest range of etiological components including labeling, overprotection, brain damage, handedness, among others that yet defy affirmation.

Andrews et al. (1983), based on their research and that of others, find little evidence to support a relationship between personality factors and neuroticism in studies of unselected groups of those who stutter. We, too, maintain that the major issue is not one of preconceived labels of neuroticism, whatever that is, but of identifying behavioral factors that characterize family relationships where stuttering is present. What is important from our viewpoint is that we attempt to understand the complex processes that occur and perhaps instigate and perpetuate stuttering.

Gottwald (1999) suggests, based on her research, that stuttering severity may be related to parent-child differences rather than to parents' absolute rate measures alone. She reports a positive relationship between child stuttering and interruptions by adults. She further identifies studies revealing that, when parents and their children speak simultaneously, stuttering increases. She also indicates that, when turn-taking rules are applied to reduce the threat of interruptions by adults, fluency is enhanced.

It seems appropriate, therefore, for us to consider the role of family within the context of how families operate as a system, given the data already gathered. In so doing, we hold to the proposition stated by Van Riper (1971) that "the greater the stress, the more likely it is that the sequencing of speech will be disrupted at a more basic level of integration" (p. 424).

Family Functioning: A Review of Major Concepts

Although many theories of family functioning have developed over the last 40 years, it is possible to identify the themes common to most of them:

1. *The presence of symptoms to characterize family conflict.* Dysfunctional behavioral patterns may

be manifest in one family member, an indication that the growth of family members in general is being thwarted. Whereas symptoms may be present in all, usually one member becomes a scapegoat. This implies a breakdown in the ability of family to share feelings and work out solutions to family problems. Despite the overt distress caused, the symptoms serve to maintain the status quo or homeostasis of the family.

2. *Homeostasis as a process that maintains family equilibrium through interaction.* Diadic or triadic interactions represent the various interpersonal and intrapersonal processes that characterize families. Each family has its own rules, which imply how each member must function for the entire family to function and survive. This adaptational process, while covertly maintaining family equilibrium or stability, actually contributes to family dysfunction. Therefore, any therapeutic attempts to modify family interaction or symptomatic behavior are frequently met with considerable resistance. Only the more functional family is likely to change its rules to satisfy the changes and needs of various family members.

3. *Family strengths and weaknesses.* Every family has tendencies to reinforce either wellness or emotional sickness, depending on the unique characteristics of the family as a whole or of one or more family members. Also implied is the ability or inability for one or more members to tolerate and cope with the strength and weaknesses of other family members. Therefore, in some families, it may be difficult for one family member to be well unless another is sick.

4. *Family communication.* The way family members communicate with each other reflects the underlying system by which the family functions. In functional families, relationships and attitudes are characterized by congruence, clarity of communication, mutual respect, love and trust, support, and encouragement. In dysfunctional families, while some aspects of these traits may be present, family communication is characterized more frequently by incongruence, distortion of meaning, projection, and conflicts that get expressed through disagreements oftentimes regarding innocuous situational events.

5. *The marital relationship.* The nature and quality of the marital relationship are prime determinants of children's behavior. Concealed or unresolved marital conflict not only influences the entire family system but may also get expressed by acting-out behavior of other family members. Such conflict also instigates projection by one or both marital partners on other family members as well. Conversely, a functional marital relationship is characterized by mutual caring and acceptance, where marital conflict gets resolved through a dynamic give and take process that appropriately excludes the children. Parental decisions regarding the children are made as a team.

Unfortunately, a sizeable number of speech-language pathologists have altered their attitudes regarding the influence of parents on fluency, according to Cooper and Cooper (1996) in their study of the opinions of 1198 speech-language pathologists, over a period of time between 1983 and 1991. The latter sample appears to reject parental causality, but apparently those interviewed did not consider the more subtle and sometimes not so subtle aspects of interaction and indirect influence such as the factors discussed earlier. The authors appear to suggest that, perhaps, a naivete exists among speech-language pathologists and there is a need to develop a cadre of specialized fluency experts in our field.

It is important to indicate that no single concept stands apart from any other; the various structures and processes overlap. Family events are multidetermined, and the configuration of the various structures and processes will determine the degree to which family dysfunction may occur. Schulze and Johannsen (1991) believe that stuttering takes place within the framework of intrafamily styles of communication and interaction. They review and outline the psychosocial and interactional variables associated with family lifestyle variables and family structure. Their perspective, while not discussed within the context of family systems per se, nonetheless is consistent with the paradigm as we see it.

Stuttering as an Identified Symptom

Our discussion of disturbed behavior and the dysfunctional family has referred to behavior and internal events considered distressing by one or more members of a family. Such distress may lead to the unwitting selection of one individual to become the disturbed "identified patient." This individual, sometimes the child, becomes a scapegoat who symbolizes the interfamily conflict. The child becomes part of a process in which attention is directed away from the underlying family conflict or other family members. We are not suggesting this is a conscious decision made by any family member, but it does imply the active involvement by all in which the child gets parental attention in any way possible. The child's response represents a homeostatic means of coping with perhaps an intolerable or distressful series of family events.

We contend that stuttering in a child may be a behavioral manifestation produced by family tensions, particularly between parents, that have not been resolved through other means. This is not to imply that the child, or for that matter the parents, necessarily is emotionally disturbed; simply that, on a continuum of emotional functioning, this particular family is functioning in the only way it thinks and knows possible, albeit dysfunctionally.

It could certainly be argued, as Andrews et al. (1983) have pointed out with regard to childhood stuttering, that "no differences in personality factors related to neuroticism have been demonstrated in control studies of unselected populations" (p. 229). Yet, we would question Andrew's implied assumption that these studies meet his criteria for "Class A facts—findings replicated in two or more research centers, there being no negative reports" (p. 226). (The reader is referred to Wingate, 1983, for an extensive and provocative discussion on the Andrews et al. paper). We do not consider the use of various personality scales reported to represent exact replications. We would further argue that the scales referred to may not necessarily measure the complex interfamilial dynamics to which we have been referring.

We hypothesize that stuttering in childhood is a complex process involving predetermined neurobiophysiological factors associated with interfamilial stress that becomes identified in the child through the disruption of communicative behavior. Although a comprehensive search of the literature in family systems theory and therapy has failed to contain any discussion or documentation of stuttering, we believe it is useful to explore the role that family environment may play in its development. In doing so, we do not presume to have discovered the multicausal answer but are merely raising several dynamic issues that we believe have relevance.

The Scapegoat and Tolerance to Pressure

We already suggested that using a child as a scapegoat may be responsible for managing roots of family tension. This may lead to disturbing secondary complications.

Let us assume that, in Family A, the 3-year-old child is showing signs of dysfluent behavior, sometimes typical in young children. Let us further assume that the parents do not appear to be particularly upset with such behavior or may ignore it, but they are wrapped up in personal, financial tensions or minimal conflict in their relationship. (Thus far, we are describing a not untypical set of circumstances in our society of the 1990s.)

Broadening this scenario, the child, as part of the family system, begins to reflect the tension or conflict with increased dysfluency and possibly other behaviors including shame, embarrassment, anxiety, and withdrawal. The focus now turns to the child, who is overtly manifesting unresolved and perhaps undiscussed parental tensions. As the parents' concern now is directed toward the child, their anxieties about themselves diminish (for the moment, anyway) and become symbolized in the child. The parents also bring into play projections emanating from their own past (regardless of a family history of stuttering or not).

As the child's dysfluency or other behavioral changes increase in severity, the parents' attitudes also change in the form of overprotection, disapproval, demands for fluency perfection, or denial in the form of "suffering in silence." What is particularly important for us to understand is that the parental attention may not be necessarily directed at the increased dysfluency per se but at the overall manifest changes in the child's behavior. Superficially, at least, this parental reaction appears to conform to Johnson's diagnosogenic theory, but not really. In the family systems theory we propose, labeling is considered only one of several possibilities.

Regardless of the nature of the parental concern, the child's tolerance to the internal or external pressure now being experienced depends on his or her own combined neurobiological predisposition and adventitiously developed capabilities. The child's coping behavior therefore is seen as an individualized and complex set of dynamic factors that may explain the many multicausal and multimodal theories in the literature reviewed earlier.

Theory notwithstanding, it is not difficult to understand how the hypothetical child's fluency development we have described may develop into the full dimension we recognize as stuttering. But we must be cautious not to presume a simple cause-effect relationship either in terms of etiological theory or developing a pattern of stuttering in the family. We hope to make evident that the family interactional process dominates and that changes of behavior are contiguous to all family members. Finally, we must consider not only the influences of an extended family and family of origin but also the possible effects of other external environmental conditions, such as loss of family income, serious physical illness of another family member, or death of a grandparent.

Stuttering and Personality

Regardless of etiological theory, most workers in the field would agree that varying combinations of dynamic factors in the environment, as the stuttering child develops, contribute generally to some difficulties in emotional adjustment. As Bloodstein (1981), following a comprehensive review of the literature, has pointed out, however, there seems to be no definitive character structure or fundamental personality traits characterizing stuttering individuals. Yet, he further reports, based on studies carried out for several years at the University of Iowa, parents of stuttering individuals tend to exhibit certain parental traits and attitudes that could contribute to the stuttering.

The Continuing Influence of the Family

We stated earlier that family relationships must be considered when attempting to understand how stuttering may be perpetuated in the young child. We also indicated that the contiguity of these dynamics can be understood without the assignment of "sick" labels to either the child or the parents. We do postulate, however, that *stuttering families* can be differentiated from *nonstuttering families* on the basis of unique family systems processes, irrespective of psychopathology per se. That is, stuttering families constitute a special and often unique combination of circumstances, reaction, conditions, behaviors, and personalities from which stuttering has evolved. In some cases, stuttering occurs as a primary instigator for effecting changes in family dynamics, whereas in others, stuttering manifests as one possible response to family conflict.

It helps to acknowledge, however, that there are probably many families from which stuttering does not emerge regardless of all the dynamics for its development to be present. We offer no explanation for this except that one or more undetermined extenuating factors differentiate these families from those in which stuttering is generated. Nevertheless, it is possible to explore how the self-image of a stuttering or "identified" child can be molded and the stuttering pattern perpetuated.

The Molding of Self-Image and Perpetuation of the Stuttering Pattern

As we consider the molding of self-image in the stuttering individual, we are clear that we refer not to a unique "stuttering personality" but to a special way in which the person perceives him- or herself.

Referring back to hypothetical Family A, we found that the identified child became more and more frustrated in the ability to communicate. The parents, in turn, responded to the best of their ability by "helping" the child. This does not mean that all their concerns are directed at the child or even that aspects of the child's development are ignored. Certainly, life continues on for the parents, including coping with their own relationship, and so the child continues on, too. Unfortunately, the child may begin to develop secondary stuttering features that are readily explained by Brutten and Shoemaker (1967).

More significant, though, is that, while the child is in the process of formulating a self-image, the stuttering becomes an inherent part of that development. How much depends on the nature, quality, and kind of family influences.

Although the empirical literature surveyed by Bloodstein (1981) and later by Ratner and Healey (1999) cannot confirm a negative self-image that is distinctive to those who stutter, few therapists would deny that the stuttering individual in time develops feelings of frustration, guilt, shame, embarrassment, rejection, and self-doubt while attempting to communicate. That the reactions of others contribute to these feelings and attitudes readily are self-evident.

We should not assume that the child we describe in Family A is condemned to a life of stuttering that precludes the positive development of other aspects of the personality and the self, despite the nature and quality of parental reaction or involvement. After all, most of us do survive to varying degrees the effects our parents' struggles have on us. It is no different for the child who stutters and who also typically grows to be a functioning adult. Little wonder that some find profound meaning in their stuttering behavior to lead them toward a professional life dedicated to solving the stuttering riddle.

What cannot be ignored, however, are the negative features of the child's communicative behavior that shape the perception that child has of self. Our clinical experiences with stuttering children and adults tell us of the domination stuttering has over all else in terms of how those who stutter see themselves and what they can or cannot accomplish in life.

Considering the child in Family A, it is important to recognize that, although early and later stuttering behavior may distract the parents from their own struggles, a homeostatic state of affairs is accomplished, at least temporarily. In time this too changes, and the child may soon cease to change the family status quo. But, even if the parents direct their attention to other matters, like the birth of another child or even their denial that a problem exists, the stuttering process nevertheless has taken hold, and, depending on the child or the nature and quality of continued family interaction, the stuttering pattern is set and a distinctive self-image established.

It is unsurprising that workers in our field find such wide variations among children and adults who stutter. We contend, however, that the abrupt cessation of stuttering or the presence of varying degrees of psychopathology can be explained by the distinctive and dynamic system that characterizes the family in which stuttering occurs and by the unique constitution and overall development of the stuttering individual. Little wonder that the vast number of experimental studies have failed to establish many definitive commonalities among those who stutter or in stuttering families, because the boundaries of homogeneous groupings are yet unclear.

Late Onset of Stuttering

While the late onset of stuttering may occur in adolescence and adulthood, its incidence is so rare as to have received little attention in the literature. Defares (1991) sees it as a part of a stress response syndrome related to specific intrapsychic preconditions and associated with trait anxiety levels. Mahr and Leith (1992), in an anecdotal analysis of four adult cases of late onset of stuttering, classify it psychogenically as a conversion reaction and describe characteristic features of the condition. Duffy and Baumgartner (1997) examined 49 adults without neurologic disease, who developed stutteringlike dysfluncies attributable to psychological factors. They found a conversion reaction, anxiety, or hysterical neurosis to be the most frequent psychiatric diagnosis. In the same study, Duffy and Baumgartner also examined 20 people with late onset of stuttering associated with neurologic disease, closed head injury, and seizure disorder and found evidence of a conversion reaction in this group as well.

The few studies available wisely refrain from generalizing their results to developed stuttering in children and avoid any explanation of a possible "sleeping beauty syndrome."

A Cognitive Learning Theory Explanation

Thus far, we have used family systems theory to explain partly the development and perpetuation of the stuttering pattern through childhood and how a stuttering self-image is shaped. We also offered several learning theory explanations that could account for the development of the phenomenon. That stuttering often continues through childhood and into adulthood could be explained readily by its self-reinforcement and reinforcement from external sources, including parental influence.

We have strongly hinted that stuttering behavior is not only an emotional process but a cognitive one as well, supported in part by diagnosogenic theory interpretations. It is possible to pursue this line of reasoning through the work of Ellis and his rational-emotive theory.

In Chapter 1, we described Ellis's theory, which contends that personality is characterized by the development of constructs, beliefs, or attitudes that are included in childhood and maintained through adult life, "and that absolutistic, perfectionistic values tend to make you feel emotionally disturbed" (Ellis 1976, p. 22). These beliefs, which he describes as irrational, are learned through a cognitive mediating process not unlike that described by Johnson, who like Ellis expands on the original semantic concepts of Korzybski (1933). Although Ellis focuses mainly on therapeutic change rather than on etiological theory or cognitive processing, we readily could apply his constructs to the development of stuttering behavior and a stuttering self-image within the context of family systems theory.

As the recipient and expression of parental conflicts and concerns, the dysfluent child soon begins to perceive himself or herself as different. Because of all the negative connotations associated with disruptive communication, feeling and believing oneself as different takes on the meaning of being worse than others. Should the parent or parents, regardless of their own relationship, have perfectionistic attitudes themselves, these are projected readily onto the child. In fact, the child's speech may not even be the issue—but merely perfectionistic expectations in general. If we also include a constitutional predisposition toward a yet undefined articulatory short-circuiting, the situation is exacerbated. Consequently, the child's developing self-image is defined in terms of "stutterer." All other aspects of the developing value system are perceived in the light of the stuttering self-image.

Should the child have the good fortune to be exposed to more positive, rational, or empirically based values, because of either changing or more positive perceptions by the parents or changes in their value system, there is a greater likelihood for the cessation of the stuttering and the enhancement of a more positive self-image. If, on the other hand, the former circumstances continue into adolescence and adulthood, the earlier irrational value system and the stuttering behavior become fixed, with or without the influence of the nuclear family. The adult then persistently perceives him- or herself in terms of "being a stutterer" and acts in other ways that individual has learned to associate with stuttering. Thus, it becomes an irrational excuse for acting remote with others, being unable to apply for a desired job, or feeling less worthy than those who do not stutter. Paradoxically, the person appears to others to be functioning adequately and in fact often does, except for that ongoing self-defeating perception. The reality is that the individual prevents himself or herself from fulfilling the personal potential that may actually exist.

While the reader may differ with the preceding explanation, arguing "look at all the stutterers who've become successful actors, singers, business executives," the author would agree that individuals, regardless of any anomaly, are able to transcend it and lead very productive lives, stuttering notwithstanding.

Therapeutic Intervention

Most workers in the field would agree that, as a result of the many experimental investigations and individual empirical case findings, no one therapeutic strategy has surfaced that could be identified as the answer to the total elimination of stuttering. In fact, it would appear that some investigations have more likely served to satisfy the individual bias of the investigator who hides behind statistical design manipulations to justify a presumably objective position and for whom a self-fulfilling prophecy is achieved. Certainly, we do not infer that all scientific studies related to stuttering should be attacked but merely that all studies must be evaluated and analyzed with greater scrutiny, with cautious avoidance of conclusive generalizations, and with less display of minutia that have little real meaning. Too often so-called objective investigations have been the subtle manifestations of deeply felt or unconscious subjective personal attitudes.

Review of Current Strategies

Although we will not discuss at length the various treatment strategies that have evolved over the last several decades, it nonetheless is useful to review the major ones before we consider the one most pertinent to the theoretical position taken in this chapter.

In an interesting study using a meta-analysis of the effects of various stuttering strategies, Andrews, Guitar, and Howie (1980) designated prolonged speech, gentle onset, airflow, and attitude techniques as the four major prevailing strategies. We have difficulty in clearly differentiating among them because ancillary treatments were included among them and seem to contaminate the attempted distinctions. A further difficulty is that Andrews et al. (1983), in a later study, refer to *five* major treatments designated in the earlier study, including precision fluency among them. Curiously, precision fluency shaping is not mentioned in the earlier study. Finally, we are troubled by the term *attitude therapy*, which in the earlier study was used to designate 12% of the studies analyzed. In their 1983 study, Andrews et al. continue to use the term, which Wingate (1983) criticizes for its vagueness.

Because of these apparent inconsistencies and the lumping together of "apples and oranges," we prefer to designate the major treatment modalities as symptom modification, fluency enhancement, and person-centered psychotherapy, for the purposes of discussion. It should be understood that, in doing so, we recognize that considerable overlap of strategies has occurred over the last 15 years, as revealed in the literature and by clinician reporting.

Symptom Modification

By *symptom modification*, we mean the reduction, alteration, or elimination of the secondary or accessory characteristics commonly associated with escape from stuttering. Among the classic strategies used have been chewing, pullouts, cancellation, gentle onset, bouncing, shadowing, prolongation, negative

practice, relaxation, rhythmic speaking, medication, hypnosis, easy stuttering, controlled airflow, and counseling associated with use of these techniques.

An inherent feature of symptom modification programs is the notion that stuttering can be controlled and that the individual is expected to live with the problem. Normally, the degree to which the person is expected to eliminate all aspects of dysfluency depends on the personal orientation of the therapist, the attitude and disposition of the client, and the nature of the therapeutic relationship.

Fluency Enhancement

We define *fluency enhancement* not so much as the reduction of stuttering behavior but as the emphasis on achieving completely fluent speech. No attempt is made to manage dysfluent speech; rather, the effort is to encourage and develop the fluent speech of which the individual is capable. The various strategies used include delayed auditory feedback, fluency shaping, cognitive retraining, systematic desensitization, medication, counseling, prolongation of sounds, token rewards, and syllable timed speech. An implied assumption of fluency enhancement therapy is that increased fluency also helps develop a more positive self-image as a nonstuttering individual, which will enhance the maintenance of fluency.

Person-Centered Psychotherapy

Person-centered psychotherapy, as we generally define it, is a process whereby a person-therapist relationship is established in which the client's inherent potential for change and growth is activated. The major assumption is that the client is responsible for his or her own destiny and has the right of choice and the ability to solve problems. Characteristic is that the client with the aid of the therapist develops personal strategies that will be personally productive. Among the methods used include family therapy, nondirective counseling, cognitive emotional counseling, transactional analysis, neopsychoanalysis, systematic desensitization, and assertiveness training. Typically, person-centered psychotherapy may include the use of combined counseling strategies, with or without symptom modification and fluency enhancement approaches.

Stuttering in Children

Consistent with the cognitive-emotional and family systems theories approach discussed earlier, with respect to etiology and the development of dysflent speech patterns, we propose a combined application with stuttering children in general. We are not convinced, however, that only a cognitive-emotional, family systems, or a combined approach is applicable to all these children. Unique family circumstances or special needs of the child would guide any creative method of choice, including the child's own expressed, even sophisticated, strategy.

Ackerman (1966), an early leader in the development of family therapy, presents a useful model that is summarized with regard to the therapist's function:

1. The therapist formulates a new network among family members, including the therapist, in which rapport, empathy, and communication play a major part.
2. Through rapport, the therapist clarifies and focuses on the major conflicts and coping behavior of family members. Through removing obstacles, disguised defenses, disagreements, and disorganized modes of thinking and behavior, the therapist attempts to clarify the conflict. Family members learn, by stages, what has been misunderstood and what the real problem is.
3. Defensive attempts by the family to deny, rationalize, and displace conflict are revealed by the therapist, ideally with affirmation by one or more members.
4. Hidden and inert interpersonal conflicts are transformed into open interactional communication.
5. Intrapersonal conflict is raised to the level of interpersonal communication.
6. The use of a scapegoat, which strengthens one segment of the family while weakening another, is neutralized.
7. Playing, in part, the role of a real parent figure, the therapist provides elements that the family

lacks but needs and the basis for emotional support.
8. Emphasizing confrontation, and to a lesser extent interpretation, the therapist penetrates and defines areas of resistance and lessens the intensity of anxieties, guilt, and conflict.
9. The therapist becomes the major figure by which the family tests reality.
10. The therapist serves as a teacher and exemplifies an ideal model, reflecting healthy family functioning.

One "Stuttering Family"

We counseled a family in which the major complaint was the "stuttering of our 12-year-old child." The family consisted of the father, Bill, a clinical psychologist; Diane, the mother, a clinical social worker; Andy, the stuttering child; and his 10-year-old brother, Dan, who had no apparent problems. Frustrated by several years of unsuccessful remediation efforts, the parental concern was that "Andy's stuttering is getting worse."

The initial interview with Andy alone confirmed a clinical picture of secondary stuttering characterized by intermittent hesitations, repetitions, and blocks with associated eye blinking and body twitching. Although Andy's pattern was severe during the loci of stuttering, he tended to be fluent approximately 80% of the time during the course of our interview. His own chief complaint was the stuttering and his inability to get along with his younger brother. He otherwise appeared to be a bright, congenial, and sensitive young person.

In a meeting of the entire family, it was immediately evident that the focus of attention was on Andy and "his problem." Bill monopolized much of the early part of the session with professional and clinical explanations of Andy's stuttering while demanding to know which therapeutic approach was to be used. He suggested that a Wolpean approach (systematic desensitization) be used (see Wolpe, 1958). It was readily apparent that Bill was unwittingly sabotaging any attempt to get at the dynamics underlying the process by which the family functioned while proving his intellectual prowess and competing with the therapist.

Any gaps in verbal communication were filled in by Diane, who declared that "there's nothing wrong with this family" and also apparently was unaware of the dynamics of family therapy. As the therapist, I was beginning to feel overwhelmed by the degree of intellectualization, rationalization, and resistance to further probing and shared these feelings with them. Although this acknowledgment was met with further resistance, their defensiveness soon dissipated as I attempted to explain what was happening.

It was further apparent that Bill, Diane, and Dan were a coalition fending off Andy and his stuttering, but no attempt was made at the time to confront them with that reality, for fear of arousing further resistance and perhaps enmity toward me. Their own fragile family network, and my lack of rapport with them, also dictated otherwise.

To counteract what I believed to be a deteriorating clinical relationship, information about the onset and perpetuation of stuttering behavior was presented. Although Bill continued to try to impress me with his knowledge and expertise, he appeared willing to listen to what I had to say about the nature of stuttering.

It should be noted that Andy's intermmitant participation and sharing of his feelings about stuttering were characterized by nearly flawless speech. Dan was less verbal and responded to me with minimal language. Virtually no verbal interaction took place between Dan and Andy.

Toward the close of the session, I was convinced that Bill or Diane would be unwilling to continue in family therapy, particularly when Bill asked what I was going to do for Andy. When we scheduled our next appointment, both Bill and Diane appeared generally impassive. Nevertheless, the entire family surprised me with their arrival at the session the following week.

Apparently, Bill and Diane felt they had benefited from the previous session and were delighted with Andy's fluency then and increased fluency during the interim. Despite their more positive attitude about participating further in family therapy, Bill and Diane continued to erect psychological barriers to my inclusion in the family network. Only Andy and Dan appeared willing to accept my participation, with their own sharing of family interactions at home. This included Dan's expressed resentment toward his parents' preoccupation with Andy and his stuttering, and Andy's feeling that the

only real attention he received from his parents was in relation to his stuttering.

These disclosures were met by defensive protestations from Bill and Diane, who declared their nonpartiality in relating to Andy and Dan. Moreover, Bill tried to impress me further with his academic and professional knowledge while still maintaining it would be best for Andy to have individual speech therapy from me. Throughout the session it was apparent that Andy's fluency was directly related to the degree of parental concealment of feelings. That is, the more Bill and Diane attempted to conceal by intellectualizing, the more dysfluent Andy became; and the more feelings they shared (which was minimal), the more fluent he became, with an associated reduction in his secondary features. When this was pointed out to his parents, it was difficult for them to take even partial responsibility.

I was not surprised when the next three family therapy appointments were canceled immediately prior to their scheduled times, and I believed I had seen the last of the family (particularly as none of the therapy fees had yet been paid). When they arrived, on time, for their sixth scheduled appointment, I said I was surprised. Despite defensive excuses for their therapy cancellations, Bill finally acknowledged that all had not been well in the family. The veil of denial began to be lifted.

He then began to express his concerns about what he described as his "mid-life crisis" and boredom with his apparently successful private clinical practice. My own self-disclosure of similar feelings and experiences drew him out further with his acknowledgment of intermittent difficulties in the marital relationship. This triggered Diane's disclosure of similar feelings about their marriage and her personal struggles with trying to be a successful wife, mother, and career woman.

Andy and Dan, obviously moved by their parents' private troubles, immediately moved to comfort them, with a pouring forth of tearful emotions by all. It was immediately evident that this was the caring, loving, and sensitive family I had originally hypothesized and psycho-pathology was not evident per se. That it had been struggling to sustain itself and survive the turbulence of modern-day life did not appear to me to be extraordinary. That the stuttering was an expression, partly at least, of the inter- and intrapersonal conflicts also seemed consistent with the reality of the family struggles.

We are not suggesting that these struggles or Andy's stuttering immediately ceased with the revelations made during the session. However, by the 16th session Andy's stuttering had virtually disappeared, his relationship with Dan had improved significantly, and although Bill and Diane continued to grapple with their own personal needs, they were able to give one another the support each needed.

At the 16th session, the family decided to terminate therapy with the understanding that a follow-up session six months hence would be arranged. Several days before this prearranged session, Andy called to inform me of the family's decision to cancel their appointment. Totally fluent, he told me his speech was "fine" and that things were going well. I wished him and his family well and did not contact them again until one year later.

In speaking with Diane by telephone, I learned that Andy's speech was essentially fluent, and although things were not always smooth for her and Bill, they had been in individual psychotherapy for the previous four months and were "learning much." The proverbial icing on the cake for me personally was the information that Andy had made a successful speech for his bar mitzvah.

What is implied from this description of a "stuttering" family is that stuttering in the family is not necessarily rooted in psychopathology, nor is it only an individual problem but a family one as well. That it is a problem involving unique and dynamic familial interrelationship processes is more likely. It should further be understood that family therapy is not a panacea for treatment even of those children who stutter mildly or moderately.

Although we have had success in treating several other "stuttering families," some have been unresponsive to a family systems approach or even counseling. Certainly, one might argue that such families are unresponsive because of deep-seated psychopathology or denial. We tend to believe, rather, that the unique processes and complex inter- and intrapersonal relationships may dictate failure or success in a family therapy approach.

Finally, we must admit that childhood stuttering may indeed have roots unrelated to family functioning.

An Individual Counseling Approach

The decision to forgo family therapy for individual counseling would be determined by consideration of the following criteria: (1) a severe degree of secondary stuttering characteristics, (2) presence of family or individual psychopathology, (3) no apparent family dysfunction, (4) confirmed or established self-image as a "stutterer," and (5) refusal by the family to be involved in family therapy.

Individual counseling for young children takes many shapes and forms and to describe them would go beyond the scope of this book. It would be most appropriate, however, to discuss a few within the context of the theories described elsewhere in the book and in particular as they might apply to the stuttering child.

Based on the criteria just listed, it is immediately obvious that the therapist is presented with a challenge more formidable than that in the case of Andy. Not only might family resistance be more pronounced, the factors perpetuate the stuttering behavior, especially the confirmed self-image problem.

Nondirective Person-Centered Counseling

Charles Van Riper (No.18), in a concise and provocative essay, describes vividly how the therapist can enter the life space of the stuttering child to understand exactly what the child is experiencing and feeling. Using nonverbal monitoring, Van Riper makes a strong case for its use over typical verbal mirroring with stuttering children who may feel too threatened by verbal interaction. Although the therapeutic outcome is not discussed, the process allows the child and the therapist to experience together all the hidden fears and avoidances associated with the child's unique stuttering pattern.

We believe that this working-through process also can be facilitated with verbal mirroring as long as the therapist is sensitive to the child's terror in communicating verbally. It is possible to integrate both verbal and nonverbal mirroring or reflection within the context of play therapy, which we do not view as a separate and distinct form of treatment. In very young children, play is more likely to be the chief medium of communication. Here again, the major determining therapeutic factor is the client-therapist relationship, through which the shame, guilt, anxiety, preoccupation, and low self-esteem associated with the stuttering behavior can be resolved.

At this point, it is appropriate to recall the classic basic principles of play therapy first described by Axline (1969):

1. The therapist must develop a warm, friendly relationship with the child, in which rapport is established as soon as possible.
2. The therapist accepts the child exactly as he is.
3. The therapist establishes a feeling of permissiveness in the relationship so that the child feels free to express his feelings completely.
4. The therapist is alert to recognizing the "feelings" the child is expressing and reflects those feelings back to him in such a manner that he gains insight into his behavior.
5. The therapist maintains a deep respect for the child's ability to solve his own problems if given an opportunity to do so. The responsibility to make choices and to institute change is the child's.
6. The therapist does not attempt to direct the child's actions or conversation in any manner. The child leads the way; the therapist follows.
7. The therapist does not attempt to hurry the therapy along. It is a gradual process and is recognized as such by the therapist.
8. The therapist establishes only those limitations that are necessary to anchor the therapy to the world of reality and to make the child aware of his responsibility in the relationship. (pp. 73–74)

Cangelosi and Schaefer (1996) and Norton and Norton (1997) describe both classical and innovative techniques in play therapy along with practical techniques even for beginning play therapists. We need to be mindful, though, that play therapy in and of itself will not necessarily be productive in the modification or elimination of the stuttering pattern and the enhancement of a nonstuttering self-image. It is likely to be effective with the young child who is either unaware of these mild dysfluencies or in families where one or both parents are obsessed with them.

The decision to use traditional play therapy, a modified verbal and nonverbal person-centered approach, or a nonplay face-to-face interactional approach certainly is determined by the age, intelligence, emotional attitude, and maturity of the child, as well as by the severity, nature, and degree of the stuttering. Further, the wise therapist must be acutely aware of the role other members of the family play, although not directly involved in the ther-apy, during the course of therapeutic intervention. Of particular importance to the therapist is the possibility that one or several family members may be deliberately or unwittingly sabotaging the therapeutic effort, which brings us to the issue of parent counseling.

Parent Counseling

Parent counseling has long been a preferred strategy used in conjunction with traditional or interpersonal approaches with stuttering children. Bloodstein (1981) includes several important aspects regarding the efficacy of parent counseling in the treatment of early childhood stuttering. Among various major admonitions to parents typically are (1) encouraging them "to refrain from reacting negatively to the speech difficulties in any way, and to see to it as far as possible that the speech interruptions are not brought to the child's attention by others" (p. 353); (2) attempting to improve the parent-child relationship; and (3) helping parents to eliminate those conditions or factors that exacerbate the stuttering behaviors, such as unrealistically high levels of aspiration.

Bloodstein cites the use of desensitization therapy as described by Van Riper (1972) as a means of assisting the child to cope better with environmental pressures at home, which presumably would be more effective when the therapist is unable to counsel the family directly. Egolf et al. (1972) involved parents directly in the therapy process in attempting to teach them a different, more positive way of dealing with their dysfluent children. Ratner (1992) provided mothers of normally fluent children instructions to slow maternal speech rate or to slow and simplify maternal speech and found that their children's speech rate and language complexity did not match maternal adjustments. While Ratner generalizes her findings to those of parents and their children who stutter, questioning the use of parent counseling as part of a regimen of indirect therapy, we would question the premise made by Ratner.

We believe that traditional parent counseling, whether used independently or in conjunction with speech therapy for the child, is most likely to be, more or less, an information-giving process that would provide us some knowledge of the dynamic relationship between parents and child. It might even, at best, give parents something different to consider regarding their communicative interaction with the child. Also, it might alleviate the guilt some parents feel regarding their role in the onset and perpetuation of their child's stuttering by not blaming them. More important, these parents need to be assisted in the understanding that the cause of the stuttering is less relevant than the role they can play as agents of change for the overall well-being of the child with the possibility also that the stuttering will diminish or vanish.

Unfortunately, much of what we suggest is difficult to accomplish in the school setting. Even with the advent of PL94-42, there has not been the full commitment of involving parents more frequently in the rehabilitative process, much less the educational one. Too often, the parents of stuttering children who need to be involved most in their therapy are the ones most resistant to participating. Also, school policy may not permit therapists more time to spend with parents unless seen by the therapist on their own time. Until the helping and educational professions together formulate a more definitive philosophy regarding the participation of the family in the child's overall education, we will continue to employ what could be considered a piecemeal approach to the child's emotional, cognitive, intellectual, and communicative growth. Unfortunately, except for isolated school districts and charter schools, our education system nationwide does not appear motivated to initiate such a drastic departure from traditional policies and practices.

Onslow and Packman (1999) describe a program (the Lidcombe Program) developed in Sydney, Australia, which focuses on providing behaviorally based speech therapy to preschool stuttering children integrated with a training program for their parents as well, to remove environmental stressors. While the reported results clearly indicate a significant improvement in the fluency of the children in the program, the effects of the parental involvement and the real changes in the parental environment are unclear. While Onslow and Packman doubt the effectiveness of the program due to environmental stressors, we suggest that a more empirically based family systems assessment would provide more definitive evidence.

Stuttering in the Older Child and the Adult

The criteria we established for our decision to counsel young children could apply to older children, adolescents, and adults, but obviously older stuttering children and adults do not share all the features characteristic of their respective problems or for that matter of their personalities and needs. In examining these differences, it is readily apparent that the older child (1) still lives at home, (2) is still in the process of self-image formulation, (3) is still involved in all of the circumstances and problems associated with prepubescent or pubescent behavior, (4) is limited in making life-affecting decisions, and (5) is still in the process of shaping an overall and distinctive personality pattern.

The adult, typically, (1) is likely to be functioning independently and no longer at home;[1] (2) has a firmly established self-image; (3) is coping with problems of school, career, or vocation, interpersonal relationships with other men and women; (4) is free to make life-affecting decisions; and (5) has an essentially fixed personality pattern.

Despite the differences enumerated, we can formulate an eclectic counseling approach suitable for either population and yet specialized to meet the needs of the stuttering individual.

Cognitive Stuttering Therapy

A rationale for stuttering therapy based on the requirement that stuttering individuals learn to accept responsibility for their communicative behavior was introduced by Rubin and Culatta (1971) and developed further by Culatta and Rubin (1973). Among the major principles initially proposed, they note that (1) speech therapy should be cognitive and direct without regard to time or symptom; (2) those who stutter must acknowledge their ability to be fluent at least some of the time and that they have the ability to be fluent all of the time; (3) individuals can have control over their dysfluency and fluency; (4) stuttering is viewed as an offensive

---

[1]In the present day United States, this is not necessarily the case, as economic conditions have frequently dictated otherwise. This obviously presents issues we discuss later.

and unpleasant behavior by most listeners and particularly the therapist, who must not conceal this attitude; (5) stuttering is self-reinforcing and provides a payoff to the individual, which must be managed in therapy; and (6) individuals misevaluate their ability to be fluent on the abstract as well as the concrete levels and are given direction to change this concept.

Culatta and Rubin have enumerated 11 principles that underscore their therapeutic approach. They are summarized in the sequential order in which they must be mastered: (1) communicating verbal content in terms of fluency and not dysfluency, (2) belief in the physical ability to be fluent, (3) self-acknowledgment of responsibility of the fluency previously achieved, (4) self-acknowledgment of the individual's own reason for stuttering and objectifying it, (5) recognition that it is valid to question reasons for dysfluency and evaluate the stuttering objectively, (6) assuming direct responsibility for fluency achieved during therapy, (7) consciously manipulating fluency, (8) predicting the nature of speech subsequent to either fluent or nonfluent speech to demonstrate control, (9) demonstration of control over dysfluency and fluency on request, (10) lengthening fluent and shortening dysfluent responses, and (11) consciously controlling fluency and dysfluency over longer periods of time.

The program developed by Culatta and Rubin appears to have a direct relationship to the cognitive-behavioral approach of Ellis, which we thoroughly discuss in Chapter 1 (Ellis et al., 1997). Although Ellis focuses on emotional disturbance, which we do not believe applies to most who stutter, his theory nonetheless is relevant with regard to stuttering behavior in general. As stated in the Preface to one of his many writings,

> people largely control their own destinies by believing in and acting on the values or beliefs that they hold. . . . People do not directly react emotionally or behaviorally to the events they encounter in their lives; rather people cause their own reactions by the way they interpret or evaluate the events they experience. (Ellis, 1977, p. 3)

Ellis further believes that the basic irrational beliefs that characterize most instances of emotional disturbance essentially are absurd and self-defeating and that the purpose of a cognitive-emotional therapeutic process "is to induce the person to recognize the absurdity of his beliefs, to relinquish them, and to adopt new more adaptive ones" (p. 3).

Moleski and Tosi (1976) compared the use of rational-emotive therapy to Wolpe's systematic desensitization therapy in the treatment of stuttering and found rational-emotive therapy to be more effective in reducing stuttering as well as accompanying anxiety and negative attitudes toward stuttering. They do not indicate, however, if any changes occurred with respect to self-image. It also is important to note that they assume stuttering to be essentially an emotional disturbance.

Regardless of the apparent differences between Culatta and Rubin's and Ellis's principles and therapeutic approaches, one major similarity is fundamentally clear—the notion that individuals need not continue to indoctrinate themselves with attitudes inculcated over a period of time and can choose a different manner of behavior through a logical thought process.

In the chapter on counseling, we discuss the use of contracting as a means of assisting the client in fulfilling goals established in therapy and practicing new modes of behavior outside the clinical environment. Shames and Florence (1980) introduced the use of contracts in their behavioral approach to stuttering therapy. Goldberg (1981) made contracts a fundamental part of his behavioral-cognitive stuttering therapy (BCST) program, through 15 major steps, beginning with extended prolongations of fluent speech and continuation through generalization of normal fluency. Since then, he has altered his approach significantly, providing opportunities for stuttering individuals to discover and develop their own strategies for developing fluency once a comprehensive diagnostic assessment is made. A significant change from Goldberg's earlier approach, which treated each client similarly, regardless of known etiology, is that the program is individually based and the individual, in a real sense, guides himself or herself toward greater fluency, with contracts still part of the program (Goldberg, 1997).

Ellis (1997) updates the self-help form first developed in 1984 to the rational emotive behavior

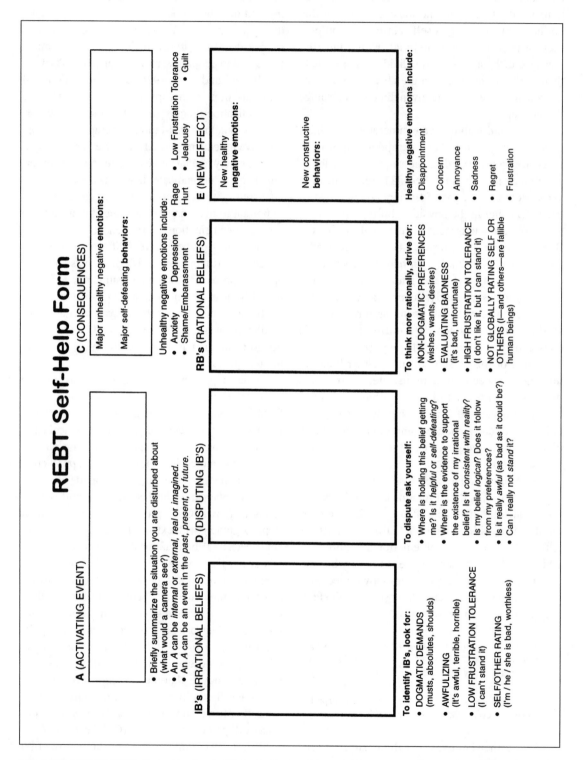

Figure 4-1. REBT Self-Help Form. (Reprinted with permission from Windy Dryden and Jane Walker, 1992, revised by the Albert Ellis Institute, New York: Albert Ellis Institute; 1996:1.)

therapy form to be used by clients as part of homework assignments, in which they record those things they feel most upset or stressed about on a particular day or throughout the week (see Figure 4–1). Such a qualitative rating scale can be a useful tool in assisting stuttering individuals to develop a more realistic attitude about their stuttering.

Synergistic Stuttering Therapy

A holistic approach, developed over many years by Bloom and Cooperman (1999), integrates components of fluency shaping, including physiological, psycholinguistic, and behavioral factors, with components of stuttering modification therapy. The latter aspect focuses on attitudinal and environmental factors. This synergistic method is individualized and involves a comprehensive assessment of the children and adults they treat. Borrowing from several different disciplines, their program appears somewhat familiar in many aspects to our approach, which is discussed next.

*Person-Centered Cognitive-
Behavioral-Emotional Approach*

We believe that a person-centered cognitive-behavioral-emotional approach can best give most stuttering individuals an opportunity to either become totally fluent, gain conscious control of their dysfluencies, and or become self-assured in their ability to communicate with others. We borrow from the authorities previously discussed, including our own philosophy and practices, to arrive at intervention principles that can best succeed:

1. *Developing the appropriate attitude necessary for active listening.* We need to be prepared for and open to understand the means by which the client copes with his or her stuttering reality. No judgment is made in the beginning regarding the individual's perhaps distorted view of self or their perception of reality, in general, although the person is aided in listening to his or her cognitive communicative message.
2. *Viewing the client as a person.* We share with the individual the belief that stuttering is not something one is, but rather represents one behavior, albeit different, among many behaviors that identify us as human. The client is helped to understand that, despite the pronounced nature and symptomotology of stuttering, we all have our own distinctly negative attributes, but that these are only one aspect of who we are.
3. *Being aware of the obstacles to active listening.* We must be prepared to acknowledge and understand our own feelings that become activated by who the client is, what is being communicated, and how it is being communicated. This means listening to our own subjective attitudes toward stuttering and not denying that listening to its distinctive features bothers, disturbs, or saddens us.
4. *Viewing ourselves realistically.* We must not confuse the struggles of any particular stuttering individual with our own life struggles and perhaps negative self-concept and need to be prepared to separate out the client's possible projections on us. This means avoiding the role of rescuer, which removes the importance of our client's active role as decision maker. It also implies tolerating our client's impatience with us when we refuse to take responsibility for our client's fluency. Only when we serve as an objective facilitator can our client make full use of the potential for change.
5. *Valuing client choice.* Because some clients may demonstrate resistance to achieving fluency or unwillingness to make the necessary commitment to such change, we must understand that any dramatic change in behavior often is fraught with anxiety or even terror. Such feelings need not be viewed as psychopathological, as the implication of achieved fluency carries with it not only dramatically different perceptions by others of the client but the client's own perception of what these changes may mean in all aspects of that person's life. We, as clinicians, may lead our client to the proverbial water but the client must chose to drink. Only if the individual is provided an opportunity to explore this resistance and its implications can the full realization of self-choice become apparent and real.

6. *Using client-therapist contracts.* The contracting procedures alluded to earlier need no repetition, except that they must be complemented by continual analysis, review, and modification through the interpersonal counseling process. Here, as therapists, we need to avoid cajoling and judging, which would only alienate the client from the particular contract and the clinician. We proceed at the client's pace with the mutual understanding that any obstacle to progress and contract elaboration is the responsibility of the client. Denial, in the form of rationalization, avoidance, and resistance is fully discussed so that the client is made fully aware of what he or she is choosing or not choosing.

7. *Using confrontation.* Confrontation can be most effectively utilized when a stuttering client attempts to hide behind irrational verbal statements of cognitively disordered thinking with respect to descriptions of self, frequency of actual stuttering, nature of the stuttering pattern, or maintaining the status quo. Sharing with the client our inability to understand the incongruency of his or her expressed communicative message or attitude places the responsibility directly on the client to clarify exactly what meaning is intended, what feeling is being experienced, or what perceived distortion of the stuttering event is made. A direct challenge to the client's perception, discomforting as it may be, nonetheless may be carried out gently, caringly, and objectively.

8. *The value of therapist self-disclosure.* Therapist self-disclosure can be an effective means of reinforcing positive behavioral change, developing a positive self-image, and extinguishing or neutralizing self-defeating behavior and attitudes. It aids the client in the realization that no one is alone in personal life struggles, albeit each is different. The client may feel comforted in knowing he or she is not "sick" or "stupid" when attempting to hide behind the rationalizations, illogical thinking, and misperceptions often associated with stuttering and the fear, embarrassment, and struggles accompanying it. To disclose aspects of oneself does not mean preoccupying the client with the struggles of one's personal life as a means of working out one's own unresolved problems. It, however, does provide a more supportive, safe, trusting, and accepting clinical environment, in which the client feels freer to explore the self-perpetuating behaviors that contribute to stuttering.

9. *Blending symptomatic strategies with counseling.* While we do not subscribe to any one symptomatic approach that helps to modify the stuttering pattern, if used at all, some degree of personal interaction is necessary. We are treating the person and not the symptom. But, when a client presents with complex cognitive, emotional, and debilitating dysfluency, we are required to follow a plan that includes a continual interweaving of both strategies. Even minimal positive changes in fluency brought about by such techniques as shaping, active prolongation, intensive smooth speech, and the like should be further reinforced by discussion of the client's reaction to the accomplishment. Occasionally, when we wish to focus more on one strategy than another, we need to allow for the inclusion of the other. This depends on the level of progress as perceived by both the client and therapist. We offer no rigid procedure to follow, because unique client needs dictate a flexible approach.

10. *Body language and paralinguistic cues.* The nonverbal and nonlinguistic features of communication will assist us in providing further clues to our client's struggle with fluency and attitudinal change, particularly when the messages are inconsistent with the verbal message given.

11. *Ancillary strategies.* We have found other disciplines provide techniques that may successfully be used with our clients, in conjunction with those already discussed. They include progressive relaxation, meditation, and visual imagery. For years, we have used vocalization in conjunction with full bodily movement to help achieve fluency. An interesting ramification of this technique is that the client for the first time may become aware of the power of his or her voice, thus adding to the individual's self-confidence as communicator.

The Client-Therapist Relationship

Regardless of the therapeutic approach used in stuttering therapy, we would agree with Cooper (1974) that the therapeutic relationship "facilitates the client's adaptation of more accurate perceptions which enable the stutterer to achieve maximum success" (p. 81). Twenty-five years later, Cooper (1999) insists that we need to attend more to emotional and cognitive components rather than on "dysfluency frequency counts" (p. 11). We would add that, because each therapeutic relationship differs by the very nature of the individuals involved, no definitive rule can be formulated governing its ongoing development. It does imply, however, mutual adaptation to moment-by-moment changes in behavior, attitude, and circumstances, thereby enjoining us as therapists to be flexible in all our responses rather than following any one predetermined course of action.

We do not wish to imply that we dispense with the overall therapeutic model we have chosen to use but rather that we make it relevant to the contracts we have negotiated with our clients. If contracts are to be broken, so be it, as long as the participants explore together the reasons and then renegotiate new ones. Recently, we had been seeing a 16-year-old young man who chose not to follow through with contracts we had formulated. Rather than enter into a discussion of what factors may have been responsible, it can be said that both parents had denied they were in any way associated with his "terrible habit." Therapy was terminated by the family following four sessions.

One further caution we need to acknowledge as therapists is that, because most of the available evidence suggests little or no pronounced psychopathology in most stuttering individuals, we should adhere to a "wellness" model in our approach. That is, we must view each therapeutic relationship in such a way so as to facilitate learning in both of us.

Finally, the relationship requires that we diligently avoid the use of the term *stutterer*, which contradicts the very mutual nature of the relationship and what we wish to accomplish in therapy. This may not be easy because the term has been well inculcated in us both personally and profes-

sionally. Those of us who resist this change in belief system must ask the questions: Why must we persist? and Of what value is the continued use of this nominal term?

Special Conditions for Family Therapy

Family therapy as a viable system of treatment for stuttering adults would be applicable only when the individual's most frequent interpersonal involvement is with other members of the family, regardless of whether the person lives at home. It is conceivable that, if family patterns in the past have been an influential part of the stuttering process, they will continue to be so. The choice by the individual to continue living at home, ostensibly for economic reasons, may also be indicative of separation and bonding needs yet unresolved.

Certainly, we need not assume these needs to be related to the stuttering dynamics, but an initial family assessment would help clarify the issue. Then it would be possible, as therapists, to determine the efficacy of continued family therapy, individual cognitive-emotional therapy, or both. Whatever the strategy, the final choice is made by the client.

Research Considerations and Conclusion

Within this chapter, we present rationales to explain etiology and therapeutic models deemed appropriate for children and adults who stutter. We do not believe that the vast quantity of research has yet corroborated a definitive etiological theory (most indications are that there is none), a characteristic stuttering personality, or even the most effective treatment model. We do not know yet why many children outgrow stuttering with no intervention or why adults suddenly become consistently fluent. There continues to be considerable controversy, too, among those who argue that no credible scientific data support the efficacy of treatment for early stuttering (Curlee and Yairi, 1997), those who believe no particular formula should dictate the quantity and quality of intervention (Packman and Onslo, 1998), the need for long-term follow-up including treatment outcome methodology (Bloodstein, 1995), and that clinicians should base their treatment on the critical analysis of all data available and "insist on treatments that have been demonstrated to be effective in well designed experimental analysis" (Ingham and Cordes, 1998, p. 17).

While our obsession with outcome data and laboratory-controlled individuals that beg to be generalized into the real clinical world and our fear that our profession shall be extinguished unless we can come up with the right numbers may have some validity, but it unfortunately jeopardizes more than our profession. Perhaps, our energies and research need to be expended to justify, with the use of vast clinical examples, that process and results cannot be measured by numbers alone and remind ourselves that enhanced communicative quality is our goal when we work with individuals who stutter.

References

Ackerman NW. Family psychotherapy: Theory and practice. *Am J of Psychotherapy.* 1966;20:405–414.

Adams MR. The demands and capacities model: I. Theoretical elaborations. *J of Fluency Disorders.* 1990;15(3): 135–141

Ambrose NG, Cox NJ, Yairi E. The genetic basis of persistence and recovery in stuttering. *J of Speech Language and Hearing Research.* June 1997;40(3):567–580.

American Speech and Hearing Association. Terminology pertaining to fluency and fluency disorders: guidelines. *ASHA.* March–April 1999; 41(suppl 19):29–36.

Andrews G, Craig A, Feyer AM, Hoddinott S, Howie P, Neilson M. Stuttering: a review of research findings and theories circa 1982. *J of Speech and Hearing Disorders.* 1983;48:226–246.

Andrews G, Guitar B, Howie P. Meta-analysis of the effects of stuttering treatment, *J of Speech and Hearing Disorders.* 1980;45:287–307.

Aronson A. *Clinical Voice Disorders,* 2nd ed. New York: Thieme; 1985.

Axeline VM. *Play Therapy.* New York: Ballantine Books; 1969.

Barbara DA. *Stuttering: A Psychodynamic Approach to Its Understanding and Treatment.* New York: Julian; 1954.

Bloodstein O. *A Handbook on Stuttering.* Chicago: National Easter Seal Society; 1981.

———. *Stuttering: The Search for a Cause and Cure.* Boston: Allyn and Bacon; 1993.

———. *A Handbook on Stuttering,* 5th ed. San Diego, CA: Singular Publishing Group; 1995.

Bloom C Sr, Cooperman DK. *Synergistic Stuttering Therapy: A Holistic Approach.* Boston: Butterworth–Heinemann; 1999.

Blum A. A neurofunctional theory of stuttering. Unpublished paper, 1984.

Brutten EJ, Shoemaker DJ. *The Modification of Stuttering.* Englewood Cliffs, NJ: Prentice-Hall; 1967.

Cangelosi DM, Schaefer CE, ed. *Play Therapy Techniques.* Northvale, NJ: Jason Aronson; 1996.

Cooper EB. Integrating relationship and behavior therapy procedures for adult stutterers. In: Emerick LL and Hood SB, eds. *The Client-Clinician Relationship.* Springfield, IL: Charles C Thomas; 1974.

———. Is stuttering a speech disorder? *ASHA* March–April 1999;41(2):10–11.

Cooper EB, Cooper CS. Clinician attitudes towards stuttering: two decades of change. *J of Fluency Disorders.* June 1996;21(2):119–135.

Culatta R, Rubin H. A program for the initial stages of fluency therapy. *J of Speech and Hearing Disorders.* 1973;16:556–568.

Curlee RF, ed. *Stuttering and Related Disorder of Fluency,* 2nd ed. New York: Thieme; 1999.

Curlee RF, Yairi E. Early intervention with early childhood stuttering: a critical examination of the data. *Am J Speech-Language-Hearing Path.* 1997;6(2):8–18.

Defares PB. Determinants of changes in trait anxiety. In: Spielberger CD, Sarason IG, eds. *Stress and Anxiety,* Vol. 13. New York: Hemisphere; 1991.

Duffy JR, Baumgartner J. Psychogenic stuttering in adults with and without neurologic disease. *J of Med Speech-Language Path.* June 1997; 5(2)(78 ref):75–95.

Egolf DB, Shames GH, Johnson PR, Kasprisin-Burelli A. The use of parent-child interaction patterns on therapy for young stutterers. *J of Speech and Hearing Disorders.* 1972;37:222–232.

Eisenson J, ed. *Stuttering: A Second Symposium.* New York: Harper; 1975.

Ellis A. Rational-Emotive Therapy. In: Binder VM, Binder A, Rimland B, eds. *Modern Therapies.* Englewood Cliffs, NJ: Prentice-Hall; 1976.

———. The basic clinical theory of rational-emotive therapy. In: Ellis A, Grieger R, eds. *Handbook of Rational-Emotive Therapy.* New York: Springer-Verlag, 1977.

———. *The Practice of Rational Emotive BehaviorTherapy.* New York: Springer; 1997.

Ellis A, Gordon J, Neenan M, Palmer S. *Stress Counseling: A Rational Emotive Behaviour Approach.* London: Cassell; 1997.

Faden AI. Iatrogenic illness: an overview with particular reference to neurologic complications. *Neurol Clin.* February 1998;16(1):1–8.

Farber SL. Genetic diversity and differing reactions to stress. In: Goldberg L, Brezaitz S, eds. *Handbook of Stress: Theoretical and Clinical Aspects.* New York: Macmillan; 1982.

Fox PT, Ingham RJ, Ingham JC, Hirsch TB, Downs JH, Martin C, Jerabek P, Glass T, Lancaster JL. A PET study of the neural systems of stuttering. *Nature.* July 11, 1996;382(6587):158–161.

Glauber IP. The psychoanalysis of stuttering. In: Eisenson J, ed. *Stuttering: A Symposium*. New York: Harper and Row; 1958.

Goldberg SA. Behavioral Cognitive Stuttering Therapy. Tigard, OR: C. C. Publications; 1981.

———. *Behavioral Cognitive Stuttering Therapy*. San Diego, CA: Singular Publishing Group; 1997.

Gottwald, SR. Family communication patterns and stuttering development: an analysis of the research literature. In: Ratner NB, Healey CE, eds. *Stuttering Research and Practice: Bridging the Gap*. Mahwah, NJ: Lawrence Erlbaum and Association; 1999.

Hahn EF. *Stuttering*. Stanford, CA: Stanford University Press; 1956.

Halpern DF. Sex differences in intelligence. Implications for education. *Am Psychol*. October 1997;52(10):1091–1102.

Hamilton V. An information processing model. In: Goldberger L, Breznitz S, eds. *Handbook of Stress: Theoretical and Clinical Aspects*. New York: Macmillan; 1982.

Ingham RJ, Cordes AK. Treatment decisions for young children who stutter: further concerns and complexities. *Am J Speech-Lang-Path*. August 1998;7(3):10–17.

Ivanova GA, Lapa AZ, Lokhov MI, Movsisyants SA. Features of stuttering preschool children. *Neuroscience and Behavioral Psyciology*. May–June 1991;21(3):284–287.

Johnson W. *People in Quandries*. New York: Harper and Brothers; 1946.

Johnson W, Associates. *The Onset of Stuttering*. Minneapolis: University of Minneapolis Press; 1959.

Kidd KK. A genetic perspective on stuttering. *Journal of Fluency Disorders*. 1977;2:259–269.

Kopp GA. Metabolic studies of stutterers: I. Biochemical study of blood composition. *Speech Monographs I* 1934;117–132.

Korzybski A. *Science and Sanity*. Lancaster, PA: Lancaster Press; 1933.

Kroll RM, DeNil LF. Positron emission tomography studies of stuttering: Their relationship to our theoretical and clinical understanding of the disorder. *J of Speech-Lang Path and Aud*. December 1998;22(4):261–270.

Leung AK, Robson WL. Stuttering. *Clinical Pediatrics*. September 1990;29(9):498–502.

Ludlow CL, Cooper JA. Genetic aspects of speech and language disorders: current status and future directions. In: Ludlow CL, Cooper JA, eds. *Genetic Aspects of Speech and Language Disorders*. New York: Academic Press; 1983.

Mahr G, Leith W. Psychogenic stuttering of adult onset. *J of Speech-Hear-Res*. April 1992;35(2):283–286.

Menzies RG, Onslow M, Packman A. Anxiety and stuttering: exploring a complex relationship. *Am J of Speech-Lang-Path*. 1999;8:3–10.

Moleski R, Tosi DJ. Comparative psychotherapy: rational-emotive therapy versus systemic desensitization in the treatment of stuttering. *J of Consulting, Clinical Psychology*. 1976;44:309–311.

Morgan RF, ed. *The Iatrogenics Handbook*. Toronto: IPI Publishing; 1980.

Murray HL, Reed CG. Language abilities of preschool stuttering children. *J Fluency Dis*. 1977;2:171–176.

Norton CC, Norton BE. *Reaching Children Through Play Therapy: An Experimental Approach*. Denver, CO: Pendleton Clay Publishers; 1997.

Onslow M, Packman A. The Lidcombe Program of early stuttering intervention. In: Ratner NB, Healey CE, eds. *Stuttering Research and Practice: Bridging the Gap*. Mahwah, NJ: Lawrence Erlbaum and Associates; 1999.

Orton ST. Studies in stuttering. *Archives of Neurology and Psychiatry*. 1927;18:671–672.

Packman A, Onslow M. What is the take-home message from Curlee and Yairi? *Am J Speech- Lang Path*. August 1998;7(3):5–9.

Poulos MG, Webster WG. Family history as a basis for subgrouping people who stutter. *J of Speech and Hearing Research*. February 1991;34(1):5–10.

Ratner NB. Measurable outcomes of instructions to modify normal parent-child verbal interactions: implications for indirect stuttering therapy. *J of Speech and Hearing Research*. February 1992;35(1):14–20.

Ratner NB, Healey CE, eds. *Stuttering Research and Practice: Bridging the Gap*. Mahwah, NJ: Lawence Erlbaum and Associates; 1999.

Rieber RW, et al. *The Neuropsychology of Language*. New York: Plenum; 1976.

Rubin H, Culatta R. A point of view about fluency. *ASHA*. 1971;13:380–384.

Schwartz MF. *Stuttering Solved*. New York: McGraw-Hill, 1976.

Schulze H, Johannsen HS. Importance of parent-child interaction in the genesis of stuttering. *Folia-Phoniatrica*. May–June 1991;43(3):133–143.

Shames GH, Florence CL. *Stutter-Free Speech*. Columbus, OH: Charles E. Merrill;1980.

Sheehan JG. Theory and treatment of stuttering as an approach-avoidance conflict. *J of Psychology*. 1953;36:27–49.

———. Conflict theory and avoidance reduction therapy. In: Eisenson J, ed. *Stuttering: A Second Symposium*. New York: Harper and Row; 1975.

Silverman FH. *Stuttering and Other Fluency Disorders*. Boston: Allyn and Bacon; 1996.

Stocker B, Parker E. The relationship between auditory recall and dysfluency in young stutterers. *J Fluency Dis*. 1977;2:177–187.

Tkaczenko OG. Tiefenpsychologische Aspekte des Stotterns [The depth psychological aspects of stuttering]. *Zeitschrift fuer Individualpsychologie*. 1990;15(4):298–306.

Tomatis A. *L'Oreille et le Language*. Paris: Editions du Seuil; 1963.

Travis LE. *Speech Pathology*. New York: Appleton-Century; 1931.

Treon M. A bi-polar etiologic stuttering threshold hypothesis and related proposed treatment approach. *Psychology: A J of Human Behavior*. 1995;32(3–4):35–51.

Van Riper C. *The Nature of Stuttering*. Englewood Cliffs NJ: Prentice-Hall; 1971.

————. *Speech Correction: Principles and Methods,* 5th ed. Englewood Cliffs. NJ: Prentice-Hall; 1972.

————. The severe young stutterer. *In Counseling Stutterers*, No 18 (pamphlet). Memphis, TN: Speech Foundation of America.

West R. An agnostic's speculations about stuttering. In: Eisenson J, ed. *Stuttering: A Symposium.* New York: Harper; 1958.

Westby CE. Language performance of stuttering and nonstuttering children. *J Commun. Dis.* 1979;12:133–145.

Williams DE. A point of view about "stuttering." *J Speech Hearing Dis.* 1957;22:390–397.

————. Stuttering therapy for children. In: Travis LE, ed. *Handbook of Speech Pathology and Audiology.* New York: Appleton-Century-Crofts; 1971.

Wingate ME. Speaking unassisted: comments on a paper by Andrews et al. *J of Speech and Hearing Disorders.* 1983;48:255–263.

Wolpe J. *Psychotherapy by Reciprocal Inhibition.* Palo Alto, CA: Stanford University Press; 1958.

Yairi E, Ambrose N, Cox N. Genetics of stuttering: a critical review. *J of Speech and Hearing Research.* August 1996;39(4):771–784.

5

Psychological Considerations for Language-Disordered Children and Their Families

Introduction

As we take on the formidable task of exploring the many dimensions of psychogenetic and social processes in the development of specific language disorders (SLD) and developmental language disorders in children, we need to set some limits and take some positions that may not satisfy the orientation of many workers in the field.

We use the term *language disorder* to describe broadly a particular behavior, regardless of etiology, following Bloom and Lahey (1978). They view language along three basic dimensions. The first is language form, in which the elements of a message, such as its shape and sound, are combined. The second is language content, which is what individuals talk about or understand relative to the message. The third is language use, in which speakers choose to speak in a particular way, depending on the listener and the context. For our purposes, we also treat the interaction of the form, content, and use of language as a complete entity, bearing in mind that each, when independently impaired at times, may be a function of diagnostic categorization. As Bloom and Lahey indicate, the emphasis must be on what children do and what they have trouble doing, so that interference in the language system may be better understood.

We shall not discuss the multidimensional nature of learning disability in children except to isolate the language component and explore its effects on the overall psychosocial development of the child. During the discussion, however, we must remain cognizant of the educational implications for, as well as the influence of, other learning disability components on the developing child. Further, our coverage of distinct categorical entities, such as mental retardation, neurological damage, hearing impairment, and autism, will be limited to the basic consideration of psychosocial effects and consistent with a generic viewpoint. To do otherwise would deflect the thrust of this chapter.

One final stipulation we make is to treat articulation disorders as a phonological aspect of language and related to all other linguistic features. In their review of the research of children with phonological disorders, Bernthal and Bankson (1981) conclude that these children, particularly those with multiple sound errors, also have difficulties in comprehension, syntax, and vocabulary.

Although the synergistic view, which implies complex interactions and interfacing among all linguistic features, is still subject to further empirical confirmation, our search of the literature has failed to justify the separation of phonology from other linguistic aspects on the basis of psychogenetic and social processes. Regardless of the philosophical positions taken here, it is hoped that considerable debate will be provoked and further empirical research inspired.

Psychogenesis of
Language Disorders in Children

It is a truism when we suggest that parents who spend much time with and give considerable attention to their children will produce healthy, productive, communicative, and independent adults. Yet, like every maxim applied to human development and in particular communicative development, the exceptions force us to modify the original rules. So-called ideal familial circumstances do not always bring about the fully functioning adult as we would wish to predict. Similarly, we often find such adults to evolve from unstable, deficient, and uncommunicative parenting.

The genesis of human communication is too complex an act to explain by a mere collection of either independent or dependent variables; but, by attempting to describe the quality of such variables and how they interrelate, we should be able to formulate postulates about its development. Toward this goal, we need to identify the most recent research findings and discuss the many relevant factors to elucidate our understanding of the problem. The most logical place to begin is with a discussion of the relationship of home environment and early language development. At this time, we shall not include children who have acquired language deviations resulting from identified physical, physiological, neurological, or sensory deficits.

Home Environment and Language Development

Several of the earlier and extensive longitudinal studies investigating the relationship of home environment and early cognitive development, done in the United States and Canada, have been compiled by Gottfried (1984a, 1984b). Citing a variety of measures employed by many authorities—including the Home Observation for Measurement of the Environment (HOME) Inventory, the Illinois Test of Psycholinguistic Abilities (ITPA), and the Bayley Scale of Infant Development (Bradley and Caldwell, 1984); the Family Environment Scale (FES), the Purdue Home Stimulation Inventory (PHSI), the Test of Early Language Development (TELD), and Variety of Experience Checklist (VEC) (Gottfried

and Gottfried 1984); the Reynell Developmental Language Scales (RDLS) (Siegel 1984); and the Bifactor Environmental Action Model (Wachs 1984)—Gottfried concludes "that assessments of proximal home environmental variables are reliable and valid indicators of the stimulation and experiences available to infants and young children" (p. 329).

He further concludes that cognitive development in young children correlates with several closely related home environment variables, among which he finds the following: (1) "Stability of home environment accounted for most of the correlations between early environment and subsequent cognitive development" (p. 336); and (2) play materials, maternal responsiveness, maternal involvement, and verbal responses to infants' vocalizations were found "to have the highest and most consistent relationships" (p. 338). A meta-analysis by Glass, McGraw, and Smith (1981) supports the findings summarized by Gottfried, with maternal involvement and responsiveness and play materials showing the highest mean correlation with the development of cognition and language. More recent studies by Huttenlocher (1998) and Duhan and Punia (1998) reinforce the contention that the home environment can be a predictor of language development, through their investigative and review of previous studies. Yet, according to Rutter and Mawhood (1991), few methodologically correct studies link language impairment and psychopathology, citing the heterogenity factor, sample bias, lack of standardized measures of behavioral responses, effects of associated impairments, and bias in clinic referrals.

The Effect of Socioeconomic Status

Although much research has revealed that children from lower socioeconomic groups demonstrate developmental lags in acquiring cognitive and language skills (Bereiter and Engelmann, 1966), more recent research has identified specific factors that would account for the delay. Based on research conducted by Bradley and Caldwell (1984); Gottfried and Gottfried (1984); Barnard, Bee, and Hammond (1984); Johnson, Breckenridge, and McGowan (1984); Siegel (1984); and Beckwith and Cohen

(1984), Gottfried (1984a) reports that children from families with lower socioeconomic status (SES) are relatively less likely to receive an intellectually advantageous home environment conducive to cognitive and language development than those from higher SES families. Differences, however, were noted strictly as a function of socioeconomic factors, regardless of other factors. The inescapable finding was that "mothers of relatively higher intelligence, as measured by vocabulary, provided a more enriched environment for their children" (p. 330).

Of particular interest was the conclusion that "middle compared to lower SES mothers spoke more to their children, were socially more involved, provided more intellectual tasks in terms of play materials, and showed consistently higher levels of caregiver responsiveness" (p. 331). An additional significant finding was that crowding in the home adversely affected home stimulation in terms of quality and quantity, thereby contributing to a cognitive and linguistic lag.

We should bear in mind, as we consider the merits of the conclusions drawn by the preceding studies, that several significant factors impinge on the nature of socioeconomic class. To begin with, lower SES mothers tend to be single parents, many of whom work and are unable to provide the necessary home stimulation and caregiving characteristics of higher SES mothers. Second, because Gottfried and Gottfried (1984) and Johnson, Breckenridge, and McGowan (1984) define intelligence as measured by vocabulary, we believe such a narrow definition fails to consider other facets of intelligence. That is, we cannot assume that lower SES mothers are necessarily intellectually inferior but only that linguistic stimulation may be lacking because of the quantity and quality of parent-child contact.

Environmental Deprivation

Abundant evidence supports the notion that early environmental deprivation is causally related to language delay. Spitz (1945, 1946a, 1946b), in his now classic study, investigated the effects of an emotionally vacant orphanage when infants were placed there at 4 months of age. Deprived of most human contact beyond the bare necessities of bodily needs, the infants essentially became developmentally retarded and susceptible to extreme emaciation (marasmus) and profound sadness (anaclitic depression). After two years, on follow-up, 37% of the children had died. Of those surviving, severe cognitive, linguistic, intellectual, and social deficits were observed. Although, we hope, such catastrophic situations no longer exist, they demonstrate how extreme disregard for infants' emotional needs can interfere with or destroy their normal development.

To a considerably lesser degree, Harlow et al. (1966) and Mineka and Suomi (1978) found short-term distress when primate infants were separated from their mothers. Although comparison of their results to those for human infants would be somewhat indefensible, Stayton and Ainsworth (1973) demonstrated that there is less short-term distress when a secure mother-child attachment is interrupted.

Bowlby (1960) attributed a variety of insults, such as linguistic, cognitive, and intellectual retardation; behavioral and socialization disorders; and disturbed interpersonal relationships, to separation from parental figures. Rutter (1983), however, found that these long-term deficits are more closely related to the degree of privation to which the child had been exposed previously, the young age at which the separation had occurred (between ages 1 and 4), the duration of the separation, and the quality and promptness of subsequent parenting.

Less obvious environmental deprivations occur in families where conditions generally are unfavorable for language development. These conditions include negative, incongruous, irrational, paradoxical, or distorted communicative interactions between family members. It is generally recognized that individual differences in language learning relate learning to various qualities associated with interpersonal relationships, particularly those involving the child and major caregiver. While there is no empirical data as such, inferences regarding the mind's ability to manipulate and encode information in relationship to the interactional process could be made.

Bilingualism

Although early references point to bilingualism as a definitive factor in the etiology of language disorders in children, it is now believed that, due to early methodological problems and cultural biases in research, positing such a relationship is not tenable. Whatever psychosocial correlates appear present in bilingual families seem more closely related to socioeconomic class.

Lambert (1977), writing on the effects of bilingualism in children, reviews the literature and suggests that bilinguals who are matched with monolingual controls actually appear to be more cognitively flexible, creative, and divergent in thought. Therefore, we would be hard pressed, given the present state of knowledge on the subject, to support the view that bilingualism per se is directly related to psychosocial maladjustment and language disorder.

Dysfunctional Family Dynamics

Because language in children typically develops and evolves within the family structure and system, it is incumbent on us to explore how dysfunctional family dynamics may interfere with and inhibit that development. Consistent with the discussions elsewhere in this text, we must consider family dysfunction along a continuum from marked psychopathology to minimal maladjustment. In so doing, however, we must bear in mind that the severity of the language disorder or delay is not necessarily contingent on the degree of psychopathology, as the child's own unique way of coping may alter the effects on him- or herself and perhaps influence the entire family system.

Unfortunately, the literature on the relationship of language development and family systems theory is disappointingly sparse. Nevertheless, it is possible to review some findings.

Cantwell and Baker (1977) found a high degree of behavior disturbance among children with language problems. In a later effort, Cantwell, Baker, and Mattison (1979) studied 100 speech- and language-delayed children, finding eight specifically language-disordered children who were diagnosed as having attentional deficit disorder with hyperactivity as defined by the DSM-IV of the American Psychiatric Association (1994). The investigators, however, did not find the psychiatric disorders to be etiological to the language disorders.

One of the most comprehensive studies was conducted by Stevenson and Richman (1978). In their epidemiological study of 705 children living in outer London, they found that of 22 children with expressive language delay, 13 (59%) had behavior problems, compared to 14% in the total population. Similarly, children with behavior problems had more than four times the expected rate of severe expressive language delay. A follow-up study of these children one year later revealed consistency in both the behavior problem and language delay. Behavior problems were characterized by immaturity, problems in social relationships with siblings and peers, and marked dependency on the mother.

The authors caution that we not assume a cause-effect relationship between disturbed behavior and communication deficits. This should be obvious, as the children studied were 3 years old, thereby obscuring any evidence of family dysfunction as a causative factor contributing to language dysfunction. It is possible that, in children who are both behaviorally disturbed and language disturbed, environmental stress may contribute to both. The evidence clearly suggests an association between behavior problems and social and family factors and that language-disturbed children come from homes with particularly adverse conditions.

Mother-Child Interactions

Earlier we reviewed the literature relating home environment in general to language development in the child, and it is clearly apparent that the mother-child interaction is the predominant feature in that relationship.

Walbert et al. (1978) used the Caldwell Inventory of Home Stimulation to assess the home environments and mother-child interactions of a language-delayed group and a matched control group of normal preschool children. Their most significant findings were that the mothers of normal-speaking children were more responsive to, more involved with, and less restrictive of their children. The mothers of language-delayed children, although generally conscientious, tended to relate to their children similarly. Missing, however, was a "dynamic verbal interchange" or a positive reciprocal communicative relationship.

These investigators were careful to note, however, that, because the children studied were beyond 2 1/2 years, it was possible that the mothers of the language-delayed children related poorly, reciprocally, in the response to the already established language delay, thereby exacerbating the language delay and the poor communicative relationship. Walbert et al. wisely avoid the temptation to assign blame for the breakdown in the communicative interaction or cite poor mother-child involvement as a causative factor in the language delay.

A major criticism is with the Caldwell Inventory of Home Stimulation, which was used to evaluate the child's environment. The scale considers only the influence of the mother-infant interaction and does not measure the effects of all family interrelationships, such as the possible effects of the marital relationship, on the mother's relationship to the child. Our criticism, however, should not detract from the overall value of Walbert et al.'s significant contribution.

Olsen-Fulero (1982) reviewed research that indicates that the mother's underlying intention gets served by the many different ways she converses with her child. Olsen-Fulero's own study demonstrates variability among mothers, especially in those behaviors most closely connected to a mother's intention. Her review demonstrates that the conversational mother who asks questions, rarely negates, and gives few directions facilitates the child's language development. Her own findings suggest that the mother who stimulates, challenges, and encourages autonomy in the child facilitates the child's cognitive development. Her study further reveals evidence of highly individualized conversational styles among mothers who interact with their children.

A major criticism of Osen-Fulero's work, which is also applicable to many other studies of mother-child interaction, is the small sample of children and mothers used.

Waterhouse (1982) studied 21 same-sex, same eye-color twin pairs and found that maternal speech patterns varied across families (mothers), reflect the child's developmental state, and reflect the mother's perception of her child. In a highly succinct and enlightening discussion, Waterhouse warns us that the complex communicative interac-

tional process between the child and mother is confounded by too many elements to draw conclusions about causality. Covariances involving genetic-familial patterns and dynamic communicative adjustments made by both mother and child might better explain the significant relationships found between mothers' and children's language performances, according to Waterhouse.

Other writers have studied the mother-child relationship with respect to language development and found significant correlations between language development and specific attributes of mothers' speech, but these attributes have been difficult to interpret (Furrow, Nelson, and Benedict, 1979; DePaulo and Bonvillian, 1978). Söderbergh (1982) confirms earlier linguistic research in his study of 3-year-old children, finding that mother-child communication, as dialogue, may contribute to positive language development, although he is cautious about drawing any conclusions.

Brazelton (1981) used split-screen videotapes of mothers interacting with their infants during the first days and weeks of life, demonstrating a dyadic communicative interaction. Unresponsive mothers were reported to be identified prior to their infants' birth.

Lasky and Klopp (1982) found that mothers of normal-language children demonstrated frequent communicative interaction in terms of expansions, reduction, imitation, use of questions, use of answers, acknowledgment, provision of information, nonverbal behavior, and use of nonverbal deixis (pointing or glancing), whereas mothers of language-disordered children infrequently demonstrated these behaviors. As was noted by previous researchers, mothers and their normal-language children seemed to be reciprocally involved in the communication process, with subtle adjustments made by the mothers in response to their children. The limited sample used in the study and the relatively older age of the babies (27 to 45 months) prevent many definitive conclusions, particularly when we consider that the first two years are of the most crucial importance in language learning.

It appears obvious that any attempt to understand the complex dynamics of the evolving language development in the child must include the mother's or the main caretaker's stimulation. As Winnicott (1965) has implied, we cannot view the infant in isolation in attempting to assess language development. Further, just as we cannot separate the child from the mother, neither can we separate the mother from her own self-concept and the attitudes that pervade her sense as a person in relation to other aspects of her life and to other persons, particularly her spouse. Mothers do not enter into reciprocal relationships with their infants untouched by prepartum personality and emotional patterns nor are they immune to the continuing influences of the child, spouse, and other children in the family.

The parents' interactions with the child and the effects on his or her language development will be influenced directly or indirectly by their own perceptions of themselves. So, too, will the mother alter her communication with the child in the continuing, changing relationship.

Therefore, what we have is a dynamic relationship in which the mother relates to her child within a complex family system, rather than in a circumscribed cocoon, a conclusion that would tax the credibility of any experimental investigation. To borrow from Winnicott, we would add that we cannot view the mother in isolation in attempting to assess language development.

Family Relationships

Virtually nothing in the literature surveyed appears to explore the effects of family relationships, the marital relationship in particular, on the development of normal or abnormal language development. Because most children do develop language, even in the midst of severely dysfunctional families, can we assume that infant language development is immune to the psychopathological processes of these families? Hardly. Even the most ardent advocate of biochemical factors in the ontogenesis of schizophrenic or autistic language in children would acknowledge that aberrant family communication cannot be disregarded.

For the present, however, we are not discussing such extremes in linguistic breakdown nor are we assuming that language disorder necessarily requires deep-rooted family pathology. We suggest that subtle and oftentimes not so subtle variations in dyadic and triadic family interactions must be considered as possible etiological factors along with the unique constitutional or genetic correlates, whatever these may be in the child. An even more complex consideration may well be the unique coping style of the family and its individual members, regardless of individual or family psychopathology per se.

In his extensive review of studies dealing with marital stress, means of coping, and its effect on depression, Ilfeld (1982) fails to identify what influences, if any, such factors have on children in the family. Based on his own major survey of more than 2,000 households sampled from a standard metropolitan statistical area, Ilfeld found marital stressors to have a strong influence on depression in the family but does not indicate specifically what effects there are on the children, much less on their language development.

Arrival of a child into a nuclear family that originally had consisted of two or three persons brings into play new factors and activates already present ones to challenge the new family. Although no documented evidence is available to isolate which factors would be etiological to faulty language development in the newly arrived child or, for that matter, the already present children, it would be helpful to identify those factors that characterize the functioning family and contribute to family and individual growth.

Fogarty (1976) has described the ideal functioning family, and we summarize his model as follows:

- The family is adaptable to and positively responsive to any change. It readily accepts any disruption and is able to move from its status quo position. This would include its response to a child with special needs.
- No one person is seen to have an emotional problem, but whatever emotional problems are present exist in the family unit and are altered by the way family members cope.
- There is a closeness and connectedness among all family members as well as with the families of origin.
- Family members solve problems by dealing with them rather than avoiding or distancing themselves from them. Never is the identity of any family member distorted by or fused with another family member. That is, each is able to maintain his or her own personal integrity.

- If a problem does arise between two family members, such as the parents, it is dealt with without the involvement of an innocent third person to judge or solve the dispute. That is, the child is not used to solve the problem that belongs to the parents.
- Individual differences are respected, encouraged, and fostered to bring out the best in each person.
- Each person is free to think and feel individually in relationship to self and to other members of the family.
  1. Each person is clearly identified and differentiated from other persons in the family. Each person is aware of what the other person gets from himself or herself and what he or she gets and needs from others.
  2. There is a recognition and awareness of "emptiness" in each other, but each is allowed the opportunity to fill his or her own void. Therefore, the child who may be struggling to solve a personal issue is not rescued by the values and judgments of others but is aided to discover personal means to deal with the problem.
  3. There is a positive emotional climate with the avoidance of what is "right" and what "should" be done. *Truth exists only in what is truly practiced* (italics mine).
  4. Healthy family functioning is directly related to and dependent on each family member enjoying other family members and the family as a whole. The problem, stated or unstated, of one family member is acknowledged and respected.
  5. Any one family member feels free to use any other family member for feedback and learning with no fear of embarrassment or criticism.

Whereas the reader may take issue with Fogarty's description of an ideal functioning family system as not being real, we would respond that the crucial element is the necessity for families to strive toward the ideal. It is the recognition of the process, not the result, that has the greatest impact.

Therapists who work with language-disordered children who have no identified organic etiological components are well aware of the wide variations among parenting and family styles. These workers, who also are knowledgeable in child development theory, would attest to the considerable range of possibilities and family circumstances under which language normally develops. Clearly, even in the most dysfunctional family, children develop language. Conversely, language-disordered children frequently have been observed in apparently functioning families. Where, then, do the discrepancies lie?

We submit that professional workers are not always privy to the subtle interactional processes among family members, particularly between mother and child. Even the most carefully thought out and objectively conducted research would be challenged to identify, in the antiseptic and experimental environment, perhaps obscure elements that either contribute to or impede language development. We do not wish to infer, however, that such research is unproductive. On the contrary, numerous studies have taken investigators into the home to identify, firsthand, the positive elements that characterize language development. But even the best-intentioned investigator could not possibly know what occurs behind closed doors after the investigator has left. Does this suggest that we ought to refrain from such investigations? Not at all. We believe it is practically possible to determine those interactional factors, albeit subtle or obscure, that could be revealed through blind self-rating instruments. These we discuss later.

The Language-Disordered Child as the "Identified Symptom"

Previously, we stated that a child could embody certain types of conflict between parents or among several members of the family and that the conflict may be manifest in a specific aberrant behavior, such as stuttering. Or, when conflict may not be present, a change in family circumstances may initiate negative behavior. Conceivably, the disruption in language development may result directly or indirectly from the child's reaction not only to obvious elements, such as a silent environment, family communication characterized by continual marital bickering, or unrealistic parental expectations, but also as a reaction to the arrival of a sibling, the mother needing to work, or a mother-father relationship that avoids conflict.

We saw a 4-year-old child whose language was characterized by severe syntactic, semantic, and phonological delay. Formal testing could not be carried out due to his marked hyperactivity, and his language comprehension was only marginally adequate. Pediatric and neurological workups were unremarkable, and the parents did not report any events indicating otherwise. Most evident during the initial contact with the child was his inability or refusal to focus on separately introduced play materials. For example, he would manipulate several toy cars for a few moments and then search for other play items. Vocalization during this time was characterized by whole single- or double-word utterances, with a distinctly higher level of content than of form.

Family therapy was initiated to learn more of the family interactional dynamics. Included were Jason (the child), his 10-year-old brother, Gavin, and the parents, Mr. and Mrs. C. The session essentially was characterized by constant interruptions by Jason, which interfered with the communicative efforts of others. His failure to remain seated during the session taxed our clinical acumen as well as our patience, but several significant facts were learned. Mrs. C had been working a day shift as a data processor for more than four years, and Mr. C worked the graveyard shift as a security guard. The family therapy session revealed that, during the afternoons, Jason was left free to do as he pleased in the home, without supervision, while his father slept. The only contact Jason had with his mother was in the late afternoon and early evening, when she felt too tired to relate to him. Other revealing family behaviors consisted of inconsistent and uncompromising differences in parental discipline; extreme guilt expressed by Mrs. C regarding her lack of attention to Jason and her anger toward Mr. C regarding his lack of attention to her and Jason; Mr. C's apparent indifference, defensiveness, and passivity in his relationship to all members of the family; and Gavin's unverbalized anger toward all.

The nature of the family communication can best be described as chaotic, which unsurprisingly resembled Jason's own dysfunctional behavior. Two subsequent family sessions differed little from the initial one, except that the family struggle to find some resolution of their difficulties was clearly evident. Although they aptly realized that Jason required more than traditional language therapy and that continued family therapy indeed would be helpful, they could not bring themselves to make a structured commitment to therapy.

This case study is one example of how interpersonal family communication and behavior in conjunction with individual personal attitudes and struggles can create a family atmosphere antithetical to normal language development in one family member. The example, moreover, points to the conclusion that no one factor within the family process can readily be assigned a major role in the development of a language disorder. It does suggest, however, that dysfunctional family dynamics could be manifested in the form of language dysfunction in the child.

The Relationship of Genetic and Psychosocial Influences

Definitive experimental evidence relating hereditary factors to the ontogenesis of language disorders has become more apparent. Ludlow and Cooper (1983) cite several descriptive case studies that have been carried out (Arnold, 1961; Luchsigne, 1970; Mattejat, Niebergall, and Nestler, 1980; and Zaleski, 1966). They conclude from the evidence from chromosomal studies that there is little scientific basis for a link between sex chromosome deficiencies and the development of language problems. Even fewer studies have attempted to establish a relationship between phonological problems and a genetic base. Ludlow and Cooper, however, report that children who are found to have some chromosome aberration also tend to have communication impairments. They cite Annell, Gustavson, and Tenstam (1970); Haka-Ikse, Stewart, and Cripps (1978); Nielsen and Sillesen (1976); and Nielsen, Sorenson, and Sorenson (1981), who report language and phonological acquisition to be delayed in 40–75% of the cases studied.

Stark, Mellits, and Tallal (1983), based on the results of their studies, do not believe we have a means to establish a direct etiology to language disorders and suggest that family studies along with standard intelligence tests, language tests, and perceptual-motor measures would help us define etiological correlates. In his study of environment, age, and organismic specificity and their effects on the cognitive-intellectual development of the child, Wachs (1984) suggests that organismic specificity may be a significant factor during the first two years "in terms of interpreting differential reactivity to the environment" (p. 320). Based on the results of an experimental investigation of 38 infants who were 11 months of age at the beginning of the study, Wachs concludes that, whereas boys and girls are equally sensitive to their environment, they are so in different ways and there is a specificity for certain environmental dimensions. The hypothesis that different individuals, regardless of sex, will react in different ways to the environment was supported with the conclusion that "genotypically based individual differences mediate the response of the individual to the environment" (p. 321) and that a bridge may be established between biological and experiential factors.

For a more thorough description of the differential responses to the environment by different genotypes, the reader is referred to the provocative work of Bodmer and Cavalli-Sforza (1976).

It has often been said that, considering all the negative influences that impinge on an infant, it is amazing how so many learn to speak. Apparently, there must be enough positive influences that foster normal language development. Because the research thus far has failed to isolate highly specific psychosocial determinants, we must continue to investigate the possibility that individual coping styles may be a significant factor in overall language development.

We are aware that, with regard to the behavior of children under severe external stress, clinical evidence suggests wide variations in response. We also are aware that some children under minimal external stress also respond along a wide continuum. Unfortunately, the lack of systematic investigation precludes us from drawing definitive conclusions, but enough evidence exists to justify some speculation.

It is evident from our earlier discussion and review of stuttering behavior in children that strong evidence suggests a genetic base for its development, and studies in the speech-language pathology literature are beginning to draw such parallels in

child language development. Garmezy (1983) leads us through a review of the literature dealing with the stressors of childhood but limits his discussion to the "psychological threat posed by loss of or separation from a parent or significant caregiver" (p. 51) and the traumatic effects of war and civil discord on children. He summarizes several different studies of resilience in children, finding some congruence regardless of methodology, conditions of stress, and type of behavioral disorder. Although Garmezy does not discuss predisposing factors as such, he alludes to the growing interest in "protective" factors, discussed by Rutter (1983) in the same text.

As others have recognized, genetic factors play a significant role in establishing individual differences in the development of and susceptibility to behavior disorders in children, according to Rutter. He discusses the effects of combined or isolated chronic and acute stressors that induce disorder. He notes: "The notion here, then, is of factors which are largely inert on their own, but which serve as 'catalysts' when combined with acute stressors of some type—to use a chemical analogy" (pp. 22–23). After the work of Brown and Harris (1978), Rutter cites catalytic factors, described as "vulnerability" variables, that tend to *increase* the effect of stressors, whereas other catalytic factors, described as "protective" variables, tend to *reduce* the effect of stressors. Much of the data reported by Rutter unfortunately applies to adults, and he wisely cautions us not to generalize too quickly to children. Nevertheless, he suggests that it would be useful to explore the effects, if any, of vulnerability and protective variables in childhood.

To parallel Rutter's concluding remarks, we believe that some children may be impeded in their language development following adverse experiences, whereas others may not. In fact, the latter may not only show resilience in not yielding "but the 'Stresses' may actually have had a positive and beneficial effect" (Rutter, 1983, p. 34). Such variables as age, sex, genetic background, temperament, problem-solving skills, and the nature of family interactions all have to be considered important to explain how and why individual differences operate. Although the direct effects of adverse experiences on language development are somewhat known, it is important that we attend to indirect effects. As Rutter notes, "Thus early events may operate through their action in altering sensitivities to stress, or in modifying styles of coping which then protect from, or predispose towards, disorder in later life only in the presence of later stress events" (p. 34).

In his comprehensive review of the literature, Leonard (1997) provides us further evidence of the possible genetic and neurobiological origins of specific language impairment (SLI) and how it is manifested in other languages. Bishop, North, and Donlan (1996) found a phenotype of heritable forms of developmental language impairment in twins using the Children's Nonword Repetition Test, claiming the test provides a definitive marker for such impairment. Konstantareas and Beichtman (1996) consider comorbidity between autistic disorders and developmental language disorders within the realm of genetic factors and infections during the prenatal, perinatal, and neonatal periods as well as neuroanatomical or neurofunctional abnormalities. While little focus is placed on psychogenic factors, in another study, Beitchman et al.(1996) found that children with pervasive language problems at age 5 demonstrated greater behavioral disturbances than subjects without such impairment.

Psychodynamic Correlates of the Language-Disordered Child

Our discussion so far has centered around general and specific psychogenetic factors contributing to language disorders in children. At this point, it would be useful to consider in more detail how language deviations manifest themselves psychodynamically relative to the major linguistic dimensions of phonology, semantics, and syntax.

In addition, we must recognize the psychological effects language disorders sometimes have on the child as well as on other members of the family. Although these effects may vary relative to a known organic base, such as a childhood brain injury, mental retardation, or deafness, or relative to a functional base, such as environmental deprivation or family dysfunction, we find many similarities as well as differences. How the child and family members cope with either a developing language

disability or an established disorder itself depends on the interrelationship among unique organismic factors within the child, the special circumstances of the family, and the attitudes of each family member. Because experimental evidence identifying these factors is not yet forthcoming, we have to rely on clinical evidence to postulate or at least speculate about such variables.

Specificity of the Disorder

The literature reveals no experimental evidence to suggest what definitive psychological effects, if any, occur in relation to specific language disorders. It is understood that original etiological-psychological factors may persist beyond the actual establishment of the disorder and be confounded by the way the child or family may respond to the language delay. Also possible is that the original etiological factors may no longer persist but that the language delay does, along with its accompanying psychological effects.

Most workers would agree that even the language-delayed child is saying some words by age 18 months and that some normal children may be saying little by 3 years of age. Therefore, the task of the speech-language pathologist is to distinguish exactly and as early as possible those children whose language represents a significant and definitive problem from those children who may be developing language somewhat later for unremarkable reasons. Moreover, it may be necessary to determine those psychological correlates that are manifestations of difficulty in conceptualizing information, difficulty in learning the language code, difficulty in applying the code conventionally, difficulty in using the code in speaking, or a late development of cognition, conventional code, and use of the code (Bloom and Lahey, 1978).

We cannot ignore, however, the evidence of the undetection of language disorders in psychiatrically disturbed children even when the child enters school, as reflected in the research of Cohen and Horodezky (1998) and Cohen et al. (1998). While language impairment had been identified previously in one sample of children, these children were more likely to be diagnosed with attention deficit hyperactivity disorder. Zalewska (1998) presents a psychological picture of children diagnosed according to the *Diagnostic and Statistical Manual-IV* (DSM-IV) as having expressive language disorders but only as one of a number of specific symptoms of a broader syndrome associated with the mother-child relationship. In perhaps somewhat strong terms, Zalewska argues that "annihilation of personal existence lies at the core of expressive language disorder" (p. 31). Perhaps, but only in the midst of an essentially silent environment or one where the child is deprived of virtually all sensory input. In their retrospective study of a sample of children and adolescents with mental retardation or developmental disabilities, Harden and Sahl (1997) found depression, posttraumatic stress, and developmental speech-language disorders in the high-functioning subjects.

Phonological Variations

Lewis and Freebairn (1997) subgrouped children with familial phonologic disorders and found that poorer oral motor coordination and productive phonology may distinguish individuals with familial phonologic disorders from individuals with phonologic disorders of unknown etiology. Rousey, one of the earliest investigators to advocate that articulation is symptomatic of a fundamental psychological disturbance, declares, "errors in articulation of consonants reflect developmental failures in personality rather than reflecting stops or arrests in the normal maturation process of speech articulation" (1971, p. 820). He appears to distinguish speech production from subsequent verbal language patterns, a proposition at variance with current thinking on language theory and development.

Representing a psychoanalytic viewpoint, Rousey refers to Erikson's infantile sexuality theory in describing the clinical meanings of misarticulated sounds. He hypothesizes the following:

- Disturbance in early and significant relationships with the father is represented by the substitution of /f/ for /θ/.
- Deprivation disturbance in the mother-child relationship is represented by distortions and substitutions of the /l/.

- The oral expression of aggression in the child is manifested in the substitution of /d/ for /ð/.
- Fixation of the child at the infantile level is represented by the persistence of a frontal lisp.
- Difficulty in early psychosexual development during the anal period is represented by the appearance of a lateral lisp.
- Anxiety characterizes the production of a strident (whistling) /s/.
- Early lack of impulse control and the inappropriate release of aggression are represented in both the consonantal and vowel /r/.
- Early fixation in psychosexual development is represented by the interchange of sounds characteristic of the oral stage of development. (p. 821)

In a later formulation, Rousey (1974) suggests that when the individual has experienced some sexual trauma, in reality or fantasy, substitution of /v/ for /ð/ may occur. He further suggests that substitution of /w/ for /r/ represents dependence on obsessional styles of thinking.

It is important to understand from Rousey's theory that "the presence of a sound articulated correctly reflects mastery of stages of emotional development" (1974, p. viii) is based essentially on years of clinical evidence but not verified by any substantial experimental data. Although some of the experimental results reported by Rousey and his colleagues suggest trends in support of certain aspects of his theory, he is careful to suggest that much more research must be done.

We would agree but, at the same time, not ignore the wealth of clinical evidence gathered to support Rousey's intriguing theory. One, in fact, need not subscribe to classic psychoanalytic theory to find some substantiation for a relationship between ego and articulatory development. Indeed, it would be difficult to treat articulatory or phonological development as an entity apart from the total organismic nature of the individual. Yet, in a later publication, which deals with the psychological factors affecting speech production, there is only a brief allusion to Rousey's theoretical development (Darby, 1981). We would hope that such an omission does not represent a total rejection of antipsychoanalytic psychiatry, as even the broad implications of Rousey's work cannot be ignored.

Regardless of psychodynamic theory, it is conceivable that dysfunctional family interrelationships, in which the child becomes the identified victim, may determine specific phonological errors, with or without other accompanying behavioral symptoms. Although at present it is difficult to make a strong case for a phonemic specificity, because articulatory-deficient children tend to have multiple errors, it is possible that the phonemic *pattern* represents the psychodynamic status of the child. Moreover, it might be useful to explore deviations in psychological development in terms of distinctive feature analysis. Most important is that we, as professionals, remain open to any possibility, regardless of previously cherished beliefs.

Syntactic and Semantic Variations

Although it would be tempting to speculate on a relationship between deviations in psychological development and deviations in the form and the content with which the child uses language, nothing in the literature investigated supports such a conjecture relative to typical language-delayed children. The difficulty in designing studies to test such relationships has been addressed by Weintraub (1981), who experimentally investigated the relationship between the use of syntax in adults and psychological defense mechanisms and found that inferences about behavior and personality can be made from analysis of the major features of free speech. He states, "We must consider . . . the fact that the frequency of occurrence of even simple grammatical structures is so dependent upon cognitive, maturational factors in preschool children that the influence of emotional variables may be extremely difficult to determine" (p. 46).

Professionals in the field generally agree that autistic children demonstrate, among other characteristics, disturbances in cognitive and linguistic processes. Although it is not our purpose here to delve into the biochemical-psychogenic conflict over etiology, we agree with Rutter (1978), among others, that many symptoms could be secondary to the primary disturbance of cognitive-linguistic impairment.

According to the DSM-IV criteria established by the American Psychiatric Association (1994) for autistic disorder, the child's language development is grossly defective, often characterized by echolalia, immediate or delayed, or reversal of first and second person pronouns, and metaphorical language. There may be a total lack of the development of language and impairment in reciprocal social interaction. Fish and Rivto (1979) report that, in some cases, babbling is retarded from the start and the child is mute. In others, both babbling and the first words may develop normally or with minimal delay, only to be arrested or to regress at the end of the second year or at the beginning of the third. In those children with more developed speech, the use of complex syntax, the formation of long sentences, and the comprehension of subtle and abstract meaning are disturbed with characteristic distortions of syntax and fragmentation of speech. Fish and Rivto also note the use of idiosyncratic terms that may be understood only if the original context of the child's association is known.

Effects of the Disorder on the Child

Regardless of the type, nature, quality, or degree of language dysfunction, the child will react to the difficulty relative to his or her unique perception of it. Secondary symptoms in the form of defenses may appear to counteract the anxiety or gain some degree of control of the anxiety. The choice of method and the quality with which the child manifests such defenses are due to a complex interaction of the child's identification with the coping style of the parent, personal developmental level, and personal unique coping style. Whereas many children with recognition and awareness of their phonological, syntactic, or semantic discrepancies readily cope and adapt with approximations toward normalcy, others are stuck in the mire of linguistic dysfunction. For these children, behavioral and personality changes occur that often obscure the earlier predisposing conditions associated with the development of the language disorder.

In their review of the literature, Cantwell and Baker (1977) found a tendency toward psychiatric dysfunction in speech-language-disordered children. Confirmation of this tendency was later reported by Cantwell, Baker, and Mattison (1979). In childhood psychosis, defensive behaviors become the most apparent characteristics of the child's illness and are basic to the actual syndromes of autism, symbiotic psychosis, and pseudoneurotic psychosis (Thompson and Havelkova 1983). Beitchman et al.(1996) found that children with pervasive speech-language problems at age 5 demonstrated greater behavioral disturbances than those 5-year-olds with no speech-language problems. Moreover, when the former sample population was examined at age 12, those with early auditory comprehension problems were found to be more aggressive and hyperactive.

Among the specific effects of language disorders of children are changes in self-concept, somatic problems, behavior disorders, and educational problems.

Stress and Coping

It would be convenient to generalize that the language-disordered child will develop a distorted self-image similar to that of the stuttering child. Nothing in the literature reviewed, however, suggests such a corollary. Certainly, the child may be conscious or made conscious of the inability to communicate appropriately by many factors, such as parental and sibling reaction or the attitude of peers and others. We are led to consider, then, how the unique personal coping mechanism operates relative to the degree of stress experienced by the child.

The coping process plays a dual function, including the regulation of emotional distress and solving the problem (Rutter, 1983). We doubt that it comes into play, relative to the child's awareness of a language deficiency, until 5 to 7 years of age, Piaget's concrete operational stage (Wadsworth, 1996). Among other things, the child now is able to compare personal linguistic functioning, in part at least, with that of others and experiences the anxiety that comes with being unable to command appropriate use of the language. Citing the work of Rose (1976), Maccoby (1983) speculates that, because the hippocampus, which has a role in behavioral maturation, does not fully mature until the age of 6 years, it is possible that the child's ability to cope may be partly connected to physiological maturation. If we add temperamental differences (presently we do not know if these are genetically or environmentally determined or both) and envi-

ronmental response as one further variable, it is apparent that no simple explanation regarding the response by the child to personal language functioning is possible.

Although not referring to language disorders per se, Rutter (1983) states the overall problem succinctly: "Intuitively, it seems that the coping process itself, in terms of active problem solving and of emotional palliation, is likely to influence outcome, but empirical data on the actual importance of coping mechanisms are still lacking" (p. 34).

Somatic Changes

A somatoform disorder is the physical expression and experience by the individual of an inability to cope successfully with psychosocial events. Although little empirical or experimental evidence suggests that the child's inability to cope with the language deficiency will be expressed somatically, it is useful to explore the possibilities. Baker, Cantwell, Mattison (1980), in their studies of 46 children with pure speech disorders and 53 children with both speech and language disorders, found that among the major complaints were those somatic in nature. We concur with Geist (1983) that it is unlikely for a linear cause-and-effect relationship, in which a complex interaction of psychological, social, and physical factors takes place, to prove more useful.

Billy, a 6-year-old boy, had been suffering asthmatic attacks for several months. On intake, he evidenced severe expressive language difficulties. The family lived on a remote farm, generally removed from social contact. Clinical testing of nonverbal performance revealed intelligence functioning to be within the norm. Cognitive receptive language also essentially was intact. Medical data, including neurological information, were unremarkable except for the asthma. The mother reported that, three years previously, at about the time Billy stopped speaking, the family was desperately attempting to save their farm from foreclosure. Although the family survived the threat to their personal and economic lives, Billy apparently was fixated developmentally in his expressive language. The mother further reported that Billy was generally ignored, except for satisfying his basic needs, during the family's struggle to maintain the farm. Hungry for attention from his mother and his father, Billy often would sit in his room picking at his toys and was generally disinterested in television. When he carried over his isolated behavior to kindergarten, his teacher initiated the referral for help.

It would be presumptuous of us to draw any definitive conclusions from this anecdote, except to suggest that while psychogenetic-social conflicts may have played a primary role in the linguistic lag, subsequent psychogenetic-social factors may have played a definitive secondary role in exacerbating the language disorder. That a somatic illness may be associated with such factors cannot be ignored.

Behavioral Problems

Profound behavioral changes in language-different children are most readily observed in autistic children. Based on his own empirical evidence and the research of others, Prizant (1983) suggests that the complex we know as the autistic syndrome, which includes deviant language, difficulties in social interaction, and compulsive and ritualistic behaviors such as echolalia, must be viewed in an interactive way. He further adds that the phenomena evidenced should be studied relative to cognitive processing and cognitive-linguistic development. Prizant appears to straddle the gap between viewing the communicative dysfunction as either a primary or secondary deficit and gives the impression of favoring a type of coping mechanism used by the autistic child. Such a mechanism is not unlike that presented by Rutter (1983), which was discussed earlier.

Although qualitatively different, the performance deficit associated with mentally retarded children can be viewed as an impairment of adaptive behavior, to a certain degree. We would agree that genetic and physiological factors set limits in these children's language acquisition and usage and ultimate language repertoire. But we cannot ignore the adventitious effects on language by their response to their own deficits.

According to Beier (1964), behavioral disturbance tends to occur more frequently in the mentally retarded than in the general population, but the degree to which the retarded child can respond to his or her own awareness of a language deficit is unclear. Certainly, the child who approximates near normal intellectual functioning is more likely to be aware of personal communicative abilities and will attempt to cope accordingly. But, even with the moderately retarded child whose language is successfully remediated, it is obvious that a modicum of awareness of the deficit can be present What effects such awareness may have on the child prior to remediation have not been revealed in the literature surveyed. One thing is certain, however, the mentally retarded child is more vulnerable to the development of unsuitable behavior than the normally endowed child in the form of anxiety, hyperactivity, and a deficient self-concept.

Some children who are unable to acquire language capability because of known neurological etiology are commonly referred to as *congenitally aphasic* or *developmentally aphasic*. They are striking in their manifestations of emotional lability, distractibility, and hyperactivity. We must be cautious, however, not to equate these children with autistic children, who present a somewhat different symptom complex.

The inability of developmentally aphasic children to process information auditorally contributes to the confusion and disorganized behavior often seen by therapists (Emerick and Hatten, 1979). When we consider, then, the constellation of primary deficits present, it is not difficult to understand the problem such a child would have in coping emotionally. Less understood is whether or not the child's coping behavior is a manifestation of the primary deficit, a secondary one, or both, as we have seen in adult aphasia.

If we add to these behavioral responses family reactions, we are confronted with a formidable challenge to sort out those elements most amenable to change. Treatment of one or more features would certainly influence the impact of the disability on the child.

With respect to more typical speech- and language-delayed children seen in school, Baker, Cantwell, and Mattison (1980) found immaturity, restlessness, short attention span, excitability, tantrums, constant climbing, and solitary behavior to be characteristic of children with both speech and language disorders. It should be noted, however, that certain methodological problems in their study, such as lack of a "normal" control group of children, sampling method, and heterogenity problems (for example, mixing dysarthric with functional disorders) preclude us from making further definitive judgments. Nonetheless, it would be difficult for us to purport that speech- and language-delayed children are oblivious to their difficulties and suggest that these children probably represent a high-risk factor for behavior disorders.

Vallance, Cummings, and Humphries (1998), using a developmental-organizational perspective to investigate problem behaviors in linguistically impaired children, found the children's impaired social interactional functioning to be the core of the development of behavioral symptomatology. Their findings seem supported by Brinton and Fujiki (1999), who also found children with SLI to have encountered social difficulties in tasks involving access, negotiation, and cooperation.

Educational Problems

Although it is not our intention to explore the vast domain of the learning-disabled child and his or her environment, it generally is agreed that language problems are common among children with learning problems. Because the ability to use language is critical to the development of other academic skills, it is not surprising that the language-deficient child, regardless of etiology, who enters school will demonstrate varying degrees of personality and behavioral problems such as poor interpersonal relationships, hyperactivity, aggression, anxiety, disinterest, anger, hostility, and selective attention difficulties. To what degree these characteristics are primary to subsequent academic underachievement or are consequential to biogenetic bases for underachievement is not yet fully understood.

Beasley's (1956) classic contribution, written more than 40 years ago, is still timely to our understanding of the child with delayed language development:

> It can be inferred that a young child who does not develop language at the usual time will bring to a language-learning situation all his previous experiences. He will have acquired certain attitudes about himself as a nonspeaker, reflecting what others think about him (funny, bad, stupid, slow, stubborn, lazy, etc.), which may act as a barrier to learning. He will also have developed certain patterns of behavior to cope with his language inadequacy, such as withdrawal, aggressiveness, apathy, or dependency, which will affect his attempts to talk. He will have been exposed to efforts employed by others to induce him to talk. These will color the way he perceives the teacher's efforts. (pp. 52–53)

Although much of what we can say, definitively or generally, about the complex internal and external forces that impinge on the child's striving toward linguistic adequacy is still within the realm of speculation and uncertainty, Beasley's elegant and lucid words deserve to be heeded. Indeed, some empirical support, although meager, for Beasley's formulations is evidenced in the Baker et al. study alluded to earlier. Evaluations by teachers of speech- and language-disordered children in their study revealed many adjustment problems, including a negative attitude toward authority, diminished academic achievement, and disruptive behavior. As speech-language pathologists, it is incumbent on us to develop more precise means to intervene appropriately when dysfunctional behavior is evidenced in language-disordered children. How this may be accomplished is discussed later.

Effects of the Disorder on the Family

In their critical review of the literature on psychiatric disorders in children, Cantwell and Baker (1977) cautiously take the position that, except in rare instances, psychiatric disorders do not cause speech and language delay. They do state, however, that in most cases psychiatric difficulties are caused indirectly by the speech and language delay.

Alluding to the methodological problems associated with the definition of psychiatric disorder, the delineation of precise types of language delays, and the determination of other related factors such as intellectual retardation and brain damage, they take the position that the parent-child interaction must be better understood. They suggest that the language-delayed child will be the most likely child in the family to "evoke disturbed patterns of parent-child interaction" because of the child's difficulty in communicating, because of individual temperament, or for other reasons. The child, in turn, will be more likely to develop emotional difficulties. Support for such conclusion is provided by Richman, Stevenson, and Graham (1982), who describe the behavioral difficulties feeding into the child-parent loop, thus affecting the sensitivity and emotional quality of the parent responses, which in turn affect the child's emotional and linguistic state.

We support such a contention but would add that a triadic or even a quadrant interaction should be considered more consistent with family systems theory. The effects of language delay on total family interaction cannot be underestimated, as any pronounced change in one family member will disrupt the equilibrium of the entire family, with each member striving to reestablish the family balance.

What is important to understand is that the family is an interaction of personalities, in which the members react to each other as individuals. Each has a particular conception of his or her role as well as a conception of the roles of all other family members. Any alteration in behavior of one member (for example, the SLI child) is viewed by other members in the light of their own personal perspectives or temperaments, which in turn will affect the original family member's perception of style. The child then will react to the way in which he or she is perceived. If the perception of one or another family member is imbued with negativism, the child will respond behaviorally in the way discussed earlier and coincidentally begin to perceive him- or herself negatively. This will further exacerbate the initial family attitude and response.

It should be made clear that this does not necessarily infer that the SLI child who reacts aberrantly does so in response to deep-rooted family psychopathology. We prefer to review dysfunctional or inappropriate family response to the child along a broad spectrum of typical family life, with the admonition that, even in the best of families, members become victims of their own peculiar attitudes and temperaments. That the child and indeed the family need assistance is obvious, but that intensive psychiatric intervention is always necessary does not represent our view.

The Reaction from Parents

Our discussion has implied that the child's language disorder has as much of an effect on parents' reac-

tions as the latter does on the child's response to the disorder, as well as on the disorder itself. Many of us are familiar with parents of language-disordered children who report that they had been told, "Don't worry, he'll outgrow his baby talk." Our concern about these families is not so much that the child undoubtedly would have benefited from earlier language therapy intervention but that the family, particularly the parents, would have been spared the anxiety, uncertainty, and confusion about the child's language competency despite the earlier reassuring imperative statement.

Parents often demonstrate an uncanny intuitive ability to recognize that "something is not right" and, because of well-intended but glib statements from professionals unfamiliar with developmental linguistic processes, begin to question their own integrity as parents, which in turn may further negatively influence their child's language development and self-concept. Weintraub (1981) reminds us that the failure of parents to interpret their child's immature language usage during the course of everyday family interaction can result in both noncomprehension and misunderstanding. We would add that such breakdowns in communication will contribute further to difficulties in the child-parent relationship.

The Reaction from Siblings

Siblings of SLI children often become forgotten members of the family and, in terms of family systems theory, the "silent identified patient." That is, while the parents are preoccupied with the other child, the nonaffected siblings may either receive less attention, become the objects of unrealistic expectations by the parents, or be made scapegoats by others.

Lefebvre (1983), discussing sibling reactions to a handicapped child in the family, cites several studies that describe how the sibling may be affected. Among the studies noted, that of Shere and Kastenbaum (1966) found emotional disturbance among nonaffected twins more often than among affected twins, with genetic endowment held constant. Lavigne and Ryan (1979) found more irritability and social withdrawal in siblings of handicapped children, before age 5, than in siblings of chronically ill children.

Therapists frequently report overindulgence of the affected child by an older sibling who understands the affected child's deficient use of language or the avoidance of interaction by the sibling with the child. Even occasional ridicule or teasing by the unaffected sibling could interfere with the affected child's attempts to cope and may contribute to the disruption of family relationships. We suggest that such behavior may be indicative of the unaffected sibling feeling a threat to his or her own place in the family or developing self-concept.

Because no studies have revealed definitively negative attitudes by siblings, we hesitate to make any generalizations about their behavior. We do suggest, however, that such investigations could be very fruitful in adding to our understanding of the psychosocial dynamics in families with language-disordered children.

Effects of Other People on the Child

Even less data are available on the negative effects that peers, teachers, and other professionals have on the child who is deficient in language. Fortunately, teachers and other professionals are more likely to have a positive effect through therapeutic and educational intervention. Nonetheless, it is useful to consider some of the evidence that suggests negative influence on the child from external sources.

The Reaction from Peers

Although very young children with language disorders may be relatively unaware of how they are viewed by their peers and unconcerned about or unaware of the discrepancy in language development, the school-age child is increasingly sensitive to the reaction of others. Thus the language-disordered child becomes vulnerable to humiliation or shame if their language proficiency is inconsistent with the unwitting norm established.

Flavel (1979) describes the growing awareness of one's image as perceived by others as part of a larger developmental process that is described as "meta-cognition." That is, the entering school-age child is beginning to develop skills at monitoring his or her own thought processes and performance. The SLI child, in our view, however, may not have developed such skills, placing the child in the situation of being vulnerable to the growing cognitive

perceptions of peers. Struggling to cope with the personal perception that "something is different" and responding to peer reaction, the child begins to behave in ways that are perceived even more negatively by peers. The child is caught in a vicious cycle of attempting to please, being unable to do so, struggling further, and incurring even further negation. In their study of social interactional behaviors of children with SLI, Brinton and Fujiki (1999) report that teacher ratings of these children found them lacking social skills, self perceptions of loneliness, and diminished peer contact.

The more pronounced the language deviation, the greater is the likelihood of negation, particularly in the case of the mentally retarded, emotionally disturbed, hearing-impaired, or aphasic child. Certainly, the degree to which the child responds and the quality of that response depend on internal factors such as temperament and individual coping mechanisms and external factors such as the family support system.

The Reaction from Teachers

Few workers would disagree that the teacher's attitude and behavior toward the SLI child may have a profound effect on the child's continuing language development.

Weinberg and Santana (1978) argue that overidentification with the child and rescuing the child from psychological and social pressures may result in insensitivity to the parents' needs and frustrations and may be in competition with them. Although these authors refer to handicapped children in general, we believe their concerns would apply to the SLI child.

Writing on the language problems of disadvantaged children, Shuy (1972) describes in vivid detail how difficult many teachers find it to cope appropriately with their pupils, either through lack of training or through frustration over their inability to handle the concomitant problems associated with language delay or usage in that population. Pleading for further research in teacher attitudes in this area, Shuy urges that special attention be given to them and that teachers be required "to develop an ability to learn how to deal with the child's language, how to listen and respond to it, how to diagnose what is needed, how to best teach alternative linguistic systems, and how to treat it as a positive entity" (p. 203). More than that, however, it is further incumbent on the teacher that differentiation be made between language that is ethnically rich and language that indeed is impaired.

We believe that the quality of response by the teacher to learning-disabled, emotionally disturbed, aphasic, hearing-impaired, and mentally retarded children who are linguistically impaired is no less important. The either overestimation or underestimation of these children's capabilities will interfere with their progressive development in language and in other behaviors. We do not question the academic competency with which the teacher helps these children, but we are concerned that the teacher may not always have the self-awareness of personal deep-rooted feelings that may emerge as projections toward these children and that may interfere with their honorable intentions (see Chapter 9 for a more extensive discussion on the issue). There is little doubt in our minds that the way the teacher perceives the child and the language disability influence the way the child perceives self and the language disability. Only further experimental study of these provocative issues can bring to light the complex nature of these relationships.

The Reaction from Other Professionals

Parents of SLI children or children who they believe to be language-disordered typically put great faith in the ability of professionals to provide the necessary information and expertise to help them and the children and perhaps to assuage their guilt over their own real or imagined responsibility for the disorder. Such faith is a formidable challenge to the professional, who is placed in the position of being all-knowing and is expected to answer to parental concerns that may go beyond the professional's level of competency.

The implication is that, as professionals, we must have a keen sense of our own specialized knowledge and a mature acknowledgment and acceptance of our limitations. To believe or do otherwise is to fault ourselves and certainly the already fragile family concerns. Glib, condescending, or authoritative-sounding responses to genuine and sometimes naive questions only obscure the real issues, delay necessary intervention, and perhaps alienate the parents from subsequent professional assistance. In any case, the language-disordered child also suffers.

In the final analysis, only appropriate referral or comprehensive differential assessment will address the needs expressed by the family. We must trust that such is the rule in real practice and that any exception is an isolated event to which we must direct our influence in affecting change.

Intervention Strategies

It is apparent to any serious worker in the field of childhood language disorders that emotional components may be difficult to separate from cognitive and symptom-based treatment strategies. In keeping within the context of this chapter and the tone of the rest of the book, however, we focus only on treatment models that are essentially psychological in nature, bearing in mind their effects on cognitive and linguistic processes.

Because it is generally understood that language develops within the framework of the interpersonal relationships among family members, the mother-child relationship in particular, we believe, as Beasley (1956) suggested, that interpersonal relationships are as important for the child without language or with disordered language. It is important, therefore, to reacquaint ourselves with the work of Cameron (1947), who Beasley quotes and who we believe needs to be recognized as one of the earliest writers on a pragmatic approach to language learning. Cameron states:

> Language habits creep so gradually into all reactions that no one can really say of a child's behavior, "Here at this instant role-taking in terms of language had its start." In play, language at first functions merely as a component or an accompaniment, but later and secondarily it acquires status as a semi-independent, equivalent form of behavior that allows its possessor to take roles first in words without deeds and then in fantasy as well. We have pointed out that language habits mold us into conformity with our culture, because language is a cultural product and highly conventionalized, and we have said that through language our covert symbolic behavior is also organized along social lines. On the other side of the

ledger is the fact that language and organized thought are together a means of enriching our potentialities for social role-taking enormously.

Talking becomes in itself not only the most effective instrument of interpersonal communication, eventually superseding all others, but also the medium through which one builds up a repertory of social roles. By learning to say what others say in context, a child learns first to express his attitudes and then by expressing these conventional attitudes appropriately, he tends actually to acquire them as his own. (p. 95)

Intervening on the interpersonal level, however, also requires that we recognize that some language-disordered children will not be responsive to a unitary approach. As Wachs (1984) points out, similar intervention approaches are not applicable to all types of language-disordered children. It is necessary, he believes, to look at the individual characteristics of each child, relative to the child's particular earlier experience, social environment, and biological differences.

We further take the synergistic position, reviewed by Schwartz et al. (1980), that phonological deficits are one aspect of total linguistic behavior and that our counseling intervention makes no distinction based on differing forms or content of such behavior. We do acknowledge, however, that individual differences, regardless of the nature of the linguistic disorder, must be considered.

Play Therapy

We typically have seen play therapy employed with stuttering children (see Chapter 4) and with language-disordered children for the purpose of resolving the child's negative feeling about self and others. We submit that play therapy has a far greater value by enhancing the linguistic competence of very young language-disordered children.

Because play constitutes a major means by which young children formulate, develop, and solidify all parameters of the linguistic process, it makes sense that we should implement therapeutic procedures to enhance these processes. The importance of the interpersonal communicative interaction between child and parent further supports our rationale for the use of play strategies to simulate such interactions.

We do not believe that play should be used only with language-disordered children who also happen to be emotionally disturbed. On the contrary, its value can be demonstrated in very young children who are language disordered, regardless of etiology, family function, or emotional adjustment. We recognize that such a viewpoint is a departure from traditionally held beliefs about play therapy, but we believe, nonetheless, that we can justify its use in a more generic way.

A Behavioral-Symptomatic-Linguistic Approach

Earlier in this book we described how play therapy may successfully be used with young stuttering children, utilizing the model originally introduced and developed by Axline (1969). With certain modifications appropriate for use with the language-disordered child, we have developed an approach based on behavioral-symptomatic principles and the principles of transformational grammar.

1. *Establishing rapport.* Utilizing play materials both familiar and unfamiliar to the child, the therapist joins the child in play, first with those materials chosen by the child. The therapist refrains from verbalization, unless the child verbalizes first, in order to establish a situation whereby the child feels in partnership with the therapist. Any threat to the status quo of the child thus can be minimized or averted to provide an atmosphere of safety in which intercommunication can occur gradually. Most important is that the child feels that a friendship is developing. All attempts at "teaching" by the therapist should be avoided at this time.

2. *Accepting the child as a person.* One of the most formidable tasks for the therapist is to avoid the trap of taking the position of the authority who knows what is best for the child. Such a position denies the child free expression of the self and the opportunity for verbal communication to occur and develop. Instead, the therapist must acknowledge and accept the child nonjudgmentally, with the understanding that the child has the capacity to change and learn. This means the formulation of a relationship in which

mutual respect naturally develops through the interchange of two people.

3. *Providing an atmosphere for feelings to be freely expressed.* As the child gradually begins to feel secure in the relationship, the opportunity for the expression of any feeling, untouched by the therapist's judgment, occurs. It is facilitated by the therapist's own expression of feelings within the context of the play situation. It further allows the therapist a better understanding of the child's present cognitive-linguistic processing behavior. Permissiveness in the relationship is not meant to imply license for the acting-out child to damage physical surroundings or for physically abusing the therapist. The therapist must respond to this child not as a parent or as a child but as another person whose personal rights have been infringed upon. We believe it is possible to set limits within the therapeutic situation whereby the child may learn the importance of mutual respect and yet at the same time not feel constraints on the expression of feelings.

4. *Reflecting the expression of feelings and thoughts.* As the relationship develops, the child feels freer in expressing feelings and thoughts to which the therapist may respond via the method introduced by Rogers (described in Chapter 1). The therapist also may use modeling techniques as described by Courtright and Courtright (1976) and Van Riper and Emerick (1984), whereby the child's play is verbalized, using appropriate transformational forms ranging from "daddy" to "daddy's coming home." Van Riper and Emerick's description of the use of expansions, extensions, self-talk, and parallel talk is particularly pertinent, so that the child is provided the full opportunity to be exposed to appropriate language usage.

5. *Encouraging child-centered choice and change making.* As the child gradually begins to recognize that expressed feelings are being accepted and to be aware of developing language usage, he or she also develops the capacity to make choices and changes appropriate to the growing self-concept. The latter we believe also positively influence the more complex use of language as the child gains more and more control over the immediate environment, albeit a clinical one at first. With direct or indirect parental support, the possibilities for even greater positive change are enhanced. We see the developing self-concept and increased language usage as interdependent, so that both must be consistently encouraged.

6. *Allowing therapy to proceed at a pace appropriate to the child.* We believe it is inappropriate, as Van Riper and Emerick have suggested, always to correct the child's misarticulations or inaccurate use of language. We never can be certain that the child is ready to be corrected, nor can we be sure if it is an effective way to enhance proper linguistic usage. A more effective approach is the use of modeling of self-correction by the therapist, vividly described by Van Riper and Emerick. Depending on the child's response to the therapist's self-correction, it is possible to determine the readiness of the child to move forward.

7. *Using language as an integral part of interpersonal relationships.* The child soon discovers that language and the personal relationship with another person are closely interwoven. Through the clinical experience, the child recognizes, on some undefined level, the effect that each has on the other.

8. *Being sensitive to multicultural language patterns.* Exciting opportunities exist for the therapist who is able to enter the world of children who are linguistically different and who may or may not have a SLI. The therapist should first attempt to learn linguistic segments from the child so that each interchange roles as both teacher and student, learning each other's patterns and helping to reinforce rapport as well.

9. *Measuring responses and taking a leadership role.* Play therapy often has been criticized for its apparent unstructured and undisciplined process, not amenable to measurement. We would agree that total permissiveness within the play therapy situation would be counterproductive in terms of language and personal enhancement. We take the position that the therapist, like the child, must take the prerogative to lead clinical events toward a positive outcome. Children appreciate adult control and direction as long as it is done with respect for the child as a person.

We do not know if the need to learn is an innate process, but workers in our field are well aware of the pleasure evidenced by children who learn to use language more effectively under direction by the therapist. Therefore, play therapy may be structured in such a way as to facilitate the counting of appropriate linguistic responses in accordance with sound behavioral principles, without infringing on the clinical interpersonal relationship.

A Social-Interactional Approach

Social-interactional approaches have achieved greater prominence over the last several years and are concisely reviewed and described by Gallagher (1996). She includes modeling, coaching, and problem-solving procedures, incorporating these with pragmatic language intervention. The use of positive peer promotion also receives major attention by Gallagher. Utilizing cooperative group experiences, less burden is placed on the child with SLI and more on the actual group itself so that all contribute to the satisfactory completion of socially sound linguistic goals. While little reference is made to the positive psychological effects on the child, the rewards are obvious.

Family Therapy

A comprehensive search of the literature through computer data banks has revealed few studies that describe the use of a family therapy approach in the treatment of language disorders in children. In their article on the effectiveness of family therapies for selected behavioral disorders of childhood as they relate to language, Estrada and Pinsof (1995) review only autism since, as they state, "it is the only pervasive developmental disorder for which there is a clear body of research involving family-oriented interventions" (p. 426). Their review of the research appears to show promise in the treatment of families coping with autism and child management skills and attitudinal improvements. Consistent with our earlier discussions relevant to the development of SLI in children, we maintain that family therapy can be used as a unitary or

complementary method to enhance language development.

More recently, Briggs (1998) outlines a four-phase process for establishing therapeutic alliances with families of children with SLI among other communicative impairments. She superimposes family therapy techniques onto speech-language therapy techniques and urges more specific information be provided in the speech-language pathology literature on how to work with families as the major decision makers on early intervention teams. Griffer (1997) proposes the use of a competency-based approach conducting family-centered assessments and the need for the development and implementation of a family systems curriculum. Such a curriculum would require the training of speech-language pathologists in family-centered principles, strategies, and techniques in the delivery of early intervention services. Positive feedback from parents accents the importance of such formal and clinical training.

Although we have worked with families in which therapy appeared to have little impact on the child's disordered language, we can report successes with other families. The following is a case in point.

Jamie R, 5 years old, was referred by the family pediatrician, a physician who was keenly knowledgeable about developmental language stages in children. On initial intake, Jamie presented with speech and language characterized by vowelized articulation with concomitant unintelligible language usage. Syntactic patterning was evident, suggesting that cognitive skills were operational to a great degree. Formal nonverbal performance tasks revealed above-normal intelligence, and informal play did not indicate the presence of emotional dysfunction.

Jamie was one of six children, of whom the nearest in age was Jill, 11 years old. Two other siblings were older adolescents, and the other two were in their twenties. Only one of them did not live at home. Mrs. R was a full-time homemaker and Mr. R was an airline executive.

The initial family therapy session, which included Jamie, Jill, and Mr. and Mrs. R, provided an opportunity to obtain the background history, including medical information. The only remarkable data to come forth revealed that Jamie was considered and treated essentially as the "baby" in the family, doted on from the earliest age by all family members except Mr. R, who often was away for days at a time on business trips. A live-in Spanish-speaking maid, who also cared for Jamie while Mrs. R attended classes at a local junior college, was said often to speak to Jamie in Spanish. Jamie reportedly understood a considerable amount of the second language, but apparently did not attempt to use it expressively.

It was hoped that the entire family could return for the second family therapy session, but conflicting schedules made that impossible. The maid, Juanita, however was now included. Although indications were apparent during the initial family therapy session, it was now clear that virtually all the participants attempted to speak for Jamie at various times. Mrs. R acknowledged that the other children did the same.

There appeared to be no underlying evidence of pronounced family dysfunction. This seemed to be a caring and loving family, the members of which were ready to do whatever was necessary to help Jamie. The author surmised that such was also the case for the absent siblings. Although Mr. and Mrs. R acknowledged that perhaps they had been contributors to Jamie's delayed language development, their concerns were not contaminated by defensive protestations. They appeared ready to do whatever was necessary to help Jamie.

Still puzzled by the apparent lack of extraordinarily negative etiological influences to account for Jamie's severe verbal expressive difficulties, we probed rather into the family interactional relationships. In doing so it was learned that Juanita had been with the family for only four years. Prior to that, Jamie had reached or surpassed developmental milestones, including the use of two intelligible words by nine months. Also, until that time, the family had had the services of a native housekeeper who had been with them many years. Her untimely death brought profound sadness to the family, which to now had not completed the mourning process.

The second session was extended one hour to allow the family, particularly Mr. and Mrs. R and Jill, to experience the pain which up to now had been concealed.

Apparently the family homeostasis had been severely disrupted upon the death of Mary (the housekeeper), resulting in a complex realignment of family members. It was not clear to me whether or not Jamie actually took on the role as the identified patient to reflect the underlying family grief, but the abrupt interruption of his developing expressive language at that time could not be ignored.

Subsequent family therapy sessions, which intermittently involved other family members, were used to facilitate the grief process, provide information about language and speech development, and provide an environment in which Jamie in particular could be allowed to communicate freely, albeit unintelligibly. Family members were provided specific guides to reinforce Jamie's correct linguistic approximations while avoiding correcting him.

To my unexpected surprise, within five months, Jamie's expressive speech and language had approached 80% intelligibility, without the benefit of traditional speech and language therapy, though he had been in kindergarten during that time. Termination of family therapy was mutually agreed on and a follow-up speech and language reevaluation one year hence revealed essentially normal speech and language consistent with his chronological age. Only w/r and th/s substitutions remained.

This case is one illustration of the exclusive use of family therapy and counseling to effect dramatic changes in a child's disordered language usage. We cannot ascertain, however, the exact elements of that process to bring about essentially normal language in the child. Obviously, all the details described plus those operating in a concealed manner were responsible.

What is pertinent to our present discussion is that family therapy does not always require a dysfunctional family per se to be successful. On the contrary, disordered language development in a child could be related to very subtle familial dynamics. Also, it must be noted that other traditional strategies certainly could have yielded similar results but without the concomitant resolution of other family issues. Most important, however, is our recognition and acceptance of the fact that it is possible for otherwise normal children to fail in their ability to acquire language normally.

Complementing our discussion of family systems, the reader is encouraged to become acquainted with the ethnographic position of Hammer (1998), who combines family systems theories with the necessity for including observable descriptions of behaviors that occur within the context of the family and child and the distinctive social environment in which they live. Not only does she insist that the family or caregivers participate as fully as possible in early intervention but urges the speech-language professional to utilize the family's skills in the enhancement of language development in the child, if impaired. Hammer believes that a family-centered approach to service delivery should remain in the control of the parents and not the therapists in the decision-making process. The ramifications for therapeutic intervention with culturally diverse populations are obvious. No longer should we impose our own professionally prescribed tactics but educate ourselves first in the linguistic and cultural environment in which we intervene.

Other Counseling Strategies

There is considerable literature on the use of counseling for parents of language-disordered children. Most has included the transmission of information to the parents about language development and training parents to use constructive communication strategies at home and to assist the child to practice assigned homework given by the child's speech-language pathologist.

The literature on the use of counseling with school-age children who are language impaired has been less fruitful, except in those cases in which the child also is emotionally disturbed or learning disabled. Unfortunately, most school speech-language pathology programs are not structured to provide, nor are school speech-language pathologists prepared to offer, counseling to the language-disordered child.

The least amount of empirical data available regards counseling in conjunction with the use of symptomatic strategies, but pragmatic approaches appear to be coming close to reconciling the two strategies.

Counseling the Parents

To counsel parents of language-disordered children effectively, it is necessary to go beyond piecemeal handouts of information to help alleviate only the language problem. We agree with Zedler (1972) that social acceptance, feelings of personal adequacy, and encouragement of individual potentialities are as important to the child as language management and, in fact, are an integral part of it.

Pressman (1983), in her study of the effects of a home-based early intervention program on parents' self-confidence and children's development, found for 30 child-parent participants that the parents' self-confidence as primary teacher of the child had increased. She also found increased stimulation in the home and in the children's intellectual development as measured by their growth in language.

Although several books published within the last 15 years have provided guidelines for the worker in special education to use with parents of handicapped children, Webster (1977) offers the practicing speech-language pathologist practical guides to developing appropriate counselor-parent relationships in working with communicatively impaired children. Molyneaux and Lane (1982) offer step-by-step procedures for working with parents of communicatively impaired children and provide the student and professional a unique interview analysis model to evaluate the effectiveness of the counselor-parent interview. Although few references surveyed reveal precise guidelines geared to counseling parents of language-disordered children, therapists can readily apply the principles described by Webster, Molyneaux, and Lane, and other researchers to whom they refer.

Finally, the role of the speech-language pathologist as counselor-educator for parents, to promote speech-language development before an interference in the process occurs, cannot be underestimated. The American Speech-Language-Hearing Association and Rossetti (1984) have addressed the need for workers in the field to counsel with mothers-to-be whose pregnancy was labeled high risk, to follow cases through their delivery, and to conduct annual follow-ups. Rosetti's general guidelines are based on the philosophic premise of the infant's right to optimum development, the need for early intervention, the responsibility of the parent as the primary programmer, the infant's need for nurturance, and the importance of "play" to the infant's development and a healthy family environment.

Counseling the Child

It is important for us to understand that counseling the school-age child or adolescent who is language delayed or language disordered does not imply that emotional disturbance must be a prerequisite condition. Language, we have seen, is learned or not learned within the context of biogenetic, cognitive, and interpersonal factors. Although we may be tempted to dismiss the language problem as an impeded stage of development, regardless of emotional components, it is more useful for us to understand the problem along a broad spectrum of human development and individual coping behavior.

We would certainly agree with Wiig and Semel (1984) that counseling would benefit the child or adolescent who needs to express feelings and attitudes about his or her deficit in order to "gain insight into the basis for the difficulties he experiences in interpersonal communication and into the causes for emotional reactions and inappropriate behavioral responses" (pp. 583–584). Equally important, in our view, is that the counseling process will actually enhance the form and content of the language behavior itself, without our necessarily working on the language independently.

We do not wish to imply that such an approach should or can be applied universally or indiscriminately. Children with neurological or organic involvement, or even those who are severely emotionally disturbed, are much more likely to respond favorably to conventional modes of speech-language therapy. In these cases, however, counseling as an adjunctive method also would be of value.

Following the broad guidelines outlined in Chapter 1 and applying principles already suggested for play therapy, it is possible to implement these in counseling with the language-impaired child, with due respect to differences in age abilities and severity of the problem. We also must be reminded that family therapy may be used to complement individual counseling procedures.

Active listening provides the opportunity to derive a clinical impression of the nature of the child's feelings, attitudes, and self-concept. Although these revelations may be not forthcoming immediately and the child may resist the relationship at first, patience on the part of the therapist

will soon nullify the resistance. Through the process of listening with empathy, openness, and awareness, the therapist feeds back to the child that which is perceived, thereby further stimulating the child's use of language.

When viewing the child as a person, the therapist's respect for the child may be manifested in the way language is used to develop the relationship. Even the child whose language functioning is severely delayed will respond nonverbally or perhaps verbally in the light of the therapist's unconditional regard.

We recently worked with a 6-year-old child who was essentially nonverbal but whose evaluative and cognitive skills were close to the norm. The child entered the office while I was munching a large, red apple. The fruit served to open up the relationship, which until then had been virtually nonexistent. Sharing the apple with the child, while imparting to her its delicious qualities, I was able for the first time in weeks to elicit two- and three-word forms along with appropriate effectual behavior. Most important, in the light of the present discussion, was the nature of the interaction, which was based on a mutual sharing of a pleasurable experience.

Often in our work with language-disordered children, we feel that, as therapists, we always must make the choices and decisions we believe to be in the best interests of the child and therapy. Unfortunately, as we emphasize the latter, we slight the former. We miss vital opportunities for language growth when we take a directive, albeit well-intentioned, therapeutic approach in which we do not provide opportunities for the child to bring his or her own world into the clinical world. The child offers us the richness of his or her experiences, which can be readily utilized within the context of our established strategies. Client choice and therapist choice need not be in conflict as long as the therapist can selectively determine which of the child's contributions are most compatible with the therapist's intentions. Therein lies the opportunity for a mutually satisfying therapeutic relationship, as well as a source for language enhancement.

With older children, particularly adolescents, the formulation of contracts will be necessary to reinforce clinical successes and ensure carryover into the child's daily life. Bearing in mind the previous discussion, only through a mutual give and take and respect for each other's ability and integrity can the contract become a constructive instrument to foster positive change. Although parental participation could well be encouraged, in many cases it must be consistent with the integrity of the child-therapist relationship. To do otherwise is to negate all the efforts that have gone into establishing the relationship and would nullify the results of therapy. Whatever the arrangements made, contract negotiation is a vital opportunity to eliminate further deficient language patterns and enhance more appropriate use of language.

Some SLI children, including those who are emotionally disturbed or delinquent, present to therapy many obstacles to language improvement. In these cases, the use of confrontation may be an effective means to help provide these children control over their own destructive, self-defeating behavior, which may be interfering with their language competency. Confrontation must occur, we maintain, in the context of a caring, nondefensive, and unconditional regard for the child, who is struggling to survive in a world perceived as threatening or rejecting. Although resistance to any kind of change, language or otherwise, may tax the emotional and intellectual limits of any therapist, these must be regarded as the child's attempt, albeit ineffectual, to cope with the present unbearable reality. Rigid, authoritarian, and judgmental attitudes on the part of the therapist will only exacerbate an already intolerable state of existence in the child and further entrench the negative attitudes toward other persons in the environment.

Used in conjunction with other strategies, confrontation can be a powerful tool not only to enhance the communicative therapeutic relationship but also to help the child realize how language can be used to achieve a more productive role for oneself in society.

Therapist self-disclosure is another technique that can be used successfully with SLI children of all ages. Thist is a way of having the child enter into the world of the therapist while losing neither personal integrity nor role identity. It is compatible with the earlier statement that the therapeutic relationship involves mutual respect in which the child is viewed and respected as a person.

Tim, a 16-year-old SLI adolescent, came from a family in which the father had been absent for 12 years and the mother was an alcoholic. Expelled from school many times, as well as in and out of juvenile hall for petty theft, Tim had other severe learning disabilities. Early efforts to help Tim with his language disability were unsuccessful until he had a therapist who was able to relate to him on his level. Sharing feelings of her own childhood struggles with Tim was instrumental in forming a therapeutic relationship in which Tim finally was able to trust an adult and start the long road toward educational and emotional adjustment, including functional language usage. Certainly, the therapeutic relationship could not have been sustained by the use of therapist self-disclosure alone, but through the judicious consideration and use of other techniques already described, positive change was possible.

Therapist sensitivity to the child's body language and paralinguistic behavior is especially important, particularly with the child who essentially is nonverbal. It is a valuable opportunity to discover cognitive processes concealed by the absence of verbal language. Although the therapist's verbalization of the nonverbal message may not always be on target, more important is the realization by the child that the therapist is trying to understand. Indeed, the child at least will be exposed to verbal language stimulation and brought into the communicative relationship.

The child who is also cognitively affected presents us with a more complex but hardly a hopeless challenge. Even this child, who may be neurologically, developmentally, or mentally impaired, nonetheless will communicate nonverbal messages that the therapist may need to decipher. In these cases it is necessary for the therapist to respond both nonverbally and verbally, if only to discover what the child is communicating. Even a minimally appropriate nonverbal or, better, verbal response by the child can be the beginning of a fruitful communicative relationship, leading to more productive language processing and functioning in the child.

We do not believe that counseling alone will bring about linguistic changes in all language-disordered children or even that enhancement of the child's self-image, personal adjustment, or emotional behavior will automatically produce age-appropriate language functioning. Conversely, achievement of normal language functioning will not necessarily produce emotionally well-balanced behavior. Empirical studies have yet to isolate all the parameters that operate in the complex cognitive-emotional-linguistic relationship. For these reasons we must not neglect the use of traditional symptomatic strategies that have become refined, particularly over the last 25 years.

It appears obvious to us, however, that a pragmatic approach to language therapy would be most compatible with the interpersonal counseling approach outlined here. Which shall receive more emphasis depends on several important conditions, including academic preparation of the therapist, sufficient intellectual competence of the child (although it should be noted that moderately low-level mentally retarded children are responsive to counseling methods), cooperation of the parents, degree and quality of neurological competence, and acceptance by and cooperation of school personnel. In the final analysis, however, the therapist must not only weigh these conditions but also consider unforeseen circumstances that may arise during therapy. Independent of all conditions, the therapist should feel free to be flexible and respond appropriately to the changing needs of the child.

Conclusion

We attempt in this chapter to draw together some of the vast body of information provided by experts from many fields to arrive at a more complete understanding of the role of interpersonal family dynamics in the genesis of childhood language disorders. Although definitive empirical research has not yet confirmed much of the clinical evidence available, we cannot ignore the significance of what already has been learned. Even more tenuous is our knowledge and understanding of all the variables inherent in the therapeutic process that in some way account for real positive change in the acquisition of language in language-disordered children.

Finally, we suggest that the establishment of an interpersonal therapeutic relationship may be fundamental to the language therapy process within the context of the unique social system of the family. How much of the process must involve counseling strategies alone, family directed decisions, or how much should depend on more traditional approaches, is yet to be determined. We attempt at least to provoke further discussion and more carefully controlled research on the matter.

References

American Psychiatric Association. *Diagnostic and Statistical Manual*, 4th ed. (DSM-IV). Washington, DC: American Psychiatric Association; 1994.

Annell AL, Gustavson KH, Tenstam J. Symptomatology in schoolboys with positive sex chromatin (the Klinefelter syndrome). *Acta Psychiatrica Scandinavica.* 1970; 71–80.

Arnold GE. The genetic background of developmental language disorders. *Folia Phoniatrica.* 1961;13:246–254.

Axline V. *Play Therapy.* New York: Ballantine; 1969.

Baker L, Cantwell DP, Mattison RE. Psychiatric disorders in children with speech and language retardation. *Archives of General Psychiatry.* 1977;34:583–591.

———. Behavior problems in children with pure speech disorders and in children with combined speech and language disorders. *J of Abnormal Child Psychology.* 1980;8:245–256.

Barnard KE, Bee HL, Hammond MA. Home environment in a healthy low-risk sample: the Seattle study. In: Gottfried AW, ed. *Home Environment and Early Cognitive Development: Longitudinal Research.* Orlando, FL: Academic Press; 1984.

Beasley J. *Slow to Talk.* New York: Teachers College, Columbia University, 1956.

Beckwith L, Cohen SE. Home environment and cognitive competence in preterm children during the first five years. In: Gottfried AW, ed. *Home Environment and Early Cognitive Development: Longitudinal Research.* Orlando, FL: Academic Press; 1984.

Beier D. Behavioral disturbances in the mentally retarded. In: Stevens HA, Haber R, eds. *Mental Retardation: A Review of Research.* Chicago: University of Chicago Press; 1964.

Beitchman JH, Wilson B, Brownlie EB, Walkers H, et al. Long-term consistency in speech/language profiles: II. Behavioral, emotional, and social outcomes. *J of the Am Academy of Child and Adolescent Psychiatry.* June 1996;35(6):815–825.

Bereiter C, Engelmann S. *Teaching Disadvantaged Children in Preschool.* Englewood Cliffs, NJ: Prentice-Hall; 1966.

Bernthal J, Bankson N. *Articulation Disorders.* Englewood Cliffs, NJ: Prentice-Hall; 1981.

Bishop DVM, North T, Donlan C. Nonword repetition as a behavioral marker for inherited language impairment: evidence from a twin study. *J of Child Psychology and Psychiatry and Allied Disciplines.* May 1996;37(4): 391–403.

Bloom L, Lahey M. *Language Development and Language Disorders.* New York: John Wiley; 1978.

Bodmer W, Cavalli-Sforza, L. *Genetics, Evolution and Man.* San Francisco: W. H. Freeman; 1976.

Bowlby J. Grief and mourning in infancy and early childhood. *Psychoanalytic Study of the Child.* 1960;15:9–52.

Bradley RH, Caldwell BM. One hundred seventy-four children: a study of the relationship between home environment and cognitive development during the first five years. In: Gottfried AW, ed. *Home Environment and Early Cognitive Development: Longitudinal Research.* Orlando, FL: Academic Press; 1984.

Brazelton TB. The first four developmental stages in attachment of parent and infant. Paper delivered at the Twelfth Annual Margaret S. Mahler Symposium; May 1981; Philadelphia.

Briggs MH. Families talk: building partnerships for communicative change. *Topics in Language Disorders.* May 1998;18(3):71–84.

Brinton B, Fujiki M. Social interactional behaviors of children with specific language impairment. *Topics in Language Disorders.* February 1999;19(2):49–69.

Brown GW, Harris T. *Social Origins of Depression: A Study of Psychiatric Disorder in Women.* London: Tavistock; 1978.

Cantwell DP, Baker L. Psychiatric disorder in children with speech and language retardation: critical review. *Archives of General Psychiatry.* 1977;34:583–591.

Cantwell DP, Baker L, Mattison, RE. The prevalence of psychiatric disorders in children with speech and language disorder: an epidemiologic study. *J of Am Academy of Child Psychiatry.* 1979;18:450–461

Cameron N. *The Psychology of Behavior Disorders.* Boston: Houghton Mifflin; 1947.

Cohen NJ, Horodezky NB. Language impairments and psychopathology. *J of the Am Academy of Child and Adolescent Psychiatry.* May 1998;37(5):461–462.

Cohen NJ, Menna R, Vallance DD, Barwick MA, Im N, Horodezky NB. Language, social cognitive processing, and behavioral characteristics of psychiatrically disturbed children with previously identified and unsuspected language impairments. *J of Child Psychology and Psychiatry and Allied Disciplines.* September 1998;39(6):853–864.

Courtright J, Courtright I. Imitative modeling as a theoretical base for instructing language-disordered children. *J of Speech and Hearing Research.* 1976;19:655–663.

Darby JK, ed. *Speech Evaluation in Psychiatry.* New York: Grune and Stratton; 1981.

DePaulo BM, Bonvillian JD. The effects on language development of the special characteristics of speech addressed to young children. *J of Psycholinguistic Research.* 1978;7:189–211.

Donahue M, Cole D, Hartas D. Links between language and emotional/behavioral disorders. *Education and Treatment of Children.* August 1994;17(3):244–254.

Duhan K, Punia S. Home environment as predictor of language development. *Psycho-Lingua.* January 1998; 28(1):45–48.

Emerick L, Hatten J. *Diagnosis and Evaluation in Speech Pathology.* Englewood Cliffs, NJ: Prentice-Hall; 1979.

Estrada AV. Pinsof WM. The effectiveness of family therapies for selected behavioral disorders of childhood. *J of Marital and Fam Therapy.* 1995;21(4):403–440.

Fish B, Rivto ER. Psychoses in childhood. In: Noshpitz JD, ed. *Basic Handbook of Child Psychiatry,* Vol. 2. New York: Basic Books; 1979.

Flavel JH. Metacognition and cognitive monitoring. *Am Psychologist.* 1979;34:906–911.

Fogarty TF. System concepts and the dimensions of self. In: Guerin PJ, ed. *Family Therapy: Theory and Practice.* New York: Gardner; 1976.

Furrow D, Nelson K, Benedict H. Mothers' speech to children and syntactic development: some simple relationships. *J of Child Language.* 1979:423–442.

Gallagher TM. Social-interactional approaches to child language intervention. In: Beitchman JH, Cuch NJ, et al., eds. *Language, Learning, and Behavior Disorders: Developmental, Biological, and Clinical Perspectives.* New York: Cambridge University Press; 1996.

Garmezy N. Stressors of childhood. In: Garmezy N, Rutter M, eds. *Stress, Coping and Development in Children.* New York: McGraw-Hill; 1983.

Geist R. Conditions with physical presentations and their psychosomatic relationships. In: Steinhauer PD, Rae-Grant Q. *Psychological Problems of the Child in the Family.* New York: Basic Books; 1983.

Glass GV, McGraw B, Smith ML. *Meta-Analysis in Social Research.* Beverly Hills, CA: Sage; 1981.

Gottfried AW, ed. *Home Environment and Early Cognitive Development: Longitudinal Research.* Orlando, FL: Academic Press; 1984a.

———. Home environment and early cognitive development: integration, meta-analysis and conclusions. In: Gottfried AW, ed. *Home Environment and Early Cognitive Development: Longitudinal Research.* Orlando, FL: Academic Press; 1984b.

Gottfried AW, Gottfried AE. Home environment and cognitive development in young children of middle socioeconomic-status families. In: Gottfried AW, ed. *Home Environment and Early Cognitive Development: Longitudinal Research.* Orlando, FL: Academic Press; 1984.

Griffer MR. A competency-based approach to conducting family-centered assessments: family perceptions of the speech-language clinical process in early intervention service delivery. *Infant Toddler Intervention.* March 1997;7(1):45–65.

Haka-Ikse K, Stewart DA, Cripps MH. Early development of children with sex chromosome aberrations. *Pediatrics.* 1978;62:761–766.

Hammer PS. Young Children's Speech Development. *Dimensions of Early Childhood.* 1998;26(2):3–7.

Harden A, Sahl R. Psychopathology in children and adolescents with developmental disorders. *Research in Developmental Disabilities.* September–October 1997;18(5): 369–382.

Harlow HF, Harlow MK, Dodsworth RO, Arling GL. Materal behavior of rhesus monkeys deprived of mothering and peer associations in infancy. Proceedings of the American Philosophical Society, 1966;(110);58–66.

Huttenlocher J. Language input and language growth. *Preventive Medicine: An International Devoted to Practice and Theory.* March–April 1998;27(2):195–199.

Ilfeld FW Jr. Marital stressors, coping styles, and symptoms of depression. In: Goldberger L, Breznitz S, ed. *Handbook of Stress: Theoretical and Clinical Aspects.* New York: Macmillan; 1982.

Johnson DL, Breckenridge JN, McGowan RJ. Home environment and early cognitive development in Mexican-American children. In: Gottfried AW, ed. *Home Environment and Early Cognitive Development: Longitudinal Research.* Orlando, FL: Academic Press; 1984.

Konstantareas MM, Beitchman JH. Comorbidity of autistic disorder and specific developmental language disorder: Existing evidence and some promising future directions. In: Beitchman JH, Cohen NJ, et al., eds. *Language, Learning, and Behavior Disorders: Developmental, Biological, and Clinical Perspectives.* New York: Cambridge University Press; 1996:178–196.

Lambert W. The effects of bilingualism on the individual: cognitive and socio-cultural consequences. In: Hornby P, ed. *Bilingualism: Psychological, Social and Educational Implications.* New York: Academic Press; 1977.

Lasky EZ, Klopp K. Parent-child interactions in normal and language-disordered children. *J Speech and Hearing Disorders.* 1982;47:7–18.

Lavigne JV, Ryan M. Psychological adjustment of siblings of children with chronic illness. *Pediatrics.* 1979;(63):616–627.

Lefebvre A. The child with physical handicaps. In: Steinhauer PD, Rae-Grant Q, eds. *Psychological Problems of the Child in the Family.* New York: Basic Books; 1983.

Leonard, Laurence B. *Children with Specific Language Impairment (Language, Speech, and Communication).* Cambridge, MA: MIT Press; 1997.

Lewis BA, Freebairn L. Subgrouping children with familial phonologic disorders. *J of Comm Dis.* 1997;30(5): 385–402.

Luchsinger R. Inheritance of speech defects. *Folia Phoniatrica.* 1970;22:216–230.

Ludlow CL, Cooper JA, eds. *Genetic Aspects of Speech and Language Disorders.* New York: Academic Press; 1983.

Maccoby EF. Socio-emotional development and response to stressors. In: Garmezy N, Rutter M, eds. *Stress, Coping and Development in Children.* New York: McGraw-Hill; 1983.

Mattejat F, Niebergall G, Nestler V. Speech disorders in children of aphasic fathers: a developmental psycholinguistic case study. *Praxis der Kinderpsychologic and Kinderpsychiatric.* 1980;29:83–89.

Mineka S, Suomi SJ. Social separation in monkeys. *Psychol Bulletin.* 1978;85:1376–1400.

Molyneaux D, Lane VW. *Effective Interviewing: Techniques and Analysis.* Boston: Allyn and Bacon; 1982.

Nielsen J, Sillesen I. Follow-up until age 2 through 4 of unselected children with sex chromosome abnormalities. *Human Genetics.* 1976;33:241–257.

Nielsen J, Sorenson AM, Sorenson K. Mental development of unselected children with sex chromosome abnormalities. *Human Genetics.* 1981;59:324–332.

Olsen-Fulero L. Style and stability in mother conversational behavior: a study of individual differences. *J of Child Language.* 1982; 9: 543-564.

Pressman S. The effects of a home-based early intervention program on parents' self-confidence and children's development. Unpublished dissertation, Rutgers University; 1983.

Prizant BM. Language acquisition and communicative behavior in autism: toward an understanding of the "whole" of it. *J of Speech and Hearing Research.* 1983;48:296–307.

Richman N, Stevenson J, Graham PJ. Preschool to school: a behavioral study. *Behavioral Development—A Series of Monographs.* 1982:228.

Rose DH. Dentate gyrus granule cells and cognitive development: explorations in the substrates of behavioral change. Unpublished doctoral dissertation, Harvard University; 1976.

Rossetti L. A longitudinal study of developmental status of high risk infants. Paper presented at the annual meeting of the American Speech-Language and Hearing Association; November 1984; San Francisco.

Rousey C. The psychopathology of articulation and voice devisations. In: Travis, LE, ed. Handbook of Sppech Pathology and Audiology. New York: Appleton-Century-Crofts; 1971.

———. *Psychiatric Assessment by Speech and Hearing Behavior.* Springfield, IL: Charles C Thomas; 1974.

Rutter M. Diagnosis and definition of childhood autism. *J of Autism and Childhood Schizophrenia.* 1978;8:139–161.

———. Some issues and some questions. In: Garmezy M, Rutter R, eds. *Stress, Coping and Development in Children.* New York: McGraw-Hill; 1983.

Rutter M, Mawhood L. The long-term psychosocial sequelae of specific developmental disorders of speech and language. In: Rutter M, Casaer P, eds. *Biological Risk Factors for Psychosocial Disorders*. Cambridge, UK: Cambridge University Press; 1991.

Schwartz R, Leonard L, Folger M, Wilcox M. Early phonological behavior in normal-speaking and language-disordered children: eveidence for a synergistic view of linguistic disorders. *J of Speech and Hearing Disorders*. 1980;(45):357–377.

Shere E, Kastenbaum R. Mother-child interaction in cerebral palsy; environmental and psychosocial obstacles to cognitive development. *Genetic Psychology Monographs*. 1966;(73):255–335.

Shuy R. Language problems of disadvantaged children. In: Irwin JV, Marge M, eds. *Principles of Childhood Language Disabilities*. Englewood Cliffs, NJ: Prentice-Hall; 1972.

Siegel LS. Home environmental influences on cognitive development in preterm and full-term children during the first five years. In: Gottfried AW, ed. *Home Environment and Early Cognitive Development: Longitudinal Research*. Orlando, FL: Academic Press; 1984.

Söderbergh R. Linguistic effects by 3 years of age of extra contact during the first hour post-partum. In: Johnson CE, Thew CL, eds. *Proceedings of the Second International Congress for the Study of Child Language*, Vol. 1. Washington, DC: University Press of America; 1982.

Spitz RA. Hospitalism: an inquiry into the genesis of psychiatric conditions in early childhood. *Psychoanal. Study of the Child*. 1945;1:53–74.

———. Anaclitic depression: an inquiry into the genesis of psychiatric conditions in early childhood, II. *Psychoanalytic Study of the Child*. 1946a;2:313–341.

———. Hospitalism: a follow-up report. *Psychoanal. Study of the Child*. 1946b;2:113–117.

Stark RE, Mellits ED, Tallal P. Behavioral attributes of speech and language disorders. In: Ludlow CL, Cooper JA, eds. *Genetic Aspects of Speech and Language Disorders*. New York: Academic Press; 1983.

Stayton DJ, Ainsworth MDS. Individual differences in infant responses to brief, everyday separation as related to other infant and maternal behaviors. *Developmental Psychology*. 1973;9:226–235.

Stevenson J, Richman N. Behavior, language and development in three-year-old children. *J of Autism and Childhood Schizophrenia* 1978; 8: 299–313.

Thompson M, Havelkova M. Psychoses in childhood and adolescence. In: Steinhauer PD, Rae-Grant Q, eds. *Psychological Problems of the Child in the Family*. New York: Basic Books; 1983.

Vallance DD, Cummings RL, Humphries T. Mediators of the risk for problem behavior in children with language learning disabilities. *J of Learning Disabilities*. March–April 1998;31(2):160–171.

Van Riper C, Emerick L. *Speech Correction: An Introduction to Speech Pathology and Audiology*. Englewood Cliffs, NJ: Prentice-Hall; 1984.

Wachs TD. Proximal experience and early cognitive-intellectual; development: the social environment. In: Gottfried AW, ed. *Home Environment and Early Cognitive Development: Longitudinal Research*. Orlando, FL: Academic Press; 1984.

Wadsworth BJ. *Piaget's Theory of Cognitive and Affective Development*. New York: Addison-Wesley; 1996.

Walbert M, Ingles S, Krirgsman E, Mills B. Language, delay and associated mother-child interactions. In: Lahey M, ed. *Readings in Childhood Language Disorders*. New York: John Wiley; 1978.

Waterhouse LH. Maternal speech patterns and differential development. In Johnson CE, Thew CL, eds. *Proceedings of the Second International Congress for the Study of Language*, Vol. 1. Washington, DC: University Press of America; 1982.

Webster E. *Counseling with Parents of Handicapped Children: Guidelines for Improving Communication*. New York: Grune and Stratton; 1977.

Weinberg N, Santana R. Comic books: champions of the disabled stereotype. *Rehabilitation Literature*. 1978;39: 327–331.

Weintraub W. *Verbal Behavior: Adaptation and Psychopathology*. New York: Springer-Verlag; 1981.

Wiig EH, Semel E. *Language Assessment and Intervention for the Learning Disabled*. Columbus, OH: Charles E. Merrill; 1984.

Winnicott DW. The theory of the parent-infant relationship. In: *The Maturational Processes and the Facilitating Environment*. New York: International Universities Press; 1965.

Zaleski T. Familial appearance of delayed development of speech. *Otolaryngologia Polska*. 1966;20:367–371.

Zalewska M. Who says, what and to whom: psychological problems of children with delayed language development. *Polish Psychological Bulletin*. 1998;29(1):19–31.

Zedler EH Social Management. In: Irwin JV, Marge M, eds. *Principles of Childhood Language Disabilities*. Englewood Cliffs, NJ: Prentice-Hall; 1972.

6

Psychological Considerations for Voice-Disordered Individuals and Their Families

---

Part I.
The Psychology of Voice Disorders in Children

Psychogenesis of Voice Disorders

Specific acoustical and physiological features of voice disorders in children cannot be readily assigned their etiological origin. They are probably the least understood of all the communicative disorders. This should not be surprising, as the human voice is the major entity through which personality is expressed. Yet the relationship between the two has mystified us for centuries and defied the best of scientific investigations.

Nevertheless, in this chapter we join the ranks of others who have attempted to make sense of that relationship. We also offer another perspective toward understanding its complexity. Our emphasis is on only the etiological correlates that are essentially psychosocial; but in its manifestation, the voice disorder also is discussed in terms of its organic as well as psychological features. It is interesting to note that *The Diagnostic and Statistical Manual of Mental Disorders,* fourth edition (DSM-IV) (American Psychological Association, 1994) has added a new category of childhood vocal tics to their classification system, but identify neither an organic-physiologic nor psychologic etiology. Nei-

ther does it identify the prevalence of other psychogenically caused voice disorders in children

Etiological Considerations

Children with voice disorders do not fit neatly into the etiological categories proposed by various investigators. More than 70 years ago, Sapir (1927) described the cultural and social factors that influence the vocal dynamics and quality in individuals. Crucial also to our understanding of how these forces affect vocalization is the recognition of the uniqueness of the vocal tract structure. We should not be surprised by Formby's (1967) findings that mothers were able to distinguish the voices of their own babies from others soon after birth.

Other investigators, namely, Wasz-Höckert et al. (1968) and Valanne et al. (1967), studied infant vocal cries and found differentiations among cries of the newborn. Also demonstrated was the ability for mothers to identify their own infants by the cry. Ostwald (1963) demonstrated differences between infants relative to their early cries by means of spectrographic analysis. He demonstrated, too, how listeners could recognize cries distinguished by need and alarm.

Moses (1954) vividly describes the vocal changes that occur as a function of the relationship between "genotypical" actions and traits and the "phenotypical" responses from others. That is, there is a relationship between the fundamental constitution and the way in which the child is attended to and protected.

Murphy (1964) discusses the origin of voice disorders in children relative to emotional conflict and confusion and in particular to the parent-child relationship. In an unpublished study cited by Aronson (1980), Barker and Wilson (1967) found that, of 153 children with voice disorders, extreme family conflict was found in 65% of their homes; and for 97 children who were considered to have normal voices, family conflict was found in only 35% of their homes.

Numerous therapists describe children who have lost temporary use of their voice as a result of isolated traumatic experiences, such as automobile accident, tonsillectomy, death in the family, or witnessing a violent event. Case (1984) discusses the complex interaction between the nervous system (the limbic system, mainly) and endocrine function and how internal or external environmental stimuli may disturb organismic homeostasis; that is, the balance among all functions of the human body. The reader is provided numerous references to explain the psychophysiological dynamics of emotion, but we caution that the relationships between these processes and vocal function are not yet entirely clear (Goodstein, 1958; Phillis, 1970; Scherer, 1972).

There appears to be little disagreement in the literature surveyed that emotional stress can affect musculoskeletal tension to induce aberrant changes in vocal usage (Aronson, 1990; Murphy, 1964; Luchsinger and Arnold, 1965; Greene, 1980; Case, 1984; Wilson 1979; Boone, 1983; and Perkins, 1983). We therefore turn to a discussion of how family dynamics may have a significant bearing on the genesis of voice disorders in children.

Dysfunctional Family Dynamics

While research has been done in the field of family therapy, in the use of family therapy for behavioral disorders in children (Estrada and Pinsof, 1995), no studies have appeared relative to voice disorders in children.

According to Van Riper and Emerick (1984), imitation and feelings of inadequacy are significant factors that may account for the development of voice disorders. To these factors, we would add not only the dynamics of the parent-child relationship but also the interplay of all members of the family. Inherent in these relationships may be the seeds for the development of voice disorders that are expressions of anger, anxiety, depression, conflict, and unsatisfied needs. Consistent with the previous discussions of family systems theory, now applied to the voice-disordered child, the cause must be searched for, not within that child's intrapsychic conflict or stressful condition, but by looking at the possible dysfunctional ways in which the entire family operates. The child becomes "symptomatic" as a result of his or her position within the dysfunctioning family system, thereby satisfying the successful emotional functioning of all other family members.

We might question why the organism unconsciously selects an abnormal vocal behavior to represent a particular dysfunctional family system. As Aronson (1980) suggests, it is possible that the child is "predisposed by personality or physiology to hyperact through a particular organ system" (p. 132). Or it is conceivable that the child's psychological and physiological adaptive mechanisms are being overloaded, forcing the emergence of vocal symptoms. One is reminded of the discussion of the etiology of stuttering. Constitutional factors appear to be taking on greater respectability today and they may well be important factors to consider in their application to voice disorders.

What is important for us to understand is that, as tension increases in a family, it either may be experienced as internal anxiety by one member or lead to conflict between two members. If a father is silently angry toward his wife, the child may express the rage through provocative vocal outbursts, perhaps leading to the development of vocal nodules. In this case, the child is manifesting the essence of a marital relationship that Kerr (1981) describes in several ways: one parent has distanced himself from the other, one parent is in conflict with the other, one parent has compromised her behavior to preserve harmony in the relationship, or both parents have united over common concern for the child—or, we would add, any combination of these may occur.

Stress in Typical Families

A constant theme throughout this book has been the notion that even the most typical family may contain roots for, or manifest behavior, producing stress. This may lead to the inception of, among other things, communicative disorders. We might expect the same conditions for the voice-disordered child. In those families that are functioning well, however, stress is not dealt with as an abstract entity but as a real thing, thereby helping to minimize its effects on all family members. In other words, the stress is less likely to be constellated in voice-disorder symptoms. The likelihood of the development of such symptoms in the dysfunctional family is obviously greater in that the child, or for that matter any other family member, becomes the unwitting victim of the unresolved family conflicts and resulting stress. It would be easy for us to cite the many family instances in which yelling and screaming are common modes by which parents communicate, and where the child adopts a similar means to communicate, with such vocal misuse leading to hoarseness. Such antecedent and resultant events need little further explanation, except that voice disorders in children do not typically follow such an obvious pattern.

Voice disorders in children are more likely to represent individualized reactions to a multitude of possible stress situations in which the vocal behavior expressed by the child is a unique form of coping strategy. Conversely, not all children will necessarily respond in the same way to identical stress-producing situations. Shipp and McGlone (1973) suggest that voice tremors that are supposed to disappear under stress may not exist at all. Siegman (1982) points out: "Whatever the explanation, individual variations in response to stress complicate matters enormously for anyone trying to develop a theoretical model of the effects of stress behavior" (p. 315). It is generally recognized, however, that, under stress, the voice will manifest definitive emotions as well as undergo various changes, resulting in either somatic or psychogenic

voice disorders. Murray, Carr, and Jacobs (1983) describe the therapeutic management of functional aphonia in five adolescents. The persistent pattern for at least four of these young people was the presence of a stressful family environment as well as maladaptive patterns in school.

Some attempts have been made to measure microtremors in the voice by means of a stress-measuring device, the Psychological Stress Evaluator (PSE; Holden 1975). Although used most extensively as a lie detection instrument, it also has been used to assess the vocal effects of stress associated with emotional disturbance. In his review of the literature on the subject, however, Scherer (1981a) cautions us that the PSE is not refined enough to justify its proponents' claims of success.

Relationship of the Somatic to Psychogenic Voice Disorders

It is not too difficult to determine and identify the presence of organic vocal pathology through typical laryngoscopic or nasolaryngeal fiberoptic examination. What is more difficult and challenging is how to manage the apparent absence of an organic or somatic condition. In such cases we have tended to lump them into categories—psychogenic, functional, psychosomatic, nonorganic.

Aronson (1990) prefers the term *psychogenic,* which he believes is less ambiguous and more definitive than the term *functional,* but he does not dispense with the latter completely. He believes that a psychogenic voice disorder generally is comparable with a functional one but is more precise and demands an explanation of causation. He believes a voice disorder to be an expression of one or more kinds of psychologic imbalance—such as anxiety, depression, conversion reaction, or personality disorder—which interfere with normal conscious control over phonation.

Although we essentially agree with Aronson's description, we would dispense entirely with the term *functional* to designate any form of voice disorder that has not been designated as organic. Our reason is that *functional* refers to an action or a process that may be operational in either organic or psychogenic voice disorders; that is, complex physiological actions involving muscular and chemical activity in conjunction with specific anatomical structures. Although we would agree with Murphy (1964), who also finds difficulty with the word, that "terms are only abstractions of the real processes" (p. 4), it is important to be able to describe precisely and behaviorally what has been abused laryngeally and how vocal structures are being misused.

For purposes of our continued discussion, then, we refrain from extensive categorization of voice disorders. We prefer to describe them relative to both their organic and nonorganic components and their mutual psychological processes.

Psychogenic Correlates

Although some voice disorders may be organic or physiological in origin, they may be maintained because of psychogenic or environmental factors. Similarly, some voice disorders that are psychogenic in origin result in organic disorders.

Monday (1983) divides functional (psychogenic) voice disorders into two categories: functional dysphonia, where there is no organic lesion in the phonatory system, and functional laryngeopathology, where vocal abuse may lead to lesions. Examples of this second category include vocal nodules, secondary laryngitis, vocal polyps, and contact ulcers. Although the psychogenic correlates of each of the major categories may be similar, it is useful to discuss them separately so that distinctive characteristics may be differentiated.

Organic Voice Disorders

The incidence of vocal nodules in school-age children is somewhat high, according to some researchers. Pannbacker (1999) provides an extensive view of the literature suggesting that the frequency of vocal nodules ranges from 15 to 35%, occuring more frequently in children than in adults. Silverman and Zimmer (1975) found that 23.4% of 162 children in kindergarten through eighth grade exhibited chronic hoarseness, and vocal nodules were diagnosed in 77.7% of the children seen by an otolaryngologist. The incidence was higher in the primary grades and occurred more in boys than in girls. This study suggested possible causes to be psychological factors, vocal misuse, and upper respiratory infection. The authors note that high expectations of performance had been expressed by parents and teachers, and a competitive spirit was apparent among the children. The children's voices were generally loud and strained, as were those of their siblings and vocal models.

Several studies cited by Aronson (1990) and Green (1989) revealed a wide and consistent array of psychological correlates in children with vocal nodules, including poor personality adjustment, problems with aggressive or assertive behavior, emotional conflict, feelings of inadequacy, and need for loud, incessant talking. Indications of problems with their parents also were revealed. In a 10-year review of public school voice clinics, reported by Miller and Madison (1984), no attempt was made to gather data on the family background of those children seen for reported voice problems. Of the 249 students examined at the school voice clinics, 40% were diagnosed as having vocal nodules, 94% of which were bilateral. Particularly interesting were concomitant problems of upper respiratory ailments, including allergies and middle ear difficulties.

Organic voice disorders, such as contact ulcers and paralysis, were found to be of low incidence in the literature currently surveyed. In their survey of the literature, Baker, Platt, and Fine (1983) report the case of a 10-year-old boy with Gilles de la Tourette syndrome, but they can offer neither a totally psychogenic or organic explanation relative to etiology. Scott and Layton (1997) in their review of epidemiologic findings related to HIV-related voice disorders in children examine the complexities involved in drawing perspectives on such children.

Relationship of Etiology to Family Response

It is obvious that no one psychological common denominator explains the occurrence of somatic voice disorders in children. One would have to make a case-by-case analysis to search for pertinent etiological factors. Explanations of factors that might maintain the problem are no easier to make. Most investigators would agree, however, that vocal abuse and misuse in conjunction with other factors would account for most of the somatic disorders described here. Case (1984) listed several forms of vocal abuse along with etiological factors that we have selected as pertinent to children. Among them are (1) yelling and screaming, (2) using hard glottal attack, (3) calling to others from a distance, (4) speaking at inappropriate pitch levels, (5) speaking excessively or abusively during upper respiratory illness or allergy, (6) vocalizing under conditions of muscular (and we would add psychological) tension, (7) vocalizing animal and toy noises, (8) participating in games involving yelling and cheering, and (9) excessive arguing with peers and family members. What is not clear is why many children who do vocalize in any one or combination of these ways do not develop and maintain a vocal pathology. We may need to consider specific predisposing constitutional factors and family influences.

It is of interest to note that several writers have reported that parents of children with diagnosed voice problems generally are unconcerned. Warr-Leeper, McShea, and Leeper (1979), in their study, reveal that parents typically felt their children's voice problems would not interfere with their education and were insignificant. The study also showed that family physicians did not usually recognize voice disorders as a problem in children. In a large study involving 1962 children (Sentura and Wilson, 1968), only 17% of the children were taken for a laryngoscopic examination by their parents, following letters describing their children's voice problems and recommending referral.

Several reasons are probable for this apparent lack of concern: (1) unlike articulation and other speech and language problems, voice problems generally do not interfere with intelligibility or communicative competence; (2) wider variations of voice usage and voice quality are more acceptable to listeners, articulation and language usage allows for little deviation before calling attention to itself; (3) parents are less well educated about the nature of voice disorders and are more likely to take on the unconcerned attitudes of their family physician; (4) public school therapists oftentimes shy away from voice therapy intervention; and (5) aberrant vocal qualities in children may reflect deep-rooted unconscious conflicts in family relationships or individual family members.

Relationships Among Use, Abuse, and Misuse

Because voice disorders rarely have much of a conscious impact on the bearer or related family members, they are less likely to cause secondary psychological reactions directly. More likely, children with somatic voice disorders will tend to make involuntary secondary physiological adjustments to compensate for the initial interference to laryngeal functioning. Such compensatory adjustments may include chronic throat clearing, speaking at a different pitch or loudness level, and faulty realignment of the vocal and resonance tract, thereby exacerbating an already unbalanced use of the voice. Notwithstanding the initial psychological, physical, or environmental conditions that may have induced the vocal pathology in the first place, continued misuse and abuse is likely. In the case of vocal nodules, a condition that originally was unilateral could become bilateral or the pathogenesis from the acute to the chronic stage may change.

The complex interplay of all these forces results in a vocal prototype characterized by constriction of the laryngopharyngeal cavity as well as excessive medial compression or longitudinal tension of the vocal folds. Asymmetrical and asynchronous vocal fold vibrating may occur, resulting in jitter, breathiness, and hoarseness or "roughness." As long as the primary conditions responsible for the voice disorder persist, it is unlikely for the disorder to change except through appropriate intervention.

Genesis of Nonorganic Voice Disorders

The paucity of substantial research to document definitive factors responsible for the development and maintenance of somatic voice disorders in children has been noted. Even less is known about the genesis of nonorganic voice disorders. Murphy (1964) appears to be one of the major original and yet definitive sources to which we must turn. Framing the disorders within the context of the parent-child relationship, he views these vocal symptoms as reflections of underlying conflicts and serving particular purposes. That is, they are viewed as secondary gains. He states:

Finally there are occasional vocal disturbances originally produced by personal stresses, which tend to persist even after the initial discomforts have been modified or resolved. A voice disorder can become self-perpetuating. A reasonable conclusion in such a case is that a kind of "physiological perseveration" is occurring. It is also likely, though, that subtle psychological determinants are at work: the voice disorder may be serving attention-getting needs; it may be a major feature of the body image; it may serve as a focus for scapegoat behavior; other secondary gains, such as hostility satisfaction, may be present. (p. 36)

Murphy's explanation would be consistent with our understanding of family systems theory, which includes the interactional processes among all family members. The child's voice disorder, then, may represent psychological disequilibrium either in the child or in the family as a manifestation of unsatisfied needs in one or in all.

Although representing a psychoanalytic viewpoint, Erikson (1963) suggests eight stages of life, three of which are pertinent to our present discussion. Failure in the second stage (ages 1–3 years) results in the child feeling inadequate, having self-doubt, and inhibiting learning basic skills like talking. Failure in the third and fourth stages (ages 4–5 and 6–7 years, respectively) results in guilt, infantile jealousy, avoidance of strong competition, feelings of mediocrity, slavish behavior, and a sense of futility. Whereas we might readily have applied Erikson's theory to our discussion of childhood language disorders earlier, it appears applicable to what several major writers already describe in children with nonorganic as well as organic voice disorders (Aronson, 1980, 1990; Wilson, 1979; Murphy, 1964). We must resist the temptation to overgeneralize our case, however, as the vast majority of the children who function psychologically in the way we have described do not develop either organic or nonorganic voice disorders. We also are familiar with children who present aberrant vocal symptoms but do not fit neatly into any of the psychogenic categories or dysfunctional families we have suggested. We could argue that such a reality can be attributed to our inability to isolate the concealed or subtle psychodynamics that escaped attention. Regardless, our task is to view each child and family objectively and without preconceived biases.

Mutational Voice

Puberty is a time of marked psychosocial and physiological changes, including acoustical and physical changes of the larynx. Generally, the adolescent is able to adapt to the laryngeal changes even though the male voice drops approximately one octave and the female voice drops three or four semitones. In some instances, persons, particularly boys, do not readily adapt or are not able to reconcile the physiological changes to the psychosocial changes. In such cases the voice may be characterized by abrupt pitch breaks that persist for months or by persistent mutational falsetto, which Kaplan (1982) defines as "psychological failure of the adolescent's voice to descend or maintain its descent to a normal adult pitch at puberty" (p. 82). The resulting high-pitched falsetto voice is described by Aronson (1980) as "weak, thin, breathy, hoarse, and monopitched, giving the overall impression of immaturity, effeminacy, and passiveness" (p. 146).

Whereas, endocrinological dysfunction may explain the persistence of the falsetto voice in some cases, its etiology generally is seen as psychogenic (Kaplan, 1982; Case, 1984: Aronson, 1990; Wilson, 1979). Unfortunately, the research evidence does not definitely describe its psychosocial dynamics, and therefore we must rely only on clinical evidence to support a psychogenic origin. Although Case (1984) describes poor self-concept and insecurity in personal relationships as factors, and Aronson (1980) alludes to weak male identification and "a neurotic need to resist the transition into adulthood" (p. 147), we still cannot be certain that such psychological factors are primary to the disorder, secondary to it, or both.

Several years ago, we evaluated a 15-year-old boy with pronounced falsetto. The initial interview revealed a young man who was effeminate, had few friends, and who essentially had avoided any participation in typical male activities. He had been under intensive psychoanalytic treatment during the previous three years for what had originally been diagnosed as a "gender identity disorder." His parents, both holding Ph.D.s in their professions, also had been in psychoanalysis because of, according to their analyst, "their role in the etiology or perpetuation of their child's arrested psychosocial development." A family interview revealed that the boy had never been seen for an endocrinological examination, which I immediately recommended. The endocrinological report revealed that their son was suffering from a severe reduction of testosterone, which was viewed as the primary source of the boy's problems. A follow-up contact made two years later revealed a young man who had made dramatic changes in his psychosocial adjustment toward a firm male identity along with a strong bass-baritone voice. His parents, too, were functioning at the peak of their professional and personal lives.

With regard to this particular case of mutational voice, we do not imply that no pertinent psychological factors were operating. More likely, there was a complex interplay of both metabolic and psychological elements that had not been appropriately considered. We would add further that psychotherapeutic intervention indeed was appropriate, but perhaps not to the extent with which it was used.

We leave to the reader the ethical, medical, and psychological implications of this case but remind ourselves of the danger of making any overgeneralization in differential vocal assessments and the need to be aware of our own theoretical biases.

Conversion or Hysterical Dysphonia

Although typically occurring in middle-aged women, conversion dysphonia has also been present in children. We would define it essentially as the partial or complete loss of voice with no apparent structural lesion or as a peripheral physiological dysfunction whereby psychological conflict or disturbance is converted into actual physical symptoms. Rammage, Nichol, and Morrison (1983) view it as a delayed shock reaction to emotional trauma. They also describe its occurrence following a throat virus or upper respiratory infection. Aronson (1990) views it as a means of blocking out emotional conflict, stress, or personal failure the individual cannot confront. In the view of Steinhauer and Berman (1983), a conversion neurosis is more likely in children with histrionic personalities, in which behavior is intense, theatrical, demanding, and superficial and the child tends to be highly excitable, irrational, and manipulative. The result is the alienation of others and interference with their interpersonal feelings.

In terms of family systems theory, we would view conversion dysphonia as a symptom not only of a deep personal emotional conflict but also as a misguided, unwitting attempt to change an existing intolerable familial situation. The differential voice assessment of such a disorder presents a formidable challenge to the voice therapist in that predisposing, precipitating, and perpetuating factors will need to be identified. In public school, this presents a considerable challenge because the school speech-language pathologist is unlikely to have access to the family environment of the child.

With respect to specific vocal symptoms, the child may present with a breathy, rough, or diplophonic voice, but abduction and adduction are normal in deep inhalation and coughing and swelling, respectively (Greene 1980). That is, the larynx may function adequately for biological purposes but not for vocalization. We will discuss the therapeutic implications of this behavior later with reference to both children and adults with conversion dysphonia.

Susan, 12 years old, was thrown from her bicycle after colliding with a moving automobile. Hospital intake revealed mild abrasions and contusions but no evidence of cerebral concussion or limb fracture. The morning following a precautionary one-night stay in the hospital, she presented with aphonia characterized by whispering only. Laryngoscopic examination revealed no visible organicity except for mild inflammation of the vocal folds due to, according to the laryngologist, a mild respiratory infection. Following two weeks of no change in her vocal behavior, she and her family were referred for a family therapy consult. Only after several family therapy sessions was it revealed that Susan's relationship with her mother had been fraught with considerable anger and resentment and that they had been competing for the attention and affection by the only male in the family, a passive husband and father. (It should be noted that Susan also was being seen during this time for individual voice therapy, which also had, for the several sessions, been unsuccessful in relieving the voice symptoms.)

Only when family communications were opened up, honestly and straightforwardly, did Susan's symptoms begin to diminish. Susan's parents were readily amenable to marriage counseling for themselves, and Susan was referred for individual psychotherapy.

This anecdote is a graphic example of how intrapersonal family conflict may play a significant part in the genesis of a psychogenic voice disorder. It must be understood, however, that such family dynamics certainly will not always result in the symptomatology described but that the interplay of several distinctive and unique personal factors could determine particular dysfunctionality.

Implications of Use, Misuse, and Abuse

Although it is clear that a direct relationship may be drawn between misuse and abuse of the voice and the development of vocal fold pathology, it is not clear how aggravation of the laryngeal mechanism may bring about vocal dysfunction in the absence of organicity. In Senturia and Wilson's 1968 study, 29 of 92 children whose larynx could be visualized revealed no discrete lesions, yet they were found to abuse their voices in any one of several ways, including screaming, yelling, excessive speaking and throat clearing, and singing. For reasons unknown, there children were apparently impervious to the development of pathology per se. We can only speculate that constitutional resilience might explain its absence. Regardless of such a variable, we support Aronson's statement that "abuse or misuse . . . is an intermediate link in the chain of causes that begins with an emotionally determined impetus to vocalize aggressively" (1980, p. 134). What, then, are the psychotherapeutic implications? Let us examine these now.

Counseling Strategies

It is important to make clear at the onset of the discussion that, while traditional modes of voice therapy have been found to be effective in the treatment of voice disorders in children, we nevertheless insist that the interpersonal relationship established between the therapist and the child is crucial to fundamental changes in vocal behavior. As Cooper (1973) points out, it is not so much a therapeutic

method used that counts as how the therapist uses it. Regardless of the method used, therapists cannot avoid, nor should they, having a direct impact on the emotional attitudes and behaviors of their young clients. Not only must we be fully cognizant of what we do and how we do it but also keenly aware of the effects and implications of our treatment.

Neither can we ignore the continuing influences and effects of the family and school environment on the child and his or her relationship to them, as such effects may well determine the therapeutic outcome. It, therefore, is unfortunate that many of us, particularly those of us who practice in a school setting, are unable to have substantial contact with the family, in order for us to provide a more comprehensive approach. These limitations, however, need not preclude our best attempts to discover through differential assessment the factors underlying the child's voice dysfunction and make do with whatever information is available to us.

It is obvious that no one approach is applicable to every child who presents with a voice disorder, nor do we know which technique works best; but we agree with Aronson (1980) that we must avoid treating voice disorders as "mechanical problems" only, particularly when emotional stress is a factor, and "voice therapy has to be tailored to the individual" (p. 194). Glaze (1996), however, employs behavioral strategies along with voice conservation and family-peer support in her work with preadolescent children with hyperfunctional voice. In her most recent survey of the literature in vocal nodules, Pannbacker (1999) concludes there is considerable variance in the treatment for children but emphasizes the importance of prevention. We would agree, but it seems reasonable, though, to combine, if necessary, the best strategies available to us in treating all voice disorders in children; emphasize those with which we feel most personally compatible; and finally, be open to learn those about which we know least.

Counseling with Parents

We already described how parents often are unconcerned with the identification and possible consequences of vocal dysfunction in their children. We would hope that such an attitude would not deter us from educating them as to the nature of their child's voice disorder.

If the child is to be helped most successfully, it will necessitate the full cooperation of the parents to ensure carryover of whatever changes we are to effect in vocal or personal behaviors. Therefore, a primary goal in counseling the parents is to provide them with information. This may be accomplished during traditional parent counseling or in family therapy, depending on the unique circumstances and needs of the family. Generally, we tend to favor a family therapy approach, if possible, so that all members of the family learn together. Reality often dictates otherwise, however, as we discussed earlier.

We developed a series of guidelines that the voice therapist might find useful as a point of departure:

1. *A description of the anatomy and physiology of the vocal tract geared to the intellectual level of family members.* This may vary, depending on the understanding of each member. Simple visual aids are particularly useful.
2. *An explanation of the actual organic conditions, if present.* If no organic condition exists, describe in the simplest way possible how hyperfunctional use contributes to aberrant vocal quality and how an organic condition may develop.
3. *A description of various forms of vocal misuse.* These, described earlier, may be elaborated on, depending on their relevance to the particular child and family.
4. *An explanation of the various environmental circumstances that may contribute to such misuse.* It is helpful to begin with a general explanation and gather from the family factors pertinent to the member's own life circumstances. Caution should be exercised so as not to inject blame, which could be counterproductive to continued parental support.
5. *A description of basic principles of vocal hygiene.* These, developed by Boone (1983, pp. 205–207), are applicable to both children and adults with voice disorders. It is important, however, that the counseling therapist not overwhelm

the family with all of the significant dos and don'ts, but determine those factors that, in the family's view, appear most pertinent. Neither the parents nor the child can be expected to make all the changes deemed necessary by the therapist immediately and should be given continued support for even modest modifications.

6. *An explanation of the overall means and goals of voice therapy if indicated.* Determination of the effective means toward these objectives must be discussed openly, with the parents and the child (if old enough) participating in the decision. General therapeutic approaches might include

> Family therapy only;
> Family therapy with individual symptomatic therapy;
> Parent counseling only;
> Parent counseling with individual symptomatic therapy;
> Individual symptomatic therapy only;
> Family therapy with individual counseling therapy;
> Parent counseling with individual counseling therapy;
> Combined individual, symptomatic, and counseling therapy;
> Individual counseling therapy only.

It is important to recognize that special or unique circumstances often will dictate the method or methods of choice and that one method may not necessarily be more appropriate than another. Regardless of choice, we believe that parent cooperation in any effort is important and necessary if permanent positive vocal changes in the child are to occur.

7. *An explanation of the role of parental assistance with the child's home practice.* Closely related to the preceding point, we believe it is unwise only to "send something home with the child" unless the parents or at least one parent is made fully aware of exactly how parent participation can best be utilized. In rare instances only (we hope) would we refrain from involving parents in the home practice, particularly if we believe they are inadvertently sabotaging our best therapeutic

efforts because of deep-rooted individual or family psychopathology.

Generally speaking, and regardless of therapeutic approach, it is wise to keep parents informed throughout the voice therapy period. It is hoped, too, that the quality of parent education would not be adversely affected by dissimilarities of clinical settings. We would take issue with those who claim that the school setting cannot provide the quality of service that so-called clinical settings provide. Therapeutic outcome, we believe, is determined essentially by the expertise of the clinical speech-language pathologist regardless of therapeutic environment, as has been demonstrated in the study by Cook, Palaski, and Hanson (1979).

Family Therapy

We already discussed how environmental stresses may lead to both organic and nonorganic voice disorders. It would seem, therefore, that family therapy would be the appropriate treatment because the family environment most likely would be the major source of the life stress. There are several advantages to this approach:

1. The voice disorder as the identified symptom may more readily be traced directly to actual family dysfunctional processes.
2. The family can learn to tune in objectively to how the child is using or misusing the voice.
3. The family members can learn how to modify their own behavior to effect positive vocal usage in the child.
4. The family also can learn how to help the child directly to use the voice more effectively.
5. The family is better able to effect changes in the extrafamilial environment, which may have been contributing to vocal misuse.

Neutralizing the Symptoms and the Behavior

Although typical family therapy focuses on modifying family homeostasis and interactional relationships among all family members to neutralize one member's symptoms and behavior, the voice-disordered child may require a somewhat different approach. It requires that attention be given immediately to the child's actions directly associated with the faulty vocal condition. The therapist attempts to elicit from the child as much information as possible regarding the need to use the present vocal pattern and the child's perceptual attitudes. The therapist must preface these attempts by encouraging all family members to share their feelings without judging the feelings of others and to be prepared to listen as openly as possible. Although an outburst of hostility may create a delicate situation, it is important for feelings to be expressed and at the same time to protect the person who does so, particularly the child.

Remember that, while vocal symptoms may be maintaining and perpetuating dysfunctional family patterns and are destructive in and of themselves, they do not lend themselves easily to direct intervention. For these reasons, it is more appropriate to identify intrafamilial relationships and interaction.

Modifying Family Homeostasis

In other discussions of family therapy, we cautioned the therapist not to get immersed in the content of what is being expressed by family members but to heed the actual process taking place. This process includes how people communicate with each other—their vocal tone, body language, and degree of participation. It tells us how parents relate to each other, how each or both relate to the child or other children, and how children relate to each other. In essence, we are given a mirror image of what actually takes place at home.

In a child-centered family in which a child has the voice disorder, it is important that the therapist is a leader who, in Minuchin's (1974) terms, must "join and accommodate" the family to create a therapeutic system. The therapist first accepts the family as it is, agreeing with the family's concern for the child, thereby gaining the trust necessary to instigate changes later. The therapist then considers the various combinations of relationships and how the elements intrinsic to them may have produced and perpetuated the voice disorder. Particular attention is directed to the latter to determine how it has operated as a homeostatic factor to maintain family dysfunction. Next, the therapist attempts to learn from family members specific circumstances and conditions that appear to bring about or are associated with an increase of vocal misuse and abuse. These may range from overall family life stress to sibling competition or to specific instances of marital discord.

The therapist then might program changes with the assistance of family or specific family members to cope with the stressors or in some cases might recommend marital couple therapy. For example, it might be more constructive to help the parents to argue their conflicts in a more congruent way, thereby reducing their loud verbal outbursts. Reduction of the latter may eliminate their need to admonish their child for "screaming all the time." Whether the therapist acts to handle the dyadic relationship between two siblings, mother-child, or father-mother or triadic relationships among mother-child-father, modifications of behavior are directed to the way they interact and the context in which these interactions take place.

Recommending changes in the style of family relating does not mean altering family values to suit our own perspectives. As therapists, we need to draw on the unrealized strengths, love, and caring that already exist to restore a healthy balance. The following case study illustrates how several of these principles may be applied.

Craig was 10 years old when bilateral vocal nodules were first discovered by the family physician. Referral to a laryngologist confirmed the diagnosis. Gentle family prodding by the public school speech-language pathologist led to the initial examination after a vocal assessment had been made. There was no way of knowing how long the condition had persisted, as the family had just moved to California from the East Coast.

The laryngologist preferred taking a conservative approach by recommending voice therapy rather than surgery, but provided the family little information other than the admonition to "help him to use his voice more softly." Craig's conscientious school therapist, however, made certain that the family was fully informed about the condition, and they learned specific ways to help him at home. Craig was enrolled in voice therapy for two half-hour sessions a week.

Craig's vocal behavior was characteristic. As an outgoing child, he screamed and yelled incessantly while playing with his friends in and outside school. According to his parents (Peter and Fay), he never stopped talking at home, and they were obviously perturbed by his shrill voice. His voice quality was generally hoarse.

After two months of voice therapy, during which time no substantial changes in voice behavior or vocal quality were evident, his therapist arranged for a parent conference. Skilled in parent counseling, she learned that Peter and Fay had made a diligent effort to follow her vocal hygiene advice, but that Craig was unresponsive to their well-meaning intentions. Clinically, his therapist had helped him obtain a balanced and healthy use of the voice, but none of this had carried over elsewhere. Recognizing that elements in the family environment were hindering all therapeutic efforts, she recommended a family therapy consultation. Somewhat hesitant at first, Peter and Fay finally agreed.

During the first meeting, their futile attempts to help Craig at home were confirmed. It was also obvious to the family therapist that their efforts were consistent with an overall pattern of rigid expectations in all aspects of behavior—everyone must eat dinner at 6:00 P.M. sharp, homework must be finished before dinner, Craig must clean his room every Saturday morning, and so forth. Peter and Fay's expectations for themselves were no less compelling. Also apparent was Fay's passive toleration of these expectations, which were rooted in Peter's strong convictions. To him, it was important that "things must always go smoothly." The family therapist also noticed how Peter needed to maintain control over the course of the session and resisted the therapist's own attempts to enter into the family process. Only when such behavior was pointed out to Peter did Fay and Craig begin to express themselves openly. Peter had much difficulty in listening to Fay's deeply felt complaint that she felt stifled by what she considered to be a "cold, clockwork atmosphere" at home but that she too contributed to such an environment. Craig complained that "home isn't fun" and that he didn't like being told "what to do all the time."

It was immediately apparent to the therapist that what had first seemed like unwitting collusion between Fay and Peter was in actuality a bond between Fay and Craig, with Peter attempting to maintain control over everything and everyone. Subsequent sessions confirmed this, and more.

It seemed clear to the therapist that although Craig's voice disorder was serving as a symptom to identify the underlying family conflict characterized by discontent, hidden anger, and resentment, Peter had also been the unidentified victim, caught up in his own unresolved conflicts with his own family of origin. Reared in a family that was obviously even more stifling, rigid, and demanding, Peter had been carrying the burden of such an influence.

Fay, on the other hand, raised in a family with two older brothers, where she had been expected to assume the stereotyped passive female role, fit the model in her present marriage but not without feelings of underlying resentment and rebellion. Her and Peter's conflict thus was based on each striving to satisfy in his or her own way unrealized needs. Craig's persistent yelling and aggressively verbal behavior was seen by the therapist as a manifestation of the silent rage felt but unexpressed by both Fay and Peter. Craig, in a very real sense, was "crying out" not only the inner family turmoil but *for* family harmony.

The therapist's major task was to help Fay and Peter relate to each other realistically and in the present, uncontaminated by past family patterns. As expressed anger began to emerge and individual frustrations came into focus, Craig's vocal behavior began to change with a reduction in vocal misuse. It was deemed important that Craig continue to attend and participate in the process, as he, too, needed to express his own frustrations and at the same time be privy to the unraveling conflicts. Individual voice therapy was resumed to enhance healthier vocal usage and help give Craig the sense of being part of the process toward overall family adjustment.

No doubt, the inherent mutual love and caring in this family were significant elements in the establishment of family harmony and growth and in the ultimate disappearance of the vocal nodules and abusive vocal behavior.

Individual Counseling Approaches

Family therapy alone may not always be possible, necessary, or in fact, the most useful method of treatment. For that matter, neither may direct vocal rehabilitation be the most effective approach. Unique, individual circumstances such as family cooperation, motivation of the child, and therapist competence will determine choice of treatment. Even among the various counseling approaches, no one approach would be deemed most effective. It, too, would be dictated by the demonstrated needs and special circumstances of the child, family, and therapist. In fact, it may be possible to combine them or even integrate one or the other with symptomatic strategies.

Play Therapy

According to Hejna (1960), among the basic principles underlying nondirective play therapy is the child's inherent need for continual growth and aspiration for self-realization. As children explore their immediate environment, they find pain, pleasure, punishment, approval, failure, and success. Some, who feel so frustrated or punished that they withdraw, feel discouraged or angry but have no viable outlet to express themselves. With respect to voice disorders, Hejna views play therapy as a natural method of releasing the child from inner frustrations, anxieties, tensions, and insecurities. As noted elsewhere in reference to the work of Axline (1969), play is a natural medium for self-expression whereby the child is given the opportunity to play out inner feelings of tension, insecurity, and so on. By their expression, such feelings are brought to the surface. Thus exposed, the child faces these feelings, learns to control them, and finally abandons them.

If the voice problems are caused or maintained by any of these emotional factors, then the vocal behavior may automatically change. If the voice problems create feelings of inferiority, play therapy might enhance feelings of greater confidence and self-acceptance and the motivation to change vocal behavior (Hejna, 1960).

In a case study described by Mosby (1970), supportive play therapy along with traditional voice therapy was used with a 10-year-old boy who had been resistive to traditional voice therapy techniques. Psychotherapy was used as a means to discover the child's underlying aggressive behavior and sought to teach him adequate coping mechanisms. Apparently Mosby's approach was successful in inducing calmer feelings, decreasing vocal misuse, and reducing the vocal nodules.

Because dysfunctional vocal behavior often is manifested in the child's typical play activities, the eight basic principles of play therapy as described by Axline (1969) are particularly applicable. The therapist

1. Establishes warm, friendly rapport with the child in an environment characterized by soft vocalization.
2. Accepts the child completely, even if the vocalization is still abusive.
3. Establishes a feeling of permissiveness so that the child feels free to express feelings, thereby minimizing the need to misuse the voice.
4. Recognizes and reflects and child's feelings, which also would reduce vocal misuse.
5. Maintains respect for the child.
6. Allows the child to lead the way.
7. Does not hurry therapy, so that a more balanced vocal pattern will emerge slowly but definitely.
8. Establishes only those limitations necessary to help the child be aware of responsibilities first to self and then to others.

Operationally, play therapy may be modified to suit the particular voice disorder and varying psychological constellation of the child. Therefore, muteness or vocal abuse will necessitate establishing differing clinical environments so that the child will be motivated to attempt a new mode of vocalization. In play therapy, as we view it, etiology is not as important as the behavioral manifestations of the child. Yet it is possible to change the latter without necessarily working directly on the symptomatology. On the other hand, the therapist should not feel constrained to adhere only to the classic principles of play therapy but also include symptom management if deemed relevant in particular cases.

Regardless of emphasis, the therapist should avoid a hodgepodge approach and have a carefully thought-out plan, including short- and long-term goals. Any modification of the plan and objectives is acceptable because we can never be certain that any clients will progress in a predictable manner. Conceivably, what may have been play therapy to begin with could evolve into direct intervention strategies.

Direct Counseling

Although direct vocal rehabilitation, which is both educational and therapeutic, typically may be effective in the treatment of voice disorders, those disorders that contain pronounced psychogenic components are less amenable to long-term change. For this reason, a psychotherapeutic approach might be a more suitable procedure. Yet we would not recommend its use with children indiscriminately, even under the guidance of psychotherapeutically trained therapists. Several, sometimes overlapping, criteria would in part dictate and qualify such an approach. They include the following:

1. *Age.* Mental age of the child would be a prime determinant, as some 10-year-olds, for example, might be more receptive than some 12-year-olds.
2. *Psychological impact of the disorder.* Some children have a strong adverse reaction to the disorder itself and will need emotional support to assist in coping with and changing the disorder.
3. *Adverse familial influences or lack of parental support.* Persistently negative factors within the home environment may not be amenable to change, so the child will have to develop ways to tolerate and counteract these influences.
4. *Presence of underlying dysfunctional psychological processes.* Pronounced stress, anxiety, poor self-esteem, and conflict associated with vocal misuse and abuse may need to be addressed before traditional strategies can be productive.
5. *Failure of traditional or symptomatic strategies.* Psychotherapeutic management, when all other strategies have been nonproductive, would appear to be appropriate even in the apparent absence of psychogenic factors.

The issue of psychotherapy has received considerable attention in the literature, with most authorities generally agreed that it should be conducted by professional psychotherapists when the voice disorder is dominated by psychopathology. Whereas some writers believe that counseling should be used only to obtain information and reduce severe distress, others prefer a total hands-off approach.

Our own perspective is based more on the appropriate qualifications and training of the therapist than on doctrinal or parochial professional territories. As far as voice-disordered children are concerned, we are not troubled by voice symptom removal per se, even when it is a manifestation of underlying psychological processes. We do believe that it should be done by a therapist who at least is cognizant of and familiar with psychopathology. After all, are any of us so bold as to prefer operating in ignorance or would we rather function with the fullest awareness possible?

The point we wish to make is that a voice disorder is not a distinct entity but a manifestation of the total being of an individual. We need at least to recognize the psychological and behavioral implications of any attempted modification of vocal function. The problem often is that, in our enthusiasm to do well, we focus on the "it" rather than on the person.

Perhaps the hesitancy of some speech-language pathologists in taking on voice-disordered children is not so much a reflection of their fear of working with these children but more an expression of an intuitive awareness of their own lack of expertise in complex psychological processes. Nevertheless, it would be useful to describe in some detail how counseling may be used by a therapist who is versed in psychological and psychotherapeutic processes.

The child with a voice disorder, be it organic or nonorganic, is in a real sense crying out for self-expression, as alluded to by Aronson (1980, 1990). We apply several principles throughout this text that may be useful in guiding our management of these children:

1. *Learning from the child the particular circumstances, personal and environmental, in which vocal misuse and abuse occurs.* The child is encouraged to share with the therapist all information deemed appropriate, including data that at first may appear irrelevant.

2. *Developing the interpersonal relationship.* An immediately effective way to reduce abusive vocal behavior is through the natural and nonjudgmental communicative relationship that should be free to develop between the therapist and the child.

3. *Giving information about the voice and its function.* Gearing information to the intellectual ability of the child, it is possible for the therapist to provide information about vocal anatomy and physiology through visual aids. At this time, it may be appropriate to describe to the child how the voice currently is being used.

4. *Helping the child take responsibility for vocalization.* Treating the voice as a separate entity is dispelled as the child is helped to understand personal control over vocalization. The child is taught that the voice itself is not expected to change so much as the *way* in which the voice is used.

5. *Dealing with emotional issues that relate directly or indirectly to vocal misuse.* As the interpersonal relationship develops, the child becomes freer in sharing feelings to which the therapist responds empathically. (See Aronson's, 1980, summary of Rogerian principles related to communication.)

6. *Allowing the child to progress at his or her own pace.* As therapists, we sometimes rush the therapeutic process in our fervor to "correct the problem." This should be avoided because it very likely represents projection, on our part, related to satisfying our own personal needs for "saving," rather than objectivity about the child's needs. It is important, however, also to be sensitive to resistance, denial, and uncooperativeness, which must be handled gently yet firmly. The child does not behave in the way described merely to spite the therapist but actually is communicating significant personal material that begs for clarification and understanding.

7. *Straying from direct discussion or management of vocal function.* During the course of the ongoing interpersonal relationship, the therapist may need to be more attentive to the self-expression of the child than to the way in which the voice may be used, misused, or abused. The therapist will have to determine how much of this can be dealt with, given his or her personal qualifications and counseling competency. If outside referral is deemed necessary, particu-

larly if powerful psychopathological issues begin to emerge, related or not to the voice disorder, the therapist may need gradually to terminate the relationship or change its clinical character. Regardless of the decision, the child should not be left to feel rejected.

8. *Helping the child communicate more congruently or with straightforward messages.* Oftentimes, the voice-disordered child has resorted to abusive vocal behavior because of the frustration in not being able to communicate clearly with those surrounding him or her. The therapist can help the child identify those feelings and attitudes held and encourage their outward expression. Thus, instead of the child needing to scream at home to gain attention, it is possible to learn to say directly to parents, for example, "I really need your attention."

9. *Helping the child recognize other personal needs, hopes, and desires that are not being satisfied.* The therapist can discuss with the child unsatisfied wishes that, in reality, may fall within the realm of possibility. The child also must be helped to understand desires that cannot realistically be fulfilled given the existing environmental circumstances and limitations inherent in being a child.

10. *Transferring interpersonal communication from the clinic to the real world.* As the child begins to gain a fuller understanding of self and uses the voice in a more open and balanced way clinically, the therapy session should be extended into various environmental situations in which new vocal behaviors and attitudes may be practiced. If screaming on the playing field had been a problem, it might be appropriate for the therapist and child to toss around a football, keeping a fair distance, in order for verbal communication to occur appropriately.

11. *Taking permanent responsibility for change.* For any vocal change to take place, the child ultimately must take full responsibility for controlling the voice in and outside formal therapy. The child must learn to take charge of any vocal situation and thereby eliminate the victim's role as a vocal misuser and abuser.

The foregoing guidelines are not exclusive to the many excellent principles and approaches already enumerated and discussed in the literature and successfully implemented (Boone, 1983; Case, 1984; Wilson, 1979; Aronson, 1980, 1990). The therapist may readily combine several strategies geared toward the individual child, including symptomatic methods. Let us consider, then, how we may integrate a symptomatic with a counseling approach.

A Counseling and Symptomatic Approach Combined

We previously inferred that it is wiser for the speech-language pathologist to counsel the voice-disordered child only when psychopathological processes are either directly or at least indirectly related to the disorder itself.

When such a relationship exists, it in fact would be almost impossible to ignore either the vocal symptom, the child's reaction to it, or the interpersonal components. Some therapists have successfully used techniques that are simultaneously psychotherapeutic and symptomatic. LaGuaite (1976) uses hypnosis successfully to reduce vocal abuse in voice-disordered children. Greene (1980) provides both general and specific methods of achieving relaxation as a means of modifying the stressors associated with vocal hyperfunction. Wilson (1979) applies the communication-centered speech therapy approach of Low, Crerar, and Lassers (1959) to group therapy with voice-disordered children.

We find that a contractual therapeutic arrangement is most conducive to the positive outcome, regardless of the methodological emphasis. That is, we ask the child to change something but it entails awareness, motivation, cooperation, and practice.

Children generally appreciate the responsibility given them consistent with directing their own vocal behavior and its modification. Although able to move at their own pace, they also are encouraged to move ahead forthrightly. Should commitment by the child to the therapeutic process lag, it is necessary for the therapist to discuss the problem openly, help the child with his or her own resistance, and try to modify the circumstances that may be hindering progress.

Sometimes the child may feel that the personal efforts to change vocal behavior are "not worth it," "too hard," "no fun," or "make me feel funny." As therapists, we must remind ourselves that these verbal expressions may be the outward manifestations of underlying feelings associated with self-concept, personal worth, or interpersonal conflict and as such demand our attention. At times, it may be necessary to support the child's need for "time-out" in order to discuss the issue further or to allow the child time to think more about it.

We have found no single explanation for the inertia that may arise in therapy. In fact, we found such children to have parents who either rigorously supervise home practice or take little or no interest in the child's voice therapy. Regardless of the degree of parental "cooperation," it is the child who must ultimately be the sole agent for positive vocal change.

We are all familiar, however, with children who may be too immature to take the kind and type of responsibility suggested here. Contractual therapy in these cases may be contraindicated, yet at the same time, we would not want to be party to continued dependency and immaturity. We would attempt, however, to strike a balance between a more directive therapeutic approach and the encouragement of more mature behavior. Some form or degree of parental cooperation likely will be necessary, but it is not our role to take responsibility for total personality enhancement and growth.

Conclusion

There appears to be sufficient evidence to suggest that voice disorders in childhood often are the manifestation of interpersonal as well as intrapersonal relationships. A specific disorder itself is rooted not so much in differential organic or nonorganic components as in the individual child's emotional state. It also is clear that the child's actual vocal quality may reflect a particular emotional state.

The presence of such nonlinear relationships presents a considerable challenge to the voice therapist, who must be well versed in traditional vocal management techniques and sophisticated in psychotherapeutic counseling. These requirements become even more vital as we turn to our discussion of voice-disordered adults.

Part II.

The Psychology of Voice Disorders in Adults

Psychogenesis

Disraeli said, "There is no index of character so sure as the voice." But, is such a statement as irrefutable as it first seems? We think not. In a provocative essay, Quan (1985) noted:

> In a purely biologic and physiologic position, the voice is controlled by muscle contractions, neural transmission, aerodynamic processes and physical resonance characteristics. In some way we control what we do to our voices, thus matching it to the way in which we want to

appear to others. On the other hand, the psychological position speaks of an inadvertent connection between the way a person uses his or her voice and their concomitant personality type. In the first example given of the purposeful control of voice, the character of the individual may not coincide with the vocal qualities that the person is choosing to emit. Thus the voice does not act as an "open window to the soul." In fact, it may even be very deceptive in personifying an opposite impression. On the other side, psychosomatic diseases have been identified as manifestations of the person's "true self." Under unconscious control, the voice may in fact show character that lies within. (p. 1)

In attempting to unravel the "several semantic and methodologic obstacles" inherent in the relationship between "normal voice and normal personality," Aronson (1980) has listed the following:

1. The difficulty in defining personality.
2. Validity and reliability problems associated with personality tests.
3. Poor definitions of voice variables.
4. Alterations of research methodologies.

To this list we would add the following two points: The psychoperceptual abilities of listeners are contaminated by their preconceived biases, thereby interfering with objectivity; and speakers who use their voice in a certain manner may be compensating by using a voice that differs characteristically from the original personality stereotype. Thus, those individuals who are essentially introverted in nature may tend toward a voice that acoustically is resonant, firm, strong, and convincing, whereas those who are essentially extroverted in nature may tend toward a voice that acoustically is thin, weak, and unconvincing. Aronson (1990), in an extensive review of the literature regarding "voice as a mirror of the personality," appears hesitant in making any generalization about any direct relationship (pp. 117–145). We would agree and add that the nuances of voice and personality are too complex to arrive at any definitive judgment.

Unfortunately, we do not yet understand the complex nature of compensatory vocal adjustments and thus we often are misled by predetermined stereotypic judgments. It appears, then, that for the moment we must study each individual's unique vocal and nonvocal personality. Such a study has special therapeutic implications, as we see later.

In Part I of this chapter we briefly alluded to the complex relationship between voice and personality relative to the development of voice disorders in children. In adults, not only are these relationships more complex, but they are manifested in a greater variety of disorders that often defy even the most astute of professionals.

As both Moses (1954) and Murphy (1964) variously describe the essence and nature of voice disorders, the development of the speaking voice is influenced not only by the speaker's feeling and attitudes about self but also by how the speaker perceives the listener's reaction to the voice. These factors combine and affect the speaker's vocal self-image, personality, lifestyle, and in some cases the vocal disorder itself. The symptoms of voice disorders develop via a process of adjustment in which the speaker is attempting to balance personal inner drives, private environment, and outer realities.

Clinically, considerable evidence suggests that stress within the individual may manifest itself vocally but also differently, as each individual has a unique means of coping both psychologically and physiologically (Scherer 1981a, 1981b). Moses (1954) postulates that the process of living involves tension from which the organism seeks release in order to reestablish homeostasis. But, if the release does not occur and homeostasis is not established, the organism will search for other avenues of release. A crucial role in the reestablishment of homeostasis belongs to the vocal mechanism, as a medium of communication. Moses expresses little doubt that the vocal mechanism is affected by tension release through the development of psychological maladjustment. But this, in turn, may result in misuse, abuse, or loss of control over the voice mechanism. Although we would not argue that all voice disorders necessarily have their genesis in psychopathological sources, emotional stress would seem to be a common denominator in most disorders of the voice. More important, then, might be our attempt to understand more fully the ongoing psychodynamic factors that characterize perpetuation of the disorder.

Gutwinski-Jeggle (1983) suggests that most voice disorders are not the result of physiological or medical problems but a manifestation of disturbance in relationships with significant others. If the client is unresponsive to traditional methods of therapy, we must look at the voice problem as symptomatic of the dysfunctional relationship or as an unconscious way of coping with other problems. Vogel and Carter (1995) appear to embrace a more holistic approach in that they view vocal dysfunction in terms of the inseparability of mind and body.

While physical dysfunction may have psychological effects, so may psychological dysfunction have physical repercussions. The outcome is a circuitous pattern in which both mind and body are affected until appropriate intervention severs the cycle.

Etiological Considerations

The physiological ramifications of stress resulting in various voice disorders, such as vocal nodules, contact ulcers, vocal polyps, spastic dysphonia, nonspecific laryngitis, and conversion dysphonia, have been described by many investigators and therapists. Rosen and Sataloff (1997) describe several physical consequences of stress on the autonomic nervous system, including the alteration of oral and vocal fold secretions that may lead to vocal fatigue. Yet objective measurements of stress have proven difficult to establish. Butcher, Elias, and Raven (1993) describe the effects of hypercontraction of both the extrinsic and intrinsic muscles of the larynx in response to emotional stress—the common denominator. They, however, find observable pathology to be inconsistent with the severity of abnormal voices described as muscularskeletal, conversion hysteria, mutational, or childlike speech (pp. 3–22). However, several tools are available that allow the therapist or researcher valid measurements of stress and the ability to relate these to vocal production.

Simonov and Frolov (1973), in the Soviet Union, devised a method based on spectrographic analysis that allowed them to differentiate degree of emotional stress in 85% of their subjects. Their studies with Soviet cosmonauts established a relationship between heart rate (beats per minute) and changes in the human voice resulting from emotional stress. In a later article (Simonov, Frolov, and Talebkin, 1975), the investigators relied on EEG measurements to determine emotional reactions. Increased heart rates were associated with increased states of stress and vocal change. Again, we must refer to the excellent review by Scherer (1981a), who reports considerable evidence to support the hypothesis that "for fairly high levels of stress and for a majority of subjects studied, fundamental frequency of the voice rises and the proportion of energy above 500 Hz in the spectrum increases" (p. 183). The difficulty in any type of systematic research, according to Scherer, is that we must study individual differ-

ences and different types of stress if we are to understand specific coping mechanisms.

The relationship between emotion and its acoustic correlates as expressed in the voice has challenged psychologists, physiologists, and voice pathologists for many years. Scherer (1981b) brings to our attention the current state of research on this complex relationship. Although it may be assumed that the human voice is affected by specific emotional conditions, we have yet to establish definitive associations between voice and the various milieus in which it is used. It would be impractical within the context of the present volume to discuss all the research that has been done in the area. It is important, however, to recognize that, until we have established definitive relationships between emotion and its vocal correlates, our efforts to establish relationships between emotion and correlates of vocal pathology could well be hampered. Regardless, we should not be prevented from forming associations between psychogenic factors and specific vocal pathologies. In doing so, we hope to avoid the dichotomy that continues to separate so-called nonorganic from organic voice disorders.

Vocal Nodules

We already discussed the psychogenic correlates of vocal nodules in children and considered the psychodynamics of vocal misuse and abuse in the disorder. Vocal nodules also is one of the most common voice disorders in adults and is similarly imbued with complex psychogenic and psychodynamic components. Clinically, common personality factors have been found in such individuals. Although Aronson (1980) views the etiology and pathology as essentially comparable for both children and adults, he suggests that there are some differences. According to Aronson, the incidence of vocal nodules is more common in women than men. These women "are talkative, socially aggressive and tense, and suffer from acute or chronic interpersonal problems that generate tension, anxiety, anger or depression" (p. 136). In describing the onset of functional dysphonia in women, House and Andrews (1994) refer to women having the inclination to "become involved in a social network in which they were overcommited, but relatively powerless" (p. 317). We would hesitate to make any generalizations, however, given the complex hormonal elements that interact with various living styles.

Greene (1980) found that, given the pronounced anxiety aspect of the personality structure of individuals with vocal nodules, there may be psychosomatic components. No systematic research is offered, however, to support that contention. The term *psychosomatic* is still fraught with controversy and problems of definition, so we will refrain from further discussion at this time. Based on her extensive clinical experiences, though, Greene has found that those with vocal nodules may not necessarily be neurotic but, rather, well adjusted. They tend to have the competitive spirit of the business executive, singer, and actor. She describes the personality type as productive, responsible, reliable, and generally gregarious.

Earlier in our chapter we referred to Case (1984) and his comprehensive list of specific types of vocal abuse and related causal factors. It is useful now to include a list of those factors more applicable to adults with vocal nodules:

1. Singing in a manner inappropriate to the actual vocal equipment.
2. Speaking in a noisy environment.
3. Coughing and excessive throat clearing.
4. Strenuous grunting with straining and exercising.
5. Smoking excessively.
6. Speaking excessively or abusively during menstrual periods.
7. Arguing intensively.
8. Talking in nightclubs or other noisy surroundings.

Although we might be tempted to paint a psychogenic portrait characteristic of adults with vocal nodules, not enough definitive evidence appears in the literature to support such a contention. Furthermore, other important factors must be considered. Based on their study of the incidence, histology, and pathogenesis of vocal cord polyps, Kambic et al. (1981) believe the distinction between vocal nodules and polyps to be a "matter of opinion." Studying 591 patients, they found that smoking and increased industrialization and air pollution, along with an excessive amount of vocal use and faulty vocal techniques, to be the major culprits. In her survey of the literature regarding vocal nodules in both children and adults, Pannbacker (1999) appears to concur with our confusion distinguishing polyps from vocal nodules.

From a therapeutic viewpoint, it would be valuable to explore and understand the precipitating factors, both internal and external, that contribute to the inception of the problem. It also is necessary to investigate and analyze the ongoing dynamic processes that perpetuate the disorder even after surgical intervention. These would include both the physiological or mechanical adjustments made by the individual to compensate for the perceived aberrant vocal quality and the psychological means by which the individual copes with the disorder. Brodnitz (1981), in his brilliant essay, emphasizes the significance of clients' own psychological reactions to their disordered voices, and we say more about this later.

One element is obvious. As in children with vocal nodules, we need to understand the stressors that continue to operate in adults with a similar condition.

Laryngeal Contact Ulcer

Laryngeal contact ulcer (LCU), like vocal nodules, is characterized by both an organic change and psychogenic factors. It appears, however, to be more prevalent in men, with many writers suggesting environmental stress as a major etiological factor. Such patients have been found to be highly competitive, compulsive, and aggressive. Case (1984) describes them "to be in their early forties, highly vocal and dynamic in verbal interactions, hard driving, perfectionist, verbally aggressive, and in professions that involve considerable vocalization" (p. 141). We have found them characteristically holding back from expressing feelings openly, tight-lipped and -jawed, and maintaining a rapid and never-ending flow of speech. They tend to resemble the Type A personality described elsewhere by Friedman and Rosenman. According to Landes (1977), American men's propensity to favor the lower pitch range to appear more masculine may account for the hyperfunctional abuse of the voice.

Negligible attempts have been made to describe contact ulcers as a psychosomatic syndrome, and although a vast body of information has been published citing relationships between gastrointestinal ulcers and stress, these findings are still inconclusive. Greene (1980) cites a study by Cherry and Marguiles (1968), who studied three patients suffering "from pharyngo-oesophagitis due to peptic acid reflux" (p. 152). They suggested that it is possible for a backward flow of peptic acid to seep into the posterior larynx resulting in inflammation and ulceration. Other clinical workers have reported the appearance of contact ulcers in association with either acute or chronic upper respiratory infections. A more recent study by Kiese and Kruse (1994), involving formal personality, psychosocial, and physical inventories, revealed a causal psychosomatic relationship in the onset of LCU. While psychosocial stressors appeared to be a dominant factor, neurologic factors could not be ruled out.

Although the relationship among all these factors remains unclear, the speech-language pathologist is challenged to discover as many as possible of those elements in order to plan an appropriate regimen of therapy. Of particular importance is the necessity to understand the coping mechanisms, both psychological and physiological, that may be maintaining the vocal disorder and how these relate to vocal misuse and abuse.

Conversion Dysphonia

Probably no other voice disorder fits the classic definition of *functional* better than that of conversion dysphonia, except that organicity sometimes is found. Bridger and Epstein (1983) define *functional* generally as a "complaint due to disordered function rather than structure" (p. 1145). We would define conversion dysphonia as a symbolic representation of psychological conflict or stress manifested through the motor or sensory activity of the vocal tract, mainly the larynx. Sometimes referred to as *hysteria dysphonia*, the person with conversion dysphonia is generally middle-aged, exhibiting excessive tension in the laryngeal area and having frequent sore throats or laryngitis (Bridger and Epstein, 1983; Kaufman and Blalock, 1982).

According to Monday (1983), it appears to occur more often in women and may be associated with a precipitating unpleasant or traumatic event. Vocal abuse or misuse may not necessarily be a contributing factor, although the patient may not have a positive attitude toward vocal usage.

Greene (1980) probably painted one of the most complete psychological portraits of such patients. They frequently are persons who demonstrate loneliness, guilt, or remorse; they develop self-pity and then vocal failure. Sometimes a fear of cancer leads to an obsessive concern over the vocal mechanism. Tension is evident in facial and postural features, and the person appears fidgety and restless and speaks rapidly. Shoulder, neck, and scalp tension produce headaches. Sometimes gastrointestinal symptoms are manifested in indigestion, poor appetite, and constipation. In extreme cases there may be anorexia, in which the person restricts the taking of food severely with the idea of relieving some former digestive trouble.

Greene also describes the presence of endocrinological factors, such as menstrual pain, headache, and general malaise in persons with conversion dysphonia. Persistent anxiety resulting in overwhelming fatigue may be accompanied by insomnia.

According to Aronson (1980), the "conversion" may be into muteness, aphonia, or dysphonia. In its extreme form (conversion muteness), the characteristic findings are "chronic stress, primary and secondary gain, indifference to their symptom, other manifestations of conversion, poor sex identification, suppressed anger, immaturity and dependency, neurotic life adjustment, and mild to moderate depression" (p. 142). There appear also to be preexisting conscious and unconscious conflicts about verbal expression of anger, fear, or sadness and a halt in communication with those individuals who are of significance to the client.

Rammage et al. (1983) also suggest that conversion dysphonia may be a delayed shock reaction to trauma. The symptoms of a rise in vocal pitch accompanied by voice breaks often appear more acute when discussing stressful events. The dysphonic individual appears less disturbed than the aphonic one and homeostasis is easier to restore. Rammage et al. also report that the individual's dysphonia often follows an actual illness such as a throat virus or upper respiratory infection. A significant corollary is that the voice symptoms appear to serve as a secondary gain. Hinsie and Campbell (1970) describe:

> secondary advantages accruing from an illness, such as gratification of dependency yearning or attention seeking . . . there are certain uses the patient can make of his illness which have nothing to do with the origin of neurosis but which may attain the utmost practical importance . . . obtaining financial compensation . . . but has acquired the unconscious meaning of love and protecting security as well . . ." (p. 316)

In an investgation of 75 female and 7 male patients, Gerritsma (1991) found distinctive personality and psychosocial factors associated with the dysphonia. In particular, Gerritsma found in the sample used, the significant presence of social anxiety and nonassertiveness in the patients. The suggestion of possible somatic factors could not be ignored but the overall results need to be viewed cautiously. The study was conducted in Germany, thus cultural as well as distinctive psychosocial factors would have to be considered.

The following case study is a classic example of secondary gain in relationship to conversion dysphonia. George T, a 55-year-old investigator for a major insurance company, did not lose his laryngitis following a bout of the flu. Soon the laryngitis was accompanied by dysphonia, characterized by a high-pitched, straining or squeezed quality. Even though the vocal fold inflammation soon disappeared, the dysphonia persisted. His laryngologist, sensitive to Mr. T's associated depression, recommended psychiatric evaluation. After several psychotherapeutic sessions, it was learned that Mr. T had been seeking an early retirement from his firm but was being denied a full retirement compensation until age 65 unless a physical disability was present. The case history also revealed that Mr. T had never been married and had been living with two older, also unmarried, sisters for many years. The psychiatrist found Mr. T to be depressed, anxious, and enraged at his employer, whom he had "put out my life for." Expression of his rage and his hurt did not appear to have any effect on the dysphonia but in fact exacerbated it, resulting in intermittent whispering. Continuing psychiatric

treatment, his psychiatrist also recommended that he receive voice therapy.

The voice evaluation confirmed that which had already been discovered. It also was possible to obtain a clear resonant voice with vowels through digital manipulation of the larynx and by having Mr. T cough or laugh aloud in a rapid CV sequence (h, ha, ha, ha, ha). This could not be carried over into single words, although he apparently assiduously practiced obtaining clear phonation on various CVC combinations. While voice therapy was essentially symptomatic, Mr. T felt the need to express long repressed feelings of regret, anger, and frustration with his life and deep feelings of inferiority. Both his psychiatrist and voice pathologist kept in constant touch, each sharing with the other information that was emerging in the two therapies.

After six months, following the initial psychiatric consultation, Mr. T abruptly terminated psychiatric treatment but continued in voice therapy. Still unresolved were deep feelings of self-effacement and anger. It was felt by both therapists, though, that voice therapy that combined symptomatic and psychotherapeutic management would be less threatening and more productive.

During the next two months of voice therapy, Mr. T was able to achieve a clear voice and balanced vocal usage on single words and short phrases. As he was appearing gradually to move toward his pre-flu voice, however, he announced he no longer desired any form of therapy.

This case study is revealing in that it reflects the complex interplay of many factors that relate to its genesis and perpetuation. The case also presented a challenge in differential assessment as several of the vocal symptoms were not unlike those associated with spastic dysphonia.

It is appropriate that we close the discussion of conversion and psychogenic dysphonia with the position taken by Scott et al. (1997), who suggest that while evidence exists to demonstrate a high degree of neuroticism, depression, and anxiety in such individuals, there is no explanation why the larynx should be the focal point of the distress. The authors go on to explain the necessity for psychological intervention and the importance of training speech-language pathologists in the use of psychotherapeutic techniques along with traditional voice therapy.

Spastic Dysphonia

The ideopathic etiology of spastic dysphonia (SD) has been a source of debate for years. The proponents for an organic basis contend that spastic dysphonia patients are not neurologically normal, but their abnormalities are not necessarily the cause of the spasticity. Aronson and DeSanto (1983) and Dedo and Shipp (1980) suggest that the majority of research done over the past 20 years points to some central nervous system involvement either directly or indirectly. Unfortunately, no conclusion has been reached about precise location. Shipp et al. (1985) report one case study that suggests neurological etiology above the larynx.

Although SD often is categorized separately from other voice disorders, Brodnitz (1976) considers the disorder to be a conversion syndrome in the vast majority of cases. In defense of his proposition, Brodnitz notes that most of these patients could sing normally, were able to isolate the onset of dysphonia as acute emotional trauma, and exhibited severe neurotic characteristics. Despite little evidence to support the view that psychotherapeutic intervention, much less traditional therapy, has any substantial beneficial effects, undetermined psychodynamic forces may yet be at work. According to Izdebski and Dedo (1981), the progression of the disorder often leads the patient to withdraw from social situations and occupations, thus resulting in severe psychological consequences. Shipp et al. (1985) has indicated that in selected cases there is probably a mechanism triggered by stress that may result in a neuromuscular imbalance involving the vocal folds.

Supporting the viewpoint of a disorder that is essentially organic in nature, Stoicheff (1983) has indicated that these patients show no remission of symptoms. It also had been determined that the onset is progressive rather than sudden and that tremor is present in some patients. Believing SD to be among the most devastating and least understood voice disorders, Stoicheff theorizes the possibility of differing etiologies for the condition. He cites the inconsistency of vocal postoperative recovery from recurrent laryngeal nerve (RLN) sectioning.

For the last 20 years, Herbert Dedo, who pioneered the technique, has used RLN in treating spastic dysphonia. He and his associates report that 92% of their patients undergoing RLN section maintained satisfactory reduction of spasticity (Dedo and Izdeski, 1983). They note, however, that RLN section should not be regarded as a cure but as a means by which the communicative functioning of most patients can be enhanced. They used subjective patient self-assessments as indices of improvement.

Aronson and DeSanto (1983), however, contend that, according to their own postoperative evaluative technique, 64% of their patient population failed to meet criteria for "successful" treatment. They relied upon pre- and postoperative evaluations by a speech-language pathologist. To substantiate these findings further, Sapir and Aronson (1985) conducted a study investigating therapist reliability in rating voice improvements after RLN section and found a high degree of reliability in sources of information on the voice effects of surgery. They also determined that future judgment of voice after RLN section should be based primarily on therapist judgment rather than on patient self-assessment.

The problem of SD takes on less clarity when we review the study by Aronson and Hartman (1981). They attempted to distinguish among three different types of SD. They found bodily tremor, diffuse neurological signs, and patterns of life stress associated with the onset of the disorders classified, along with essential tremor. While the authors claim their results are inconclusive, they suggest that, although psychogenic factors may not be necessarily responsible for vocal stoppages, they "well may serve to precipitate or exacerbate an incipient neurologic disorder" (p. 59). More recent investigations appear to add to the psychogenic versus neurologic dilemma. Milutinovic and Kosanovic (1990) found no evidence of neurologic disease in 15 of 22 patients diagnosed with SD but also found signs of organicity in 7 subjects. The authors suggest that SD, in some cases, may be the initial symptom of an organic lesion within the CNS that has yet to appear clinically. Lieberman and Reife (1989) present one case of a 23-year-old male psychotic patient with combined choreoathetoid dyskinesia and SD associated with clinical and electromyographic (EMG) signs of muscle denervation. They suggest the possibility of basal ganglia involvement and the peripheral neuromuscular system. The latter appears to support Dedo's work discussed earlier. Silverman and Hummer (1989), who evaluated 20 subjects identified as having SD and described their speech as lacking fluency, suggest the possibility of a fluency disorder not unlike stuttering with similar phenomenological, symptomological, and etiological elements. Finally, Pennington (1998), in a very limited study involving one patient diagnosed with SD, used hypnotherapy successfully to improve vocal performance.

There is little question that, regardless of etiology or premorbid personality, the distress brought about by the disorder may have a profound effect upon the person's career and marital and social life. Emotional responses may range from anger to withdrawal and, in extreme cases, definitive personality changes may occur. Although surgical intervention appears to be the major treatment of choice, there is sufficient evidence to suggest some form of psychotherapeutical aid, even though the latter has not been found to be a panacea of treatment. It is obvious we must continue to rely on symptomatic, subjective and individualized strategies until definitive outcome studies dictate otherwise.

Laryngectomy

In the last three decades, numerous advances have taken place to assist our understanding of the anatomic-physiological factors and modes of treatment for laryngectomy. As a life-saving procedure for carcinoma of the larynx, the far-reaching psychological ramifications for the individual so afflicted has received less attention. Fontaine and Mitchell (1960) are among the earliest writers to refer to the emotional and sexual problems brought on after laryngectomy. In the past decade more authorities have referred to the profound psychosocial implications of such a tragedy.

It has been established that heavy cigarette smoking and excessive intake of alcohol are the two most critical agents responsible for the development of cancerous lesions in the larynx. It has been further suggested by other investigators that tobacco and alcohol abuse are addictions that have associated features of personality disturbance, anxiety, and depression (Wallen and Webb, 1975). These

may be a response to an inability to cope effectively with life stresses. Discovery by such individuals that they have cancer and must have laryngeal amputation to survive is likely to have some profound effect on them, although little research has been done to document this.

Weisman (1979) and Weisman and Worden (1976–1977) found that, among cancer patients in general, those who were more emotionally disturbed tended to be withdrawn and disengaged from others. Less disturbed patients characteristically confronted the problem by accepting the situation, taking firm action, and seeking medical help. Although not referring to cancer to the larynx specifically, Weisman has described four psychosocial phases related to the stage, treatment, and progression of cancer: existential plight, accommodation and mitigation, recurrence and relapse, and deterioration and decline.

It would appear obvious that removal of the larynx will have a profound psychological impact, although the effects may differ with respect to the sexes. For the male, amputation is akin to castration, which could be equated to the loss of manhood, as the larynx, next to the penis, represents masculinity both symbolically and figuratively. For the female, loss of the larynx could well represent disfigurement and the associated distortion of the persona or self-image. In their study, Weinstein, Vetter, and Sersen (1964) found that women between the ages of 20 and 70 years rated the tongue as their most important organ, but no distinction was made between that and the larynx. We contend that the two would be equivalent, as both organs are integral for purposes of communication in human species.

Most important in our roles as speech-language pathologists is how we attempt to aid such individuals in coping with their loss and the implications of readjustment. We have referred elsewhere to Tanner's (1980) incisive essay on loss and grief as they relate to the communicatively disordered, but he makes only fleeting reference to amputation as an aspect of loss of self. Surprisingly little data are available in the literature surveyed about the mourning process in families where laryngectomy has occurred, but as we discuss presently, an explanation is possible.

Several studies in the present decade contribute to our understanding of how laryngectomized individuals and their families cope. Richardson et al. (1989) examined the relationship between social environmental variables and psychological, physical, and speech dysfunction following laryngectomy in 60 patients. They concluded that interpersonal support from family and friends was strongly associated with improved psychosocial and physical function but less of an association with speech adjustment. Devins et al. (1994) collected data from interviews of 51 patients to determine the psychosocial impact of "perceived stigma" from laryngectomy. They found that perceived stigma and intrusiveness of illness were related to psychosocial well-being and emotional distress (p. 608). In their study of depression following laryngectomy in 63 men, Blood et al. (1993) found that those who demonstrated internal control also scored as better adjusted and had fewer communication problems. In their comparative study of laryngectomized patients and those who received only radiotherapy, Byrne et al. (1993) found the former sample to be more depressed, with associated poorer communication skills. Stams et al. (1991) also conducted structured interviews with 51 laryngectomized patients, and found that preoperative visits by fellow laryngectomized individuals predicted later quality of life. The investigation also revealed that poor psychological adjustments were related to length of time in the hospital following surgery, complaints of lack of social support, and changes in lifestyle. Changes in self-concept also predicted both psychological adjustment and quality of life. Not surprisingly, the extent of social support predicted the use of esophageal speech.

Several excellent sources are available relative to pre- and postoperative counseling with laryngectomized individuals and their families (among them Salmon, 1979; Reed, 1983; and Keith et al., 1977, and Kommers, Sullivan, and Yonkers 1977, viewing the laryngectomee's home environment as a crucial determinant toward maximizing rehabilitation success), but most are essentially information rather than psychodynamically oriented. Unfortunately, in a later study by Zeine and Larson (1996), a survey to determine if preoperative and postoperative counseling services had improved since the 1977 study by Keith et al., revealed that little change had been made to improve the situation. The need for patient and family education cannot be underestmated. Despondt and Gehanno (1995) provide an extensive review of the benefits of patient education along with the rationale for continued family, social, and professional rehabilitation. The management of issues associated with socioculturally different populations also are discussed.

While providing information is extremely important, a proper interpersonal counseling relationship with the patient and the spouse could help resolve many of the problems that arise, particularly postoperatively.

In a retrospective study by Kommers and Sullivan (1979), answers to a comprehensive questionnaire given to 45 wives of laryngectomized men indicated a definite "need for improved family counseling both before and after surgery" (p. 411). Of those wives interviewed, 60% reported shock, fear, panic, and denial on first learning of cancer, and 50% noted that their husband's personality or attitude had changed immediately following surgery. They were either depressed or irritable. Although not addressed specifically, the mourning period appeared not to be prolonged. A possible explanation for this may be that, with the acquisition of alaryngeal speech, considerable psychological readjustment is likely to occur.

This should not nullify the need for family counseling or family therapy to help the client and spouse work through the myriad of personal, family, and social problems that could ensue. Salazar-Sanchez and Stark (1972) used a crisis intervention model involving a speech pathologist and social worker, applying interventive and preventive strategies with laryngectomized individuals and their families. Ideally, the speech pathologist who is skilled in counseling would be the most appropriate person to assume the major task because of the greatest frequency of professional contact. In their investigation of counseling needs of male and female laryngectomized persons, Salva and Kallail (1989) conclude that more and improved pre- and postoperative counseling was needed. There were gender differences regarding feelings about surgery, emotional support systems, and perceived usefulness of information given by counselors. Greene and Mathieson (1991), who interviewed 30 patients and their spouses regarding quality of life and the psychological state of the spouse, found that spouses experienced higher levels of depression, tension, and fatigue than their partners. These results appear consistent with our earlier analyses of spouses' emotional state following CVA and TBI.

In some cases, individual counseling for the laryngectomized patient is recommended even though alaryngeal speech may not yet be fully established. Fullest use of a speech aid is well justified in such cases, even if to be employed only temporarily for interpersonal communication in therapy as well as at home and socially. (Our position is that a speech aid should be used whenever alaryngeal speech or inserted devices are unfeasible or as an adjunctive aid for even proficient alaryngeal speakers.) Counseling does not have to be singled out from traditional alaryngeal voice therapy and, as we suggest all along, should be integrated within the total therapeutic process. Anand and Anand (1997) found that the use of art therapy with over 100 patients, covering a period of 14 years, served as a significant diagnostic and therapeutic tool in enhancing psychosocial adjustment.

It would appear that quality of life is probably the most valuable enhancement that can be achieved with the individuals we have been describing. In this light, Maas (1991) developed a quality of life model to help the individual deal with the psychosocial, speech, vocational, and other aspects in assisting the person to think more deliberately about complication following surgery. Maas distinguishes two types of problem-solving strategies: coping and solving. Maas's model resembles somewhat, the ethnographic intervention model of Hammer, discussed earlier.

Finally, we should not underestimate the value of New Voice Clubs, which can serve as powerful support groups for the patients readjusting and reentering into life. Whatever the therapeutic support, either formal or informal, the individual can be helped to find a new meaning in life despite the specter of cancer to which he or she may yet be vulnerable.

Counseling Strategies

It appears appropriate and logical following the previous discussions that a psychotherapeutic approach to the treatment of voice disorders in adults is in order. Perhaps *psychotherapeutic* is not the best word to describe exactly how we can most effectively manage our clients. In essence, we must decide how much of a holistic practitioner we choose to be. Or we might consider, as Brodnitz (1981) maintains, that, for us to "normalize" vocal function, it is necessary that we "respect the 'Gestalt' of the voice" (p. 24). Most important, however, is our understanding that we, as voice therapists, are not seeking a change in the client's essential being but only a change in which the client uses the various parts of self to vocalize. As Cooper (1973) has correctly cautioned us, "all voice types in one fashion or another represent to the individual a commitment to the cultural norms of the society and/or to the stereotypes the individual has regarding the voice for a given person, position, and situation" (p. 50). Thus, it appears reasonable, as Cooper suggests, that vocal rehabilitation requires a variable approach with varying emphasis on either the mechanics of production or on what he describes as "vocal psychotherapy."

Because vocal change is our chief objective, much will depend on what we perceive as necessary to change and what our clients deem important to modify. The two may not always be compatible. Can we be certain that we always know best what must be changed or can we be open to the client's personal perceptions of what can realistically be modified?

As one of our graduate students so aptly put it:

it may be easier for the therapist to see that certain changes can only benefit the client than it is for the client to believe such a thing, let alone to feel it on all conscious and unconscious levels. After all, a major survival activity throughout life is to "get your act together," and if this can be done while being genuine, it is certainly more powerful. But most of us rely on at least a few stopgap measures to help us present to the world what we feel is an acceptable front. This front becomes an armor defending us against the threat of being discovered to be truly what we fear we are. Creating in others a desire to shed that burdensome armor is some of the art that therapists must develop throughout their professional careers. People naturally "compensate" and it takes powerful motivation to make them want to give up that compensation. (TeSelle, 1985)

We view voice therapy as a reciprocal arrangement between therapist and client whereby adaptation is made by each to suit the needs of the client as they occur during the therapeutic process. An individual counseling approach appears to be a most appropriate treatment to satisfy these requirements.

Individual Counseling

Counseling, a both therapeutic and educational process, should be flexible enough to fit the objective reality of the clinical situation and the therapeutic relationship. Consistent with the earlier discussion in this chapter, we make no distinction between identified organicity or lack of it when psychological components are present and obvious. We do not infer that differential assessment should be omitted. On the contrary, it becomes all the more important and significant if we are to consider vocal pathology as part of a total human process.

One further consideration is pertinent to our discussion. We prefer to style our therapeutic approach to the person and not to the particular voice disorder identified. One exception to this rule, however, is the treatment of laryngectomy, which we believe to have unique characteristics so as to require special attention.

Guidelines for Intervention

We developed several guidelines that, when considered in the context of basic counseling principles covered earlier and elsewhere, can serve to lead us appropriately toward healthier vocal usage for the person. Similarities of therapeutic guidelines for both children and adults obviously overlap and are intentional. We have chosen as well to integrate

whatever symptomatic treatment is necessary within the context of our approach but not to dwell on specifics, as they are covered elsewhere in this and other books on counseling.

The Case History Process

The case history may provide us with important data, but more significant is the knowledge gained through the actual interactional dialogue with the client. What is valuable is not what has happened in the past per se, but how the client perceives what has occurred. Maintaining an open-ended discussion may also give us an immediate visual and acoustical picture of vocal usage, as well as the present feelings and self-image attitude of the client.

The Differential Assessment

Also interactional is the means by which we determine the effectiveness or ineffectiveness with which the client vocalizes. We also wish to discover the possible presence, if any, of pronounced organic components that may demand immediate medical attention. We prefer using the vocal analysis profile format of Perkins (1971), who considers the various components of voice as either dependent or independent functions. His discussion of the concept of constriction fits neatly with our encouragement of the client to talk about the stress associated directly or indirectly with his or her vocal usage. The performance of the oral-maxillary facial examination provides an opportunity to stimulate the expression of feelings concerning each element of the procedure. We thus can derive some notions of how the client reacts to various vocal changes that occur and those that do not. Such a process will help set the stage for the course of therapy that is to be determined.

The Interpersonal Relationship

As the free flow of communication between the client and the therapist develops, the client is more likely to drop the psychic defenses that may be associated with vocal abuse and misuse. Likewise, it will be easier for both to identify obvious and subtle connections between faulty vocal habits and various emotional components. This interaction further allows the therapist to learn more about the client than ordinarily would be revealed through a rigid case history and vocal examination.

The Uniqueness of the Individual

The therapist needs to maintain a flexible approach that will suit the particular person being treated and not the identified vocal disorder. For that matter, it is conceivable that one individual with vocal nodules could be more like another individual with nonorganic dysphonia than one with vocal nodules. It also is necessary for the therapist to be attuned to differing client needs; for example, the financial necessity to remain in a dead-end job, powerful resistance to terminating a destructive and stressful marriage, need of the professional voice user to go beyond a vocal range that is physiologically abusive. It is not our role to intercede in even the consideration of such decisions but to assist the client in at least understanding the dilemma, should the issue arise, and perhaps indirectly suggest further counseling assistance. We cannot avoid the problem, however, if it relates directly to vocal management.

Client Responsibility

A major goal in voice therapy is to educate clients that they have within themselves the ability to change many, if not most, of the features that contribute to vocal misuse and abuse. Client resistance to making such a choice may be embedded in deep-rooted psychopathology or needs associated with the maintenance of a particular vocal image. Regardless, we must again avoid taking the position of "rescuer" and facilitate self-direction if permanency of vocal change is to occur.

Vocal Personality Factors

Although the relationship between personality characteristics and vocal style is yet unclear, it is the therapist's responsibility to determine, in concert with the client, how the latter perceives self in relationship to personal vocal style. It then is necessary to determine if the client needs to maintain a particular vocal style to enhance a favorable perception of self, especially if the former is lacking. The clinical challenge for change is quite formidable because it may involve a metamorphosis of individual behavior and personality. The reader is referred to the more comprehensive discussion of this issue by Cooper (1973).

Therapeutic Congruency

Most therapists are well aware of voice clients who ostensibly seek help for their voice disorder but actually have a different agenda. Some profess the desire to follow all of the advice their therapist has to offer regarding vocal change. In actuality, though, they may put up barriers to the implementation of such changes. Others immediately ventilate pent-up feelings regarding self-esteem, life struggles, and emotional conflict. These individuals resist taking too close a look at their problems on a deeper level and simultaneously reject management of the vocal symptoms.

Such seemingly paradoxical attitudes offer a considerable challenge to the therapist, who must now sort out with the client exactly what is desired. Although a nondirective counseling approach may be in order, a more direct and gently confrontive approach could be implemented effectively. The client must be helped to decide what direction to take, with clarity and openness in interpersonal communication being maintained. Irrational and unproductive attitudes need to be exposed and recognized as inhibitors of further progress. Unsurprisingly, some such clients who are able to make this breakthrough carry these new communicative behaviors into personal relationships with significant others in their lives. Whereas dramatic changes in vocal usage may occur for a few, others may still require considerable symptomatic management.

Combining Symptomatic with Psychotherapeutic Management

We already mentioned that no one therapeutic approach is appropriate for every client and that symptoms cannot readily be distinguished from vocal functioning or human behavior. Therefore, therapists need to be flexible enough to respond to whatever components arise or are evident in any one moment or extended period of therapy. Also, we must be aware that having our clients do vocal exercises necessitates an understanding of how they are responding psychologically to them. Correspondingly, any positive change in vocal behavior should be viewed in the context of the client's vocal perception of psychological behavior.

Although this overall approach may appear to resemble a potpourri of therapeutic tactics, such is not the case at all. Based on the initial assessment, voice therapy for a particular individual must have short- and long-term objectives but be amenable to change as new data are discovered during the process. That is, therapy should be diagnostic in nature, responsive to the needs of the client, yet integrated so that both client and therapist are aware of how all the elements interact. In this way "elocutionary"-type voice therapy, whereby voice is regarded as a distinct entity separate from the person, can be avoided.

Contracting

As with voice-disordered children, but perhaps even more so with adults, it is necessary for both client and therapist to be on the same track if a positive outcome is to be realized. That is, voice therapy is characterized by a process of negotiation whereby each successive step is understood by both parties and appropriately carried out. Any obstacles to continued progress must be analyzed and removed and adjustments in therapy made, if necessary, for therapy to succeed.

Contracts between client and therapist will vary in their design, formality, and organization, depending on the particular therapeutic circumstances, nature of the voice disorder, and specific client needs. In most cases, the contract can be a mutually agreed-on verbal commitment to a series of appropriate therapeutic steps. For others it must be a written commitment to meet the expectations deemed suitable by both client and therapist, Whatever arrangement is made, the contract should be treated not as an end in itself but as a viable means to enhance the interpersonal relationship, encourage

congruency, and ensure a positive therapeutic outcome for the client.

Special Counseling Problems

The therapist must be particularly conscious about some aspects to therapy with the voice-disordered person. One involves touching the client's neck or shoulder, which for some clients could be misinterpreted as a sexual advance. To nullify such a perception, the therapist must explain fully the purpose of such touching or physical manipulation and ask the client permission to do so. Obviously, we need to respect the client's wishes if such actions are refused.

Transference and countertransference, if they occur, must be kept in objective perspective and should be discussed openly. Although unlikely to emerge in most cases, instances whereby dramatic positive vocal and personality changes occur may trigger them. Therefore, any departure from the formal clinical environment to external environments where carryover can be more objectively observed must be considered carefully.

Persistent resistance to the modification of vocal behavior despite full acquiescence by the therapist to the client's wishes must be interpreted to be deeply rooted psychodynamically. If unresolved, the therapist must take steps to recommend gently outside referral to either another therapist or psychotherapist. The therapist well grounded in the theory of psychopathology will know best when and how to deal with "difficult" clients.

Conclusion

We have demonstrated that voice disorders in adults, like voice disorders in children, cannot be separated from the person. In adults, however, the psychodynamic factors are more complex both etiologically and intrinsically to the specific disorder. Our attempt has also been to approach treatment based on the individual uniqueness of the client and not on the disorder. Most important, however, is that we not neglect all the therapeutic tools we have available to us regardless of our biases. To quote Brodnitz (1981), we need not allow the "products of our gadget-happy times . . . to interfere with the integration of vocal use as a unified function" (p. 25). Yet, at the same time, we have to recognize that even the gadgets have value in our holistic approach to the client.

References

American Psychological Association. The Diagnostic and Statistical Manual of Mental Disorder, 4th ed. (DSM-IV). Washington, DC: American Psychological Assocation; 1994.

Anand SA, Anand VK. Art therapy with laryngectomy patients. *Art Therapy.* 1997;14(2):109–117.

Aronson A. *Clinical Voice Disorders.* New York: Thieme Stratton; 1980.

———. *Clinical Voice Disorders.* 3rd ed. New York: Thieme Stratton; 1990.

Aronson A, DeSanto L. Adductor spastic dysphonia: three years after recurrent laryngeal nerve resection. *Laryngoscope.* 1983;93:1–8.

Aronson A, Hartman DE. Spastic dysphonia as a sign of essential (voice) tremor. *J of Speech and Hearing Disorders.* 1981;46:52–58.

Axeline VM. *Play Therapy.* New York: Ballantine Books; 1969.

Baker EL, Platt JA, Fine HJ. Tic de Gilles de la Tourette: survey of the literature, case study and reinterpretation. *Clinical Psychology Review.* 1983;3:157–178.

Barker KD, Wilson FB. Comparative study of vocal utilization of children with hoarseness and normal voice. Paper presented at the convention of the American Speech and Hearing Association; 1967.

Blood GW, Dineen M, Kauffman SM, Raimond SC, et al. Perceived control adjustment and communication problems in laryngeal cancer survivors. *Perceptual and Motor Skills.* 1993;77(3, Pt. 1):764–766.

Boone DL. *The Voice and Voice Therapy,* 3rd ed. Englewood Cliffs, NJ: Prentice-Hall; 1983.

Boone DL, Mc Farlane SC. *The Voice and Voice Therapy,* 5th ed., Englewood Cliffs, NJ: Prentice-Hall; 1993.

Bridger MWM, Epstein R. Functional voice disorders: a review of 109 patients. *J of Laryngology and Otology.* 1983;97:1145–1148.

Brodnitz FS. Spastic dysphonia. *Annals of Otology, Rhinology and Laryngology* 1976;85:212–213.

———. Psychological considerations in vocal rehabilitation. *J of Speech and Hearing Disorders.* 1981;46:22–26.

Butcher P, Elias A, Raven R. *Psychogenic Voice Disorders and Cognitive Behavior Therapy.* San Diego, CA: Singular Publishing; 1993:3–22.

Byrne A, Walsh M, Farrelly M, O'Driscoll K. Depression following laryngectomy. *British J of Psychiatry.* 1993;163:173–176.

Case JL. *Clinical Management of Voice Disorders.* Rockville, MD: Aspen Systems Corp,; 1984.

Cherry J, Marguiles SI. Contact ulcer of the larynx. *Laryngoscope.* 1968:78.

Cook JV, Palaski DJ, Hanson WR. A vocal hygiene program for school age children. *Lang-Sp-Hear Services in Schools.* 1979;10:21–26.

Cooper M. *Modern Techniques of Vocal Rehabilitation.* Springfield, IL: Charles C Thomas; 1973.

Dedo H, Izdebski K. Intermediate results of 306 recurrent laryngeal nerve sections for spastic dysphonia. *Larygoscope.* 1983;93: 9–16.

Dedo H, Shipp T. *Spastic Dysphonia.* Houston: College-Hill Press; 1980.

Despondt J, Gehanno P. Laryngectomized patients' education and follow-up. *Patient Education and Counseling.* 1995;26(1–3):33–36.

Devins GM, Stam H, Koopermans JP. Psychological impact of laryngectomy mediated by perceived stigma and illness in transiveness. *Canadian J of Psychiatry.* 1994;39(10):608–616.

Erikson EH. *Childhood and Society,* 2nd ed. New York: W. W. Norton; 1963.

Estrada AV, Pinsoff WM. The effectiveness of family therapies for selected behavioral disorders of childhood. *J of Marital and Fam Therapy.* 1995;21(4):403–440.

Fontaine A, Mitchell JCE. Oesopahgal voice: a factor of readiness. *J of Laryngology* 1960;74:870.

Formby D. Maternal recognition of infant's cry. *Develop Med Child Neurology.* 1967;9:293.

Gerritsma EJ. An investigation into some personality characteristics of patients with psychogenic aphonia and dysphonia. *Folia-Phoniatrica.* 1991;43(1):13–20.

Glassel WL. A study of personality problems and vocal nodules in children. Paper read at the American Speech and Hearing Association Convention; San Francisco; 1972.

Glaze LE. Treatment of voice hyperfunction in the pre-adolescent. *Lang-Sp-Hear Services in Schools.* 1996;27(3): 244–250.

Goodstein LD. Functional speech disorders and personality: a survey of the research. *J of Speech and Hearing Research.* 1958;1:359–376.

Graham M. *The Clinician's Guide to Alaryngeal Speech Therapy.* Boston: Butterworth–Heinemann; 1997.

Green G. Psychobehavioral characteristics of children with vocal modules: WPBIC ratings. *J of Speech and Hearing Disorders.* 1989;54:306–312.

Greene MCL. *The Voice and Its Disorders,* 4th ed. Philadelphia: Lippincott; 1980.

Greene MCL, Mathieson L. *The Voice and Its Disorders,* 5th ed. San Diego, CA: Singular Publishing; 1991.

Gutwinski-Jeggle J. Psychognen dysphonien asl beziehungssturungen: Moglichkeiten und Grenzen ihrer logopadischen behendlung (Psychogenic vocal problems as relationship disturbances: possibilities and limitations for treatment by speech therapy). *Praxis de Psychotherapic and Psychosomatik.* 1983;28:43–53.

Hejna RF. *Speech Disorders and Nondirective Therapy*. New York: Ronald Press; 1960.

Hinsie LE, Campbell RJ. *Psychiatric Dictionary*, 4th ed. New York; Oxford University Press; 1970.

Holden C. Lie detectors: PSE gains audience despite critics' doubt. *Science*. 1975;190:359–362.

House AD, Andrews HB. Life events and difficulties preceding the onset of functional dysphonia. *J of Psychosomatic Res*. 1994;32(3):311–319.

Izdebsk K, Dedo H. Spastic dysphonia. In: Darby J, ed. *Speech Evaluation in Medicine*. New York: Grane and Stratton; 1981:609–618.

Kambic V et al. Vocal cord polyps: incidence, histology and pathogenesis. *J of Laryngology and Otology*. 1981;95: 609–618.

Kaplan SL. Mutational falsetto. *J of the American Academy of Child Psychiatry*. 1982;21:82–85.

Kaufman JA, Blalock PD. Classification and approach to patients with functional voice disorders. *Annals of Otolaryngology and Rhinolaryngology*. 1982;91:372–377.

Keith RL, Shane HC, Coates HL, Devine KD. *Looking Forward: A Guidebook for the Laryngectomee*. Rochester. MN: Mayo Foundation; 1977.

Kerr ME. Family systems theory and therapy. In: Gurman AS, Kniskem DP, eds. *Handbook of Family Therapy*. New York: Brunner/Mazel, 1981.

Kiese CH, Kruse E. Contact ulcer of the larynx: a psychosomatic disorder? *Folia-Phoniatrica*. 1994;46(6):288–297.

Kommers MS, Sullivan MD. Wives' evaluation of problems related to laryngectomy. *J of Communication Disorders*. 1979;12:411–430.

Kommers MS, Sullivan MD, Yonkers AJ. Counseling the laryngectomized patient. *Larygngoscope*. 1977;87: 1961–1965.

Laguaite JK. The use of hypnosis with children with deviant voices. *International J of Clinical and Experimental Hypnosis*. 1976;24:98–104.

Landes BA. Management of hyperfunctional dysphonia and vocal tension. In: Cooper M, Cooper MH, eds. *Approaches to Vocal Rehabilitation*. Springfield, IL: Charles C Thomas; 1977.

Lieberman J, Reife R. Spastic dysphonia and denervation signs in a young man with tardive dyskenesia. *British J of Psychiatry*. 1989;154:105–109.

Low G, Crerar M, Lassers L. Communication centered therapy. *J of Speech and Hearing Disorders*. 1959;24: 361–368.

Luchsinger R, Arnold GE. *Voice-Speech-Language*. Belmont, CA: Wadsworth; 1965.

Maas A. A model for quality of life after laryngectomy. *Social Science and Medicine*. 1991;33(12):1373–1377.

Mathieson CM, Stam HJ, Scott JP. The impact of a laryngectomy on the spouse: who is better off? *Psychology and Health*. 1991;5(2):153–163.

Miller SQ, Madison CL. Public school voice clinics, Part II: Diagnosis and recommendations—a 10-year review. *Lang-Sp-Hear Services in Schools*. 1984;15:58–63.

Milutinovic Z, Kosanovic R. Contribution to the understanding of the etiology of spastic dysphonia. *Folia-Phoniatrica*. 1990;42(2):98–100.

Minuchin S. *Families and Family Therapy*. Cambridge, MA: Harvard University Press; 1974.

Monday LA. Clinical evaluation of functional dysphonia. *J of Otolaryngology*. 1983;12:307–310.

Moore P. Voice disorders. In: Shames G, Wing E, eds. *Human Communication Disorders: An Introduction*. Columbus, OH: Charles E. Merrill; 1982.

Mosby DP. Predominant personality characteristics of 25 children with voice disorders. Paper read at the American Speech and Hearing Association Convention; 1967; Chicago.

———. Psychology versus voice therapy for a child with a deviant voice: a case study. *Perceptual and Motor Skills*. 1970;30:887–891.

Moses P. *The Voice of Neurosis*. New York: Grune and Stratton; 1954.

Murphy AT. *Functional Voice Disorders*. Englewood Cliffs, NJ: Prentice-Hall; 1964.

Murray SC, Carr ME, Jacobs V. Functional aphasia in the child and adolscent: therapeutic management. *Lang-Sp-Hear Services in Schools*. 1983;14:260–265.

Ostwald PF. *Soundmaking*. Springfield, IL: Charles C Thomas; 1963.

Pannbacker M. Treatment of vocal nodules: options and outcomes. *Amer J of Sp-Lang Pathology*. 1999;8(3): 209–217.

Pennington A. Two hyprotherapy studies. In: Syder D, et al., eds. *Wanting to Talk: Counseling Case Studies in Communication Disorders*. London, UK: Whurr Publishers; 1998:185–207.

Perkins W. Vocal function: a behavioral analysis. In: Travis LE, ed. *Handbook of Speech Pahtology and Audiology*. New York: Appleton-Century-Crofts; 1971.

———, ed. *Voice Disorders*. New York: Thieme Stratton; 1983.

Phillis JA. Children's judgments of personality on the basis of voice quality. *Developmental Pscyhology*. 1970;3:411.

Quan K. The Relationship of Voice to Personlaity. Unpublished paper. San Francisco State University; 1985.

Rammage LA, Nichol H, Morrison MD. The voice clinic: An interdisciplinary approach. *J of Otolaryngology*. 1983;8:315–318.

Reed CG. Surgical-prosthetic techniques for laryngeal speech. *Communicative Disorders: A Journal for Continuing Education*. 1983;8:109–124.

Richardson JL, Graham JW, Shelton DR. Social environment and adjustment after laryngectomy. *Health and Social Work*. 1989;14(4):283–292.

Rosen DC, Sataloff RT. *Psychology of Voice Disorders*. San Diego, CA: Singular Publishing; 1997.

Salazar-Sanchez V, Stark A. The use of crisis intervention in the rehabilitation of laryngectomees. *J of Speech and*

Hearing Disorders. 1972;37:323–328.

Salmon SJ. Pre- and post-operative conferences with larygectomized and their spouses. In: Keith RL, Darley FG, eds. *Larynectomee Rehabilitation.* Houston: College-Hill Press; 1979.

Salva CT, Kallail KJ. An investigation of the counseling needs of male and female laryngectomees. *J of Comm Disord.* 1989;22(4):291–304.

Sapir E. Speech as a personality trait. *Am J of Soc.* 1927;332: 192–205.

Sapir S, Aronson A. Clinician reliability in rating voice improvement after laryngeal nerve section for spastic dysphonia. *Laryngoscope.* 1985;93:200–202.

Scherer KR. Judging personality from voice: a cross-cultural approach to an old issue in interpersonal perception. *J of Personality.* 1972;37:215–221.

———. Vocal indicator of stress. In: Darby JK, ed. *Speech Evaluation in Psychiatry.* New York: Grune and Stratton; 1981a.

———. Speech and emotional states. In: Darby JK, ed. *Speech Evaluation in Psychiatry.* New York: Grune and Stratton; 1981b.

Scott GS, Layton TL. Epidemiologic principles in studies of infectious disease outcomes: pediatric HIV as a model. *J of Comm Disord.* 1997;30(4):303–324.

Scott GS, Dreary IJ, Mackenzie K. Functional dysphonia: a role for psychologists? *Psychology, Health, and Medicine.* 1997;2(2):169–180.

Sentura B, Wilson F. Otorhinolaryngic findings in children with voice deviations. *Annals of Otology, Rhinology and Laryngology.* 1968;77:1027–1041.

Shipp T, Izdebski K, Reed C, Morrissey P. Intrinsic laryngeal muscle activity in spastic dysphonia patient. *J of Speech and Hearing Disorders.* 1985;50:54–59.

Shipp T, McGlone RE. Physiologic correlates of acoustic correlates of psychological stress. *J of the Acoustic Society of America.* 1973:53–63.

Siegman AW. Nonverbal correlates of anxiety and stress. In: Goldberger L, Breznitz S, eds. *Handbook of Stress: Theoretical and Clinical Aspects.* New York: Macmillan; 1982.

Silverman EM, Zimmer CH. Incidence of chronic hoarseness among school-age children. *J of Speech and Hearing Disorders.* 1975;40:211–215.

Silverman FH, Hummer K. Spastic dysphonia: a fluency disorder? *J of Fluency Disorders.* 1989;14(4):285–291.

Simonov PV, Frolov MV. Utilization of human voice for estimation of man's emotional stress and state of attention. *Aerospace Medicine.* 1973;44:256–258.

Simonov PV, Frolov MV, Talebkin VL. Use of the invariant method of speech analysis to discern the emotional state of announcers. *Aviation, Space and Environmental Medicine.* 1975;46:1014–1016.

Stams HJ, Keepmans JP, Mathieson CM. The Psychosocial impact of laryngectomy: a comprehensive assessment. *J of Psychological Oncology.* 1991:9(3):37–58.

Steinhauer PD, Berman G. Anxiety, neurotic and personality disorders in children. In: Steinhauer PD, Rae-Grant Q, eds. *Psychological Problems of the Child in the Family,* 2nd ed. New York: Basic Books; 1983.

Stoicheff ML. The present status of adductor spastic dysphonia. *J of Otolaryngology.* 1983;12:311–314.

Tanner DC. Loss and grief: implications for the speech-language pathologist and audiologist. *ASHA.* 1980;22: 916–928.

TeSelle N. Voice: mirror of the soul. Unpublished paper, San Francisco State University; 1985.

Toohill RJ. The psychosomatic aspects of children with vocal nodules. *Archives of Otolaryngology.* 1975;101:591–595.

Valanne E, Vuorenkoski V, Partanen TJ, Lind J, Wasz-Hockert O. The ability of human mothers to identify the hunger cry signals of their own newborn infants during lying-in period. *Experientia.* 1967;23:768.

Van Riper C, Emerick L. *Speech Correction: An Introduction to Speech Pathology and Audiology,* 7th ed. Englewood Cliffs, NJ: Prentice-Hall; 1984.

Vogel D, Carter J. *The Effects of Drugs on Communication Disorders.* San Diego, CA: Singular Publishing;1995:31–143.

Wallen V, Webb V. A study of background characteristics and traits of laryngectomees. *Military Medicine.* 1975;140: 532–534.

Warr-Leeper GA, McShea RS, Leeper HA. The incidence of voice and speech deviations in a middle school population. *Lang-Sp-Hear Services in Schools.* 1979;10:14–20.

Wasz-Hocket O, Lind J, Vuorenkoski V, Partanen TJ, Valanne E. The infant cry: A spectrographic and auditory analysis. *Clinics in Developmental Medicine.*1968;29 Spastics International Medical Publications in Association with Heinemann Medical.

Weinstein S, Vetter R, Sersen E. Physiological and Experiential concomitants of the phantom. VRA Project No. 427, final report. New York: Albert Einstein College of Medicine; 1964.

Weisman A. *Coping with Cancer.* New York: McGraw-Hill; 1979.

Weisman A, Worden J. The existential plight of cancer: significance of the first 100 days. *International J of Psychiatry in Medicine.* 1976–1977;7:1–15.

Wilson DK. *Voice Problems of Children,* 2nd ed. Baltimore: Williams and Wilkins; 1979.

Wilson FB, Lamb MM. Comparison of personality characteristics of children with and without vocal *nodules* on Rorschach protocol interpretation. Paper read at the American Speech and Hearing Association Convention; 1973; Atlanta.

Zeine L, Larson M. Pre- and post-operative counseling for laryngectomees and their spouses: an update. *J of Comm Disord.* 1996;32(1):51–71.

7

Psychological Considerations for Congenitally and Degeneratively Involved Individuals and Their Families

Cleft Palate

Cleft Palate in Children

Although cleft lip and palate is only one of a wide variety of craniofacial anomalies, we have chosen it for selective attention because it is the most likely to fall within the province of the working speech-language pathologist. Also, it generally is the least severe of the craniofacial deformities physically and the most amenable to reconstructive surgery and habilitative intervention.

The occurrence of cleft lip and palate at birth generally requires the attention of a variety of specialists representing plastic surgery, pediatrics, otology, speech-language pathology, dentistry, audiology, and psychology. Ideally, these professionals act as a team to guide the afflicted child and the family through an oftentimes agonizing series of surgical procedures and feeding, hearing, speech-language, dental, and upper respiratory problems.

Because of the interplay of many aspects of development and associated complications, it is uncertain if intelligence falls below the norm in cleft palate children. It is evident that because language generally is more slow to develop and because of the other special problems noted, generalizations about mental development may be difficult to make (McWilliams, 1982).

One would expect the psychosocial problems to be a natural concomitant to all of the developmental aspects evident, and that the child's speech and language would either influence or be influenced by psychosocial factors. Let us, therefore, explore this issue.

Psychosocial Correlates

No definitive evidence appears to support the view that cleft palate children are necessarily more emotionally disturbed than other children. Starr (1980) investigated the relationship between facial attractiveness and behavior in 49 10-year-old and older subjects with cleft lip and palate and found no statistically significant relationships between the attractive and less attractive group. Starr used the six behavioral scores of the Missouri Behavior Problem Checklist to measure ratings of self-esteem and attitudes toward the cleft. It was suggested that, because of good lip repair, the likelihood of negative ratings by naive judges was contraindicated.

Richman and Millard (1997) analyzed longitudinal behavior ratings for 44 children (aged 4–14 years) with cleft palate (CLP) only and examined the relationship of speech, hearing, and facial disfigurement at age 9 in predicting behavioral characteristics and school achievement. Their results indicated increasing levels of social inhibition over age for girls with CLP but less so for boys. There also were increasing levels of conduct problems for older girls with CLP but less for boys.

It appears that physical attractiveness can be an important variable in the judgments made by others. Langlois and Stephen (1977), in their study of the effects of physical attractiveness and ethnicity on children's behavioral attributes and peer preferences, found that attractive children were perceived as being smarter and better liked than unattractive children by elementary school age peers. The effects of facial disfigurement on teachers' perception of the intellectual ability in children with cleft palate were investigated by Richman (1978), who found that teachers tended to rate children with noticeable disfigurement as less intelligent than those with relatively normal facial appearance.

In a later study, Harper, Richman, and Snider (1980) studied teachers' ratings of school behavior of 124 10- to 18-year-olds with two types of disability with varying degrees of disfigurement. They matched cleft palate and cerebral palsy groups in terms of sex, age, IQ, grade level, and socioeconomic status. They also used the Missouri Behavior Problem Checklist and found subjects with cleft palate to be more impulsive than those with cerebral palsy. Those subjects with mild physical impairment in either category demonstrated greater impulse inhibition than more severely impaired subjects. The authors caution us to reserve any definitive conclusions found because of methodological problems of sampling test standardization and teacher bias. That children with cerebral palsy, because of their disability, are less likely to act out also has to be considered a contaminating factor.

Children with cleft palate certainly would be more susceptible, one might believe, to the effects of the primary deformity as well as to all of the secondary consequences of the defect. Indeed, some might be emotionally disturbed, but these children are more likely to have been affected by inadequate self-coping behaviors, family responses, poor or delayed medical and nonmedical support, or any combination of these.

Generally, however, children with cleft palate are fortunate to have the advantage of multidiscipline intervention support. This would mitigate against disturbed emotional behavior and in fact would give strong impetus to their overall growth and development. Regardless of these opportunities, however, the child and the family must still endure the reality of the birth defect itself—the often frequent hospitalization and surgery, speech or language problems, and the sometimes distorted views others have of an infant deformity.

Some mothers and fathers in particular must cope initially with the shock of who they have created. They may find it extremely difficult to admit their unspoken feelings that "you or I or we have created some sort of a monster." These self- or outer-directed recriminations only add to the frustrations these parents have in facing the reality before them. It may well be that the resultant speech or language problems, but not the cleft lip or palate per se, contribute more to adjustment problems. The initial impact of such a birth, however, cannot be ignored.

A greater incidence of mental retardation among children with cleft palate has not been borne out by the empirical literature. McWilliams and Smith (1973) have reported that, although intelligence may tend toward the lower end of the normal range, it does not appear as a definitive problem. If these children do test lower at the preschool level, as Musgrave, McWilliams and Matthews (1975) have found, it is more likely to be a function of the contaminating influences noted in the Harper, Richmond, and Snider study and perhaps of the test instruments themselves.

Family Influences

A child who is to develop psychosocial adjustment problems is likely to do so as a manifestation of the way the family responds to and subsequently copes with the initial physical trauma. Drotar et al. (1975) delineate five stages of adaptation by parents to the birth of a child with a deformity. These are not unlike the stages of grief described elsewhere in this text in that they include (1) the initial shock and disbelief, (2) denial, (3) anger, (4) adaptation, and (5) acceptance. How parents successfully move through these stages and what effects they have on the child is dependent on several interrelated factors, including

1. The mental health of individual family members.
2. The nature of the marital relationship.
3. The ability to cope with stress.
4. The quality and degree of the deformity.
5. The nature of and degree to which the family receives information about the deformity and its possible sequelae.
6. The effectiveness of the habilitation team.

Despite our clinical inclination to identify the difficulty with which families respond to the child and the deformity, the research thus far clearly indicates that parents generally can cope quite successfully with the many implications and complications associated with the defect itself (Tiza and Gumpertz, 1962; Goodstein, 1968; McWilliams, 1970). Regardless of these generalizations, however, we must take care not to ignore the real concerns, anxieties, and despair presented by individual families. As Lutz (1978) advises, based on his extensive experience with cleft palate families, many are not able to cope without significant counseling assistance from professional members of the team.

Brantley and Clifford (1980) investigated maternal reactions of 200 mothers, 97 of whom had children with cleft lip-palate and 103 who had physically normal children. Using factor analyses in three factors—maternal positive affect, paternal positive affect, and parental anxiety—they found that mothers of physically normal children scored higher in terms of positive affect than mothers of the cleft lip-palate children. These findings must be interpreted cautiously because the parental assessments were retroactive and the mothers' reactions were likely to be projections on their part; that is, reactions related to their own perception of themselves as mothers. The latter reported less positive affect for both themselves and their spouses. Although there was greater parent anxiety about the future and upper-class mothers of the children with cleft lip-palate were affected more negatively, the mothers' projected feelings onto the fathers were more evident when they felt that they were not in control of their own lives. The results are somewhat weakened by the lack of standardization of the assessment scale used.

Among the concerns parents have, however, as indicated by Weachter (1959) and cited by Goodstein (1968), are (1) the appearance of the child, (2) the efficacy of surgery, (3) the development of speech, (4) spousal reactions, (5) sibling reaction, (6) family of origin reactions, (7) mental development, (8) financial burdens, and (9) the possibility of cleft palate in subsequent children. All these concerns, we believe, become interwoven with the various stages of adaptation, as outlined earlier, but may be minimized by the way in which families are assisted in gaining knowledge and understanding of the problems of cleft lip and palate.

Counseling the Family

Throughout this book we insist that providing information to the family about the nature of the communicative disorder is a fundamental aspect of the counseling process and necessary to the development of the interpersonal therapeutic relationship. It is of no less importance in assisting the families of children with cleft lip and palate.

Lutz (1978), among others, has clearly described the immediate necessity for providing information about many aspects of the problem. Bradley (1960) questioned 43 parents of children with cleft palate and found that these parents preferred receiving information and counseling directly from skilled professionals rather than from nonpersonal sources such as visual or auditory materials.

Spriestersbach (1961) delineates several basic concerns that parents felt were most important about which to be knowledgeable. Among them were (1) what they must do as parents, (2) information about surgical intervention, (3) cosmetic and physical aspects of the deformity, (4) prognosis related to survival, (5) understanding their own reactions to the child, (6) concomitant future difficulties, and (7) nature of speech and language problems. Lutz summarizes other important areas about which parents have concern: information about possible hearing impairment, future personality and social adjustment of the child, educational problems, vocational expectations, and marriage prospects.

It is obvious that no one member of the professional team could possibly provide all the answers to these parental concerns. On the other hand, it would make little sense for the parents to be bombarded with information from even a few of these professionals. One solution to this dilemma was found by a professional team of which we were a member in a large Midwestern city.

Serving in the roles of both speech pathologist and counselor, we had the responsibility of gathering the impressions from other members of the team after the child and parents were initially seen by all. Although the pediatrics member was the first to provide some answers to the family's immediate concerns, the decision to pace the amount of subsequent information to be provided was left to us. Monthly team assessments afforded families opportunities to raise pertinent issues of concern, saving them from professional overload. If a major concern was related to surgical procedures, the plastic surgeon was available to give more definitive information. If any member of the team felt that the family as a whole were unable to cope, the family was referred to us for informational counseling and, if needed, adjustment counseling. Rarely did family members report that they were out of touch with the team; and although they sometimes felt overwhelmed by the input of several professional disciplines, they welcomed the information provided them.

Our experience with more than 150 families of children with cleft lip or palate over a period of three years tended to confirm data, reported by Goodstein (1968) and others, that although parents of cleft palate children often have anxious concern about their child, their level of adjustment ultimately was not substantially different from that of parents of unaffected children. Conceivably, the effectiveness of the team of which we were part could explain the low level of adjustment problems, but there were plenty of instances of parents and families who needed intensive psychotherapeutic counseling. We would hesitate to state, however, that such instances would be any different for 150 families of children with no physical problems.

We cannot minimize the importance of providing families the best that modern habilitation programs have to offer. As Goodstein (1968) notes, "it is important to identify those parents, who because of their own needs can benefit by special counseling help, or who, because of their own psychological inadequacies, are unable to provide emotional support for their children" (p. 208).

The use of family counseling or family therapy as the treatment of choice is not as clearly defined, particularly with very young children who have a cleft palate, as for families of other communicatively disordered. Marital discord that is revealed after the birth of a child with a cleft palate is best handled, however, within the context of couple counseling. If adjustment and attitude problems are observed in cleft palate families with other children present, we would prefer a family systems approach. Such an approach also would be beneficial for families in which the child with a cleft palate has been shielded from the realities of his or her condition and the suppressed feelings of the parents. That the child be able to participate actively in the therapeutic process would be a prime prerequisite.

Ricky L, age 7, was born with a bilateral cleft of lip and palate. In a family with two older brothers, Bobby, 12, and Micky, 15, Ricky had been through a series of surgical procedures that had required extensive hospitalization complicated by severe upper respiratory infections and feeding problems.

The parents, Connie and John L, had requested a counseling consultation, ostensibly because they did not feel they could cope with Ricky's responses to the taunts of his peers at school. He often was in tears at school or at home, and Ricky's articulation and schoolwork had regressed. For Connie and John, it was an additional situation to tax their already strained limits.

Although they had had the best of what the modern team approach could offer, Connie and John had not come to terms fully with their years of struggle. After having shielded Ricky from their own unresolved grief and having insulated him from experiences they felt would aggravate his feelings of vulnerability, they had come to realize that their own attitudes perhaps were exacerbating an already intolerable situation. Because this was an essentially functional family, the parents needed little prodding to face the issues they had concealed for so long—the harsh realities of the earlier struggles and, perhaps more important, the prospect of further cosmetic repairs.

Probably the most positive elements for productive solution to their difficulties was the support and love they all gave to each other, the above-average intelligence of each family member, Ricky's caring and understanding teachers, a highly competent speech-language pathologist who had been working with Ricky at school, and the continued expert medical care under the supervision of Ricky's pediatrician.

Individual Counseling

A few children with cleft lip or palate would probably benefit from individual counseling in conjunction with speech-language therapy, as often the speech-language pathologist has the most professional contact with the child. We do not wish to imply that the child need be emotionally disturbed per se for us to intervene psychotherapeutically. Often just merely the supportive, caring, and accepting attitudes expressed by the therapist may suffice to help any of those children with their associated struggles.

The therapist who has worked with a child who has difficulty in managing appropriate velarpharyngeal competence, continues to flare the nostrils, or is unable to maintain plosian for /b/, /p/, /t/, /d/, /g/, and /k/ is well aware of the frustration and self-effacement underlying the child's attempts.

The decision to intervene psychotherapeutically often is dictated by the child's own inclination, albeit subtle, to reveal personal concerns. Further, it would entail the support of the family; and if such intervention is to be carried out in school, it would require a liberal acceptance and approval by the appropriate administrative personnel.

We believe it is possible to weave counseling strategies among the traditional symptomatic procedures commonly employed by speech-language pathologists. Each can be mutually beneficial as long as the technique in and of itself does not become of sole importance. The therapist must be flexible enough to shift strategies in response to the changing needs of the child. Even with the young school-age child, feelings about appearance and lack of intelligibility might interfere with the implementation of speech-language techniques only. Unless these feelings are allowed to surface, they may continue to intrude on successful resolution of the speech or voice problem.

We do not suggest that all school-age children with cleft lip-palate necessarily are aware of their unintelligibility or for that matter suffering from feelings of inferiority or rejection. As counseling speech-language pathologists, we must refrain from projecting our own sympathetic feelings and attitudes about disfigurement and hypernasal speech and voice on the child, who may be coping quite well with all of the difficulties.

Randy is an intelligent and well-liked 10-year-old boy who apparently had adjusted satisfactorily to his repaired unilateral cleft of the lip and palate. Although his speech still is characterized by nasal snorts and imprecise articulation, despite having had pharyngeal flap surgery, he nevertheless relates well to his peers and performs successfully in school. He takes in stride the knowledge that he is to have cosmetic surgery for his lip within three years and in fact looks forward to it, knowing that his appearance most likely will improve. His supportive and caring family contribute, no doubt, to his feelings of adequacy and competence in all of his endeavors.

Randy's well-meaning school therapist had helped Randy make significant improvement in his intelligibility, and because he appears to be "so well-adjusted" feels safe in probing for possible remaining areas of concern. His resistance to her attempts to "counsel" and his desire to "work on my speech" is greeted, fortunately, with undefensive support by her and her realization that she had intruded inappropriately. His therapist is mature enough to acknowledge how much Randy had taught her.

We cite this example not to imply that children like Randy are totally free of any interpersonal difficulties, particularly those surrounding a repaired cleft lip-palate but to caution that counseling in many cases may be contraindicated. In this case, we do not question the counseling competence of the therapist per se but, more important, cite the value of recognizing when and when not to intervene psychotherapeutically.

Probably the greatest value in counseling parents of children with cleft lip-palate or these children themselves is to help them cope, not so much with their own reactions but with the attitudes and reactions of others. Whether expressed or unexpressed, these may present obstacles to the overall adjustment of the family and more specifically to the habilitation of the child. How well counseling is managed early in the child's life will certainly influence his or her passage through adulthood. It is to this period we shall now turn.

Cleft Palate in Adolescents and Adults

Those of us who work with adults who carry the literal and figurative scars of cleft lip-palate from childhood must first acknowledge that many, if not most of them, have blended successfully into the mainstream of society in every aspect. This does not mean that they are necessarily immune to the environmental pressures that impinge on all of us but that they have the fortitude to establish a viable place for themselves in their living environment. We need only look to those who have become productive members of the theatrical, helping, business, teaching, and legal professions to confirm our viewpoint.

Our concern here, then, is with those who have fallen between the proverbial cracks and who, because of early ineffectual habilitative management, negative family influences, other environmental factors, racism, or any combination of these, are fixated at the inter- and intrapersonal struggles of their childhood years. Unfortunately, the lack of any substantial experimental research in the area of adolescents and adults with cleft lip-palate forces us to rely only on our personal clinical experiences and speculative assumptions. Nevertheless, it is important that we value the insights gained from working with our adolescent and adult clients so that our understanding of the problem can enhance all of our subsequent therapeutic efforts.

Psychosocial Correlates

In a literature, one study stands out as providing us a clue to a feature that is pertinent to adolescents and adult adjustment: physical appearance and self-esteem. Starr (1982) administered the Physical Attractiveness Scale and Self-Esteem Scale to 67 persons with repaired cleft lip-palate, age 19–33. Physically attractive subjects tended to rate themselves higher in self-esteem than subjects who were less attractive. No differences between the two groups were found with regard to sex, educational attainment, or type of cleft. Starr concludes that there is a relationship between self-perception of physical attractiveness and self-esteem. He suggests that the lack of differences with respect to type of cleft could be explained by the effectiveness of plastic surgery to reduce facial disfigurement.

Our difficulty with this study is the assumption implied with the Physical Attractiveness Scale that physical attractiveness is an objectively measured variable. It would have been useful to have had independent judges rate physical attractiveness and compare these measures with the ratings of the cleft lip-palate subjects. But that would not have eliminated the problem of subjectivity. We cannot disregard, however, the importance of cosmetic appearance, which as presented in the media, is the passport to success in all areas of endeavor.

There appears to be no definitive evidence to suggest that adolescents and adults with cleft lip-palate have serious personality and social problems beyond those of a comparable non-cleft lip-palate population. We would need to make a case-by-case study to determine the degree to which the "deficit" itself and the attitude developed about it had influenced the personality and social development, as well as other aspects, of the person's life.

Ralph is a self-referred, unmarried 52-year-old retired postal worker who was born with a unilateral left complete cleft lip and palate. Repair of the cleft lip and palate had taken place over several operations that began during his first year of life and ended at age 12. He suffered a concussion at age 9 when he was hit by a car. On intake he reported that there was no immediate or lasting effect on his speech and language. He also had open-heart surgery when he was 43 and again at age 50. He was in speech therapy for most of his elementary and some of his high school years.

His decision to seek out speech therapy at age 52 was based on a longtime desire, and he feels now that he had retired he has the time to do so. Although friends and relatives tell him his speech is acceptable, he feels that his "mushiness" will prevent him from finding a part-time job and expresses fear of not being understood by others. Clinical impressions reveal otherwise, as his overall intelligibility approaches 100%. Although nasal emission and hypernasality are evident, he compensates remarkably well, considering his limited velopharyngeal closure. Formal and informal psychological testing reveals above-normal intelligence but emotional insecurity, anxiety, and attitudes of inferiority and self-effacement. He sees his life as a failure, but after learning of the need to have coronary bypass surgery, decided it was time to make "something more of my life."

On the surface, Ralph appears to have led a relatively quiet, introspective, and private life, but beneath is revealed a man who has never been able to accept the reality of his cleft lip and palate. He never thought he could do anything vocationally beyond sorting mail and had found this activity excruciatingly boring. He volunteered that his heart condition had been a message to him to live life more fully, and that although he feels that the "cards are still stacked against me" is determined to make whatever changes are necessary.

The profile illustrated by Ralph is representative of the complex psychodynamic factors that probably operate in some adults with cleft lip-palate. Certainly, as professionals, we are unlikely to have the opportunity to intervene with such individuals but should be cognizant that they do exist and recognize the reality of the suffering silence. Some adults with a cleft palate who ostensibly refer themselves for speech therapy actually are crying out for help with their overall adjustment difficulties.

Individual Counseling

Counseling the adolescent or the adult individual with repaired cleft lip-palate essentially is no different from counseling other communicatively impaired individuals. The adult who stutters or who still maintains a deficient language pattern frequently presents the therapist with negative attitudes concerning self-worth and self-image that may be continuing to hamper that person's total life adjustment.

The individual with repaired cleft lip-palate who continues to cope unsuccessfully with listener-observer perceptions of hypernasality, oral-facial deformity, or compensatory facial distortions while speaking obviously requires counseling intervention. Some individuals, in fact, may struggle with their self-concept and -image, although they may no longer have visual or acoustic features that call attention to the observer. These individuals apparently are fixed in the attitudes held at an earlier age, even though speech therapy and corrective surgery have successfully removed all signs of the original conditions.

Most important for the counseling therapist, then, is to attend to the individual's present negative attitude about self regardless of the actual physical reality. Therapists certainly have no control over how people in their clients' environments will respond to them, but individuals with a cleft lip-palate have the potential to change their own attitudes toward and perceptions of themselves. It is important to acknowledge, however, situations in which a client may be prevented from job advancement because of a supervisor's unenlightened or personally distorted image of physical differences. Generally we can do little to alter that person's projections and attitude except perhaps in only special instances. More often we can only help the client either adjust to the present job situation, try to change it, or move to another job.

Regardless, the client must be helped to understand that he or she is not inferior and that one cannot allow the inferior attitudes of others to restrain oneself from developing the full potential of one's capabilities. After all, many of us throughout our lives are often forced to cope with situations and circumstances that seem terribly unfair, yet we must refrain from wallowing in self-pity if we are to effect a more positive resolution for ourselves.

Similarly, adults with cleft lip-palate must learn to separate the physical reality of the deformity from all of the other positive potentials and assets they possess. Too often such individuals burden themselves with all of their perceived liabilities, thereby obscuring all else they may have going for them in their lives. It is a task, however, that demands personal courage and tenacity, because attitudes ingrained over many years resist the best of individual and therapeutic efforts.

Although little research evidence supports the notion of a "handicapped personality," the cleft lip-palate deformity may stimulate maladjustment, which in turn may be reinforced by others in the afflicted person's environment. We must bear in mind also that the iatrogenic factor, described elsewhere, may be operating as well. As professionals, it is important that we, too, perceive our clients as persons and refrain from conceptualizations with labels. To do otherwise will only distract us from focusing on the necessary elements that will foster positive changes in our clients' attitudes and behaviors.

In addition to the psychological and interpersonal dynamics operating in adolescents and adults with cleft lip-palate are those speech and voice components that continue to interfere with communication. Although the former may appear to be the overriding issue, we must not ignore the importance of employing traditional speech and voice therapy practices to alter distorted articulation patterns and hypernasal voice.

Ralph, described earlier, within a period of six months, was able to improve significantly both his articulation and voice to the point where he no longer felt these interfered with his life. Although he had not had speech or voice therapy since junior high school days, his motivation and willingness to practice new patterns helped bring new meaning to his life. In his case, the counseling aspect per se appeared to play a complementary role as he made rapid and continuous progress. He became a better speaker through the interplay of successful compensatory speech and voice skills and the modification of self-effacing and self-defeating attitudes. It appears that, although counseling was a contributory factor, speech and voice therapy had intrinsic psychotherapeutic value as well. To have focused merely on altering fixed attitudes would not likely have satisfied all of his goals.

Conclusion

Children and adults with repaired cleft lip and palate are a population who, in metropolitan areas, have had the advantage of the full range of habilitative intervention. Unfortunately, this is not the case in many of the rural areas of the United States. We still see children who have received little or only superficial medical, habilitative, and educational attention. A case also may be made for Native American children, who still are denied access to proper and complete medical care. They cannot be ignored either and also require counseling but in accordance with a highly defined paradigm that would apply to cleft palate and SLI children as well.

Although research has failed to identify definitive problems of personal maladjustment in the cleft palate population, it has pinpointed the necessity for being cognizant of the possibility for emotional components and interpersonal problems. Although these can significantly affect the overall social, intellectual, cognitive, and communicative development of the individual, counseling alone cannot resolve all the difficulties this population must face. Only when counseling is used in conjunction with other methods of management can the full potential for any individual with cleft lip-palate be realized.

Cerebral Palsy

Cerebral Palsy in Children

The profound significance of the birth of a child with cerebral palsy is well known. Cerebral palsy represents a wide constellation of neurological features characterized by paralysis, incoordination, weakness, and involuntary athetotic or spastic movements, often involving the entire body, along with sensory-perceptual and medical problems.

But even more significant are the severe developmental, social, and psychological implications that typically accompany and complicate the initial neurological state. Lefebvre (1983) reports 60% of these children to have defective vision, and 50% are said to have borderline or below-average intelligence. (We hesitate to fully accept the intelligence figure because intellectual growth easily can be influenced by any one of a combination of the accompanying deficits.) Lefebvre notes that nearly half of the children born with cerebral palsy are also hearing impaired, communicatively disordered, and dysphagic. Seidel, Chadwick, and Rutter (1975) found cerebral palsied children with normal intelligence to be more vulnerable to psychiatric problems than nondisabled children and those with more extensive brain damage to be three times more vulnerable to psychiatric illness. Rutter, Graham, and Yule (1970), in a carefully controlled study, found that, although environmental factors such as the parents' reactions to the disability had some influence, the neurophysiological impact was much greater and revealed a distinctive primary neuropsychiatric effect.

Most important to the present discussion, however, is the recognition of the devastating and overwhelming impact, either directly or indirectly, of this complex syndrome on the emotional growth of the child. We need also to understand how the child's emotional responses may affect the condition itself. This is determined greatly by how the family and social milieu impinge on the child. As suggested by Buscaglia (1975), the person who is disabled will be influenced by society to "limit his actions, change his feelings about himself, as well as affect his interaction with others. The degree to which he is influenced will depend on the strength, duration and nature of the judgmental stimulus" (p. 15)—and, we would add, the quality and consistency of habilitative intervention.

As speech-language pathologists, we have a very special role to play, as it is only through communication, be it verbal, nonverbal, or argumentative, that the disabled individual can begin to establish the personal relationships necessary for continued growth and, indeed, survival.

Psychological Correlates

Surprisingly, not much literature focuses on the adjustment problems and personality factors for the child with cerebral palsy, perhaps because of the overriding concern by most caregivers for the child's other seemingly insurmountable handicaps.

Sigelman, Vengroff, and Spanhel (1984) performed a Life-Function Analysis on 14 major impaired populations. Through a comprehensive literature search they gathered statements concerning limitations in functioning related to the 14 con-

ditions of impairment. Among the 1,222 statements of limitation found for cerebral palsy, the following percentages for each of the major life functions were determined: mobility, 44%; communication, 30%; health, 14%; social-attitudinal, 6%; and cognitive-intellectual, 6%. Interestingly, among all 14 major impairment groups, social-attitudinal statements were represented least in the literature surveyed in cerebral palsy, whereas communication problems were among the most frequent. Therefore, if we add social-attitudinal statements to communication statements, together they represent more than a third of all statements made about cerebral palsy.

The results of the Sigelman, Vengroff, and Spanhel study should be viewed cautiously, in that their findings are based on literature covering all age groups with cerebral palsy and, further, may represent more the academic interest of the writers rather than of the actual reality of the person with cerebral palsy. Nonetheless, we cannot ignore the major concern about combined social-attitudinal communication factors.

Richardson (1969) insists that cerebral palsy cannot be defined in a unitary fashion. Impairment in motor functioning will affect and be affected by sensory, behavioral, intellectual, and social elements. Because of these physiological limitations, these individuals are hindered from participating in the active process of socialization. Thus, the stage may be set for further alienation and negative reactions to their disability.

Gardner (1973) describes the profound psychological and physical frustrations of these children, particularly when at birth they are unable to have a normal interaction with their parents. Deprived of a satisfactory interaction, they develop feelings of low self-esteem and evolve into a social world with which they feel little relationship. The range of reaction may extend from extreme rage to a self-imposed exile to an alienating world. Recognizing early that they are abnormal, they consider that their physically impaired body is perceived by others in terms of rejection.

Shontz (1984) advances contradictory propositions that (1) the "psychological reactions to the onset or imposition of physical disability are not uniformly disturbing or distressing and do not necessarily result in madadjustment" and (2) "reactions (favorable or unfavorable) to disabilities are not related in a simple way to the physical properties of the disabilities" (p. 128). He reports little systematic evidence to support the notion that psychiatric disturbance occurs any more frequently within the disabled population than with the population in general. Also lacking, according to Shontz, are any definitive studies relating degree of physical disability to personality. Among the four affirmative propositions put forth, Shontz suggests that there is no simple cause-effect relationship between the actual physical disability and a predictable adjustment reaction. He also suggests that environmental influences and the perceptions of others will have as great an effect on the psychological reactions of the disabled person as that person's own internal perception. It is the interaction of these two major perceptions that must therefore demand our attention.

Perhaps the most controversial of Shontz's propositions is that the disability itself is only one factor affecting the individual's total life situation and that it may be minor relative to other influences. He goes on to suggest it is possible that "when a disability opens up opportunities for learning, challenges the person to achieve successfully, in short promotes ego growth, it is a source of growth and ultimate maturity" (p. 130).

In the light of Shontz's constructs, we must be cautious not to overinterpret, because he refers to physical disability in general. Certainly, the implications for other forms of disability discussed elsewhere in the text and for cerebral palsy must be considered, Shontz, in fact, stresses the importance of viewing and understanding the physically disabled person as a unique individual in the light of that person's particular life context.

Family Influences

It is obvious that the earliest familial reaction to the birth of a child with cerebral palsy involves the response of the parents to the child. In a study involving 30 pairs of twins, one of which in each pair had cerebral palsy, Shere (1957) found that social and emotional maladjustment was not directly caused by the cerebral palsy itself but that the child's aberrant behavior pattern was related to the parental response and attitude toward the child. Such findings appeared to receive support in the postulates put forth by Shontz.

Unfortunately, few definitive studies have been done about the mother-child interaction immediately following birth or in the infant's early stages of life. No mother, even one who previously has successfully reared children, is prepared to cope with a child who has difficulty sucking, feeding, and swallowing. Not only must she deal with these problems but cope with the child's overall bodily reflexive patterns, which are foreign to her. Richardson (1969) discusses the parents' preoccupation with the child's overall bodily appearance and function, which becomes intensified the more the focus is on the child. This may be the parents' way of attempting to cope with the situation or perhaps to convince themselves of the actual reality.

In Chapter 5, we discuss the significance of the complex interpersonal relationship in the development of speech and language and socialization in the normal child. Because the mechanisms of feeding and sucking are related to the earliest vocal cries of the infant and because the mother may never become proficient in feeding her cerebral palsied child, there is some reason to believe that normal speech and language will be hindered. A further confounding influence may be the mother or father's negative responses, either covert or overt, to the child's behaviors, as suggested by Shere and Kastenbaum (1966). Contributing to the disruption in the developmental process is the hospitalization for complicated illnesses, resulting in separation from the mother and father. An additional factor that exacerbates the ongoing trauma in the family is the nature of the doctor-parent communication. Quine and Rutter (1994), in their investigation of parental satisfaction with medical communication when their child is diagnosed with cerebral palsy or other congenital anomaly, found that more than half of the parents were dissatisfied with the communication. The data collected revealed three major components of dissatisfaction: lack of communication once the disability is identified, lack of a sympathetic approach in communicating information, and absence of full disclosure to reduce anxiety.

Support systems for parents of children with cerebral palsy are not always adequate for several reasons. Medical necessities often preclude attention to family adjustment reactions. Friends and extended family members not living in the home frequently distance themselves from the "birth tragedy," projecting their own fears and unresolved conflicts concerning life's traumatic events or physical disabilities. So, the family is left to cope in whatever way is possible. A strong marital bond certainly would have a very positive influence on the overall adjustment process, which in turn would contribute to the child's overall well-being. A weak martial bond, on the other hand, could be fraught with reciprocal recrimination and blame, adversely affecting, directly and indirectly, the child's development. In their study of family and maternal influences on perceptions of children's adjustment to cerebral palsy, Perrin, Ayoub, and Willett (1993) conclude that family interactions are important to the psychological adjustment of the child.

The stress created by the birth of a child with cerebral palsy can be better tolerated by a family that is essentially functional; that is, one in which all present members have established a sense of their own individual identities and, in Maslow's words, have "self-actualized." They are individuals who, in Hill's (1958) description, can cope with the crisis by temporarily limiting their own personal ambitions and working cooperatively to develop positive goals. A Polish study by Pisula (1998) reveals that, for mothers of cerebral palsy in particular, the physical disability is the greatest source of stress.

In being able to separate themselves from the child, parents are better able to see their child as a unique person who, although requiring considerable special attention from them, has the potential to achieve some degree of independence. They are able to relate to the child without overprotecting him or her, thereby reducing the common likelihood of helplessness and dependency. This is not to suggest that the child will not suffer the "slings and arrows of outrageous misfortune." All of the unselfish caring, love, and concern for the child will not alleviate the ever-present multihandicapping nature of the disability, but they can help to prevent many of the secondary disabling effects of poor physical and mental adjustment patterns. Most important is that a functional family can inspire the autonomous development and creative potential of the child, notwithstanding the permanent disabling features.

In terms of family systems theory, the child with cerebral palsy should not become the identified symptom to represent a family pattern of conflict avoidance. In dysfunctional families, an inordinate amount of attention devoted to the child can be used as an excuse by the parents to avoid quality time with each other and allows the family energy to be dissipated. As Versluys (1984) points out, although secondary gains for the patient, such as attention, love, and care, may be apparent, the child also, unfortunately, is taught avoidance of responsibility and dependency. In this way the child gains an inordinate amount of power over the family.

Whatever speech and language difficulties directly related to the initial disability are present, these may be readily exacerbated by the ever-present dysfunctional family process, as we discussed in Chapter 5, on language disorders.

Featherstone (1980) offers a complete description of marital stress resulting from sadness, anger, fear, and fatigue. She describes both the undermining and the strengthening of faith in the marital union that can occur as a result of the stress experience, The disabled child thus can threaten the fabric of even a relatively solid marriage, by provoking powerful feelings, by representing the uneasy symbol of shared failure, by requiring changes in the family structure or system, and by fostering the basis for ongoing conflict.

Probably the most profound effect on the child and the overall family system are the grief reactions experienced in particular by the mother and father. Among the many theories advocated to explain the shock, disbelief, and denial of parents faced with the crisis of having a disabled child, Solnit and Stark (1961) advance the idea that the mother is mourning the loss of the expected healthy child and realizes the fear of having a damaged child. For mothers experiencing guilt, sorrow, mourning, anger, and apprehension, the warm nurturing relationship with a child may be disrupted or perhaps never initiated.

Because we already describe the mourning process elsewhere in the text, we need not repeat it here except to suggest that the denial stage may have the most intense influence. Denial in and of itself should not be viewed negatively, however, because, as we have seen, it may aid the family in coping with its new reality and in time help propel it to a more productive stage. Only when the disability, regardless of its severity, is seen as a family and not an individual dilemma can family members begin the process of adaptation and growth. Positive parental self-perception as well as positive perception of the child undoubtedly enhance the child's own self-perception and in turn contribute to the future well-being of all.

Counseling the Family

Previously we discussed the importance and significance of providing the family information about the nature of disabling events that, among other results, affect the communicative functioning of the individual. The birth of a child with cerebral palsy demands no less.

Typically, the pediatrician or the neurologist has the task of explaining the nature of the child's disability and the profundity of its implications. Such a responsibility places a great burden on the physician, who generally is looked up to as the expert who will be able to predict the outcome of such a devastating event. Naturally, too many intrinsic and extrinsic factors make such a determination impossible, yet the family, particularly the parents of the child, are justified in expecting some explanation. Both callous, unfeeling, and glib input or unrealistic, overoptimistic, and vague explications are equally ineffectual in satisfying the immediate concerns of the parents. They want and need the caring, understanding, and honest support of their physician, who is willing to listen and answer as many of their concerns as is professionally and humanly possible. Physicians need not burden themselves with perpetuating their "deity" image and can do themselves and the parents a great favor by referral to appropriate counseling professionals. One other complicating factor is the time limitations put on the physician by the restrictions that are characteristic of many managed care organizations.

Mitchell (1981), who studied 152 families in New Zealand, drew up a composite statement based on major concerns of these families:

As the parents of a handicapped child we want all those various professionals who deal with us to treat us with openness, honesty and sensitivity. While the pressures of a handicapped child in our family is never easy to come to terms with, please recognize that we have good support from our family and friends and that we are not emotionally incapacitated by our problems. Some of us, however, do need counseling, especially when we first find out about our child. Meeting other parents helps us to adjust, so please put us in touch with each other.

Above all, perhaps, what we want is information—up to date information on how we can help our child. Information on the services that are available to us, and information on the benefits to which we are entitled.

The professionals we find most helpful are those who see us often and offer us practical advice. Although we may find some problems in attending parent training courses, don't underestimate our willingness to take part—especially if they are based in our local community and provide us with ideas relevant to our child.

When it comes to school, please remember that we would like our child to attend a regular school—provided special help is provided.

Finally we are articulate parents. Not all of us are able or willing to share our concerns with others. Some of us feel that we have a long-term problem that other people don't really understand. (pp. 65–66)

Most provocative about Mitchell's statement is that it reminds the professional that parents of children with cerebral palsy can be remarkably resilient in their period of crisis and stress, and as long as they know that some support is forthcoming, they and their children not only can survive but thrive. The reader will find the publication edited by Eisenberg et al. (1993) particularly useful in that beyond its comprehensive coverage of medical aspects of cerebral palsy, psychological and other background information critical to its' study are also included.

Although the child with cerebral palsy is a family issue, we support the contention made by Thurer (1984) that it is also a "woman's issue." As Thurer states in her provocative essay about the mothers of these children,

These women often struggle with a relentless grind of caring for an individual who may require feeding, dressing, toileting, frequent medical supervision, and constant supervision. Of course men may be involved in these tasks, but typically it is the female parent who is in charge of vigilantly overseeing the child's care. Sometimes these mothers have no respite. (p. 293)

Family counseling can be most effective when it also focuses on the issues that relate directly to the feelings and attitudes of the caregivers as well as the practical problems with which they must cope. They include the following:

1. Assisting the parents in working through their grief reaction, feelings of anxiety, guilt, depression, and hopelessness. Support must be given for their own psychological needs and their communication and parenting skills. This includes helping them recognize that their feelings are normal and acceptable.
2. Enhancing their self-esteem to help them feel that they have control over their lives and assisting them to become more assertive in their interaction with professionals.
3. Concentrating on strategies to assist their involvement in the education and treatment of their child and in establishing goals that are consistent with the child's potential as well as with their own family values and expectations.
4. Helping the parents cope with unexpected stressful or crisis situations involving the child, such as serious illness and hospitalization, orthopedic surgery, or behavior problems.
5. Assisting the parents in dealing with their own marital relationship, particularly when it is being affected either directly or indirectly by the child.

Family counseling is not necessarily the only method of choice and in fact may be more productive when combined with parent support groups. The latter can alleviate the family isolation and remind the parents that they are not alone in their struggles. In addition, families can give aid and comfort to each other, sharing common problems. It is not unusual for such families to discover their own strategies and management procedures. Even the most expert professional cannot possibly know all that would benefit the family. The common sharing of even the most minute details of daily problems and of "things that work" can add immeasurably to the overall functioning and adjustment of the family.

Although family therapy as a treatment choice for the family of a child with cerebral palsy has received scant attention in the literature, it may be most appropriate for those families with able-bodied children as well. Even so, families with no other children would benefit from a therapeutic approach that includes the participation of the parents and the child. We believe it is extremely important for the child to feel a vital part of the family, regardless of the verbal communication deficit and physical disability. Although active participation may be negligible, the child nonetheless has the opportunity to communicate nonverbally what, heretofore, may have been inappropriate or impossible. Family therapy in fact may be the most effective means of encouraging "individuation" in all family members, particularly the child, as described elsewhere in this text by Minuchin, Jung, and others. We would define *individuation* as a life process in which the individual moves toward establishing a sense of personal uniqueness, distinction, and individuality apart from others. For the child with cerebral palsy, it also means the growing self-concept of feeling important in and having a role in life.

Individual Counseling

Whereas counseling procedures for children described elsewhere in this book may be applicable to children with cerebral palsy, the special physical and emotional circumstances of these children demand a somewhat modified approach. Too often these children are ignored psychotherapeutically, with emphasis being directed at the educational and therapeutic aspects of habitation. Although educational and therapeutic approaches contain strands of psychotherapeutic elements, we believe it is important to identify the latter and maximize their use either independently or in conjunction with other strategies.

We have seen how play therapy can be used to facilitate speech and language development as well as enhance the emotional and interpersonal development of the child. For the child with cerebral palsy, it is an opportunity to explore physically in a prone or sitting position the immediate environment, unencumbered by the restrictions of a wheelchair. It allows the child to develop physical, communicative, and educational skills by providing an opportunity to modify that environment. Such a process is consistent with the goals of the physical therapist, who, according to Anthony (1980), is concerned with restructuring the child's impaired skills, teaching new physical skills, and modifying the immediate environment to conform more appropriately to the child's level of physical skill. Most important, we believe, is the opportunity for the child to develop a sense of autonomy, personal integrity, and physical control (within limits, of course). The speech-language pathologist skilled in the use of the speech-related physical therapy techniques advocated by Bobath and Bobath (1972) or Rood (cited by Gillette, 1969) can add further to the child's overall development. Fortunately, today there exist techniques like neuromuscular electrical stimulation and dynamic bracing along with innovative physical therapy strategies to decrease spasticity (Scheker, Cheser, and Ramirez, 1999).

We recognize that children with cerebral palsy who manifest the most severe features of their athetotic, spastic, rigid, or ataxic involvement would be hampered in their quest for physical control. We maintain, however, that speech-language pathologists can adjust their strategies to conform to the physical realities of their young clients and enhance whatever potential does exist. Again, the nature of the interpersonal relationship itself, regardless of severe physical disability or even treatment mode, may be a crucial element in fostering positive changes in most aspects of the child's development.

Speech-language pathologists can be successful only insofar as they have the support and can operate in conjunction with the parents, psychiatrist, physical therapist, psychologist, or rehabilitation counselor, among others. To function otherwise in the capacity we advocate could breach the boundaries of ethical and professional responsibilities. It nonetheless is important for us to be and feel secure in our request for cooperation and remain steadfast in our therapeutic convictions.

We need to recognize these same considerations in counseling the older child with cerebral palsy. Regardless of mainstreaming in the classroom, speech-language pathologists in the schools often are given the major responsibility for responding not only to the speech-language needs but to the psychosocial needs as well. In fact, it is not unusual for the latter to be part of the child's IEP (individual educational plan). How responsive the speech-language pathologist must be to these needs perhaps is moot, as children with cerebral palsy may make

little distinction in the material they wish to share or in the behaviors they manifest in speech-language therapy. What is important is that the therapist be prepared to cope with whatever emerges. To focus only on the child's speech and language needs while the child is expressing other needs as well would be to invalidate the child's most crucial concerns. After all, no other professional may be available so often to respond holistically to the child.

The challenge, as we see it, is to be as totally responsive to the child as possible while not abrogating our major responsibility as agents of communicative habilitation. We believe it is possible to integrate traditional strategies with counseling strategies in such a way that the child's overriding needs—namely, interpersonal communication and adjustment—are met.

One important way to accomplish this is to bring the child to a certain degree of body relaxation through inhibition of reflex activity and normalization of body tone, as advocated by the Bobaths. The resistance techniques of brushing and icing as advocated by Rood or the use of progressive relaxation techniques may not only facilitate more intelligible articulation but also help to alleviate exacerbated body tension brought on secondarily by anxiety and psychological stressors. For extensive discussion of these and other techniques, the reader is referred to the writings of Payton, Hirt, and Newton (1977). Our major concern is that these physically manipulative exercises are carried out not in terms of doing something *to* the child but in terms of doing something *with* the child. Implicit, then, is the development of a therapeutic relationship involving mutual trust, empathy, critical listening, and nonjudging that we describe elsewhere. Such an approach encourages the child to develop a greater degree of personal control while extending the limits of the physical disability.

Providing opportunities for the child to express personal concerns about and reactions to perceptions of him or her by others in the child's immediate environment could be conducive to removing some of the barriers to more effective personal and interpersonal communication.

If we are to be significant caregivers in the cerebral palsied child's life, it is our responsibility to help alleviate the inner turmoil and suffering borne by such a child. If, on the other hand, we believe that we cannot assume such a role, then it behooves us to help the family obtain the assistance needed by the child.

Cerebral Palsy in Adolescents and Adults

The plight of the adult with cerebral palsy attempting to become part of the mainstream, although significantly reduced, has not yet been fully acknowledged and dealt with even during this enlightened period of the 21st century. Unlike the assistance provided when they were younger, adults often lack the benefit of professional assistance to aid them in developing the social skills and opportunities to relate successfully with able-bodied or even with other disabled persons in their environment. Relying on case examples, Heller, Alberto, and Meagher (1996) review the psychological and environmental factors affecting 8–16-year-old students. Among the factors identified are motivation, self-concept, social-emotional problems, pain, fatigue, and absenteeism.

Livneh (1984), based on a comprehensive review of the literature on the origins of negative attitudes toward people with disabilities, developed a classification system that encompasses several sources of these attitudes. We outline them here, but recommend that the reader refer to the Livneh article and the extensive list of references cited for a more definitive discussion.

There are twelve major categories, which we summarize as follows:

1. Negative attitudes, based on social and cultural conditioning and expectations, toward disabled individuals.
2. The effects of early childhood influences on the development of adult stereotypic attitudes and standards.
3. Complex psychodynamic systems responsible for creating unrealistic expectations and conflicts when relating to disabled persons.
4. The igniting of unconscious anxiety in the able-bodied person, as the result of perceiving the disability as God's punishment for committing sin or as an excuse for committing a future evil act.

5. Confusion and anxiety in able-bodied persons, brought about by being unprepared for the unstructured social, emotional, and intellectual relationship with the disabled person
6. The development of negative attitudes exemplified by a fundamental aesthetic-sexual antipathy toward visible disfigurement.
7. The threat to the able-bodied person's own conscious and unconscious body image or concept kindled by the presence of the physically disabled person.
8. The stereotypic and inferior status associated with being part of a minority group, thereby reminding the able-bodied person of his or her transient existence.
9. The anxiety associated with death identified with disability, thereby reminding the able-bodied person of his or her transient existence.
10. Discriminatory practices against the disabled person as a result of prejudice-provoking behaviors, such as being dependent, fearful, and insecure.
11. Specific negative attitudes related to the visibility, severity, and functional ability of the disabled person.
12. Negative attitudes fostered by such demographic factors as sex, age, socioeconomic status, and educational level as well as personality-connected factors in the able-bodied person, such as ethnocentrism, authoritarianism, self-concept, aggression, ego strength, and degree of self-insight.

Psychosocial Correlates

It is not unusual for children with cerebral palsy to progress into adulthood with continuing difficulties in their overall communicative functioning, as well as problems of social-emotional adjustment, as long as negative attitudes toward them prevail. Among the more profound problems for these disabled adults are those of sexual dysfunction and adjustment and the relationship of these factors to self-concept. Although it would be inappropriate to discuss this issue at length, the reader is referred to the more extensive coverage by Diamond et al. (1984).

Regardless of even the most diligent rehabilitative efforts earlier in their lives, the adult with cerebral palsy continues in the struggle with problems of self-identity, body image, and feelings of inadequacy, frustration, and resentment. The limits of their tolerance often are taxed to the extreme in their attempts to become independent and self-sufficient—and many do, despite all the socioeconomic barriers they still must confront.

We said earlier that the personalities of individuals with cerebral palsy do not differ from the personalities of able-bodied individuals except for the consequences of the family system of which they are part. An individual who was overprotected by parents as a child might find difficulty, as an adult, in practicing independence and self-sufficiency. Yet, it is conceivable for such an individual to respond conversely; that is, to strive desperately for independent action and be convinced of becoming self-sufficient.

Some adults with cerebral palsy were reared in families in which the disability had been denied and where, as a child, the individual was expected not only to learn self-sufficiency but also to take on responsibilities unrealistic for even an able-bodied child.

Seth was such a child. From the earliest age, his father refused to accept the reality of his son's combined athetotic and spastic physical involvement. He could not tolerate having a son, an only one at that, who would not be able to do everything an able-bodied child could do. Seth's mother, a passive, morose, and often sickly person, could do little directly to counter her husband's dominating and dictatorial attitudes and actions. Seth's ambulatory ability was all the more reason for his father to exact from him complete obedience and expect him not only to care for himself at the earliest age but to take on major household chores. Tearful protestations were met with physical and mental abuse characterized by strap whippings and ridicule about his "laziness."

School was a welcome respite for Seth, who was bright and, although severely dysarthric, highly communicative. He ingratiated himself with his teachers and a succession of school speech-language pathologists. His thirst for learning was unquenchable but he resented his father's authoritarian control over when and how much to study. Performance of the necessary household chores had to come first, always.

Family vacations, which generally consisted of long backpacking treks in the Sierra Mountains of California, offered Seth little relief from the demands of his father, who expected him to be able to keep up with the pace of his parents. Torturous as these physical exertions were for him and despite his quadraparesis, Seth rarely protested but deeply resented his father's demands. His mother, because of her own physical malaise, never accompanied them.

At 15 years of age, Seth also was expected to work after school and during weekends in order, in his father's words, to "pay for his own keep" and help support the family. (It should be noted that Seth's father was a gainfully employed commercial artist who earned a salary sufficient to support the family.) Seth's priorities essentially were ranked in the following order: go to school, clean the house, do 2 hours of homework every weekday, and work at least 16 hours a week. Whatever little time remained for play and recreation was spent breaking into car lots at night, hot-wiring the cars, and driving them around. These often were solitary ventures because Seth had few friends to join him in his nightly escapades.

On graduation from high school, Seth left home to take a one-room flat and continued to work part-time while he attended a junior college. His meager earnings and social security payments, although barely enough to help support him, were sufficient to help him sustain his independence. The once weekly dinner visits to his parents soon ceased because he no longer wanted to wash all the dishes as condition for invitation to dinner.

Seth, having no friends and no essential support system to help give him guidance for the future, felt generally lonely and found solace only in caring for younger wheelchair-confined children with cerebral palsy while ingratiating himself with their parents. In a very real sense, he was soon treated as a member of the family without the demands previously made on him by his own family.

One child with which he was particularly close moved to a small rural community. That gave Seth the impetus to move there as well, since the city in which he had lived offered little for him. By now Seth was 21 years of age and obtained part-time employment in a plumbing supply business while continuing to attend a junior college. He soon entered into a homosexual relationship with his 15-year-old friend, apparently with the knowledge of the child's single parent.

Troubled by guilt, confusion, and uncertainty about his life, he sought psychotherapeutic assistance by a clinical psychologist to whom he revealed the extent of his homosexual relationship and his personal torment. Bound by what was an infringement of state law concerning sexual encounters with minors, the clinical psychologist reported Seth to legal authorities, who quickly arrested him. Despite the protestations of the child's mother and son, Seth was forbidden to see either her or her child again and ordered to participate in group therapy sessions with abusive parents.

Initially, Seth felt alienated from the group and resentful that he was being perceived as a child molester, but because of a compassionate and understanding group therapist, Seth became an active participant in the group. He finally found a forum in which he could share himself and at the same time receive the support for which he had hungered all of his life. As Seth noted in a personal communication with us, "They're the first people in my life who really understand what I must go through being palsied."

This anecdote is a poignant illustration of the dilemma in which some individuals with cerebral palsy might find themselves. While not totally physically incapacitated, Seth strove to enter the mainstream of life of the able-bodied but found rejection or little support. Conversely, neither could he identify fully with those who were more severely disabled, except as a caregiver or protector. Ironically, he was labeled a child molester instead. Sexually rebuffed by able-bodied women and unable to establish relationships with women who were more physically disabled than he, few options appeared open to him.

His own father's dogmatic, authoritarian, and excessive expectations certainly must be considered an influential factor in Seth's overall psychosocial development. Although one might argue that, by such parenting, Seth learned independence at an early age, we would add, At what cost? Obviously, any expression of his own free will was stifled early by an abusive father who could never accept Seth's disability. Such denial contributed further to his inability to establish his self-identity and was a factor in preventing him from belonging anywhere. In perpetual desperation, Seth reached out to those with whom he felt he would be accepted, with little consciousness of his actions.

Seth's legal punishment for the "crime" he committed might be questioned by many of us, and although he appeared to derive substantial rewards from the group therapy experience, it raises serious ethical, legal, and moral issues about society's understanding and treatment of the adult with cerebral palsy.

Individual Counseling

Too frequently, as in the case of Seth, persons with cerebral palsy also fall within the proverbial cracks of the best intentioned habilitative programs. Seth never received any substantial counseling except by his last high school speech pathologist, who was skilled in psychotherapeutic management and had the support of her special education supervisor. Unfortunately, her contact with Seth was too brief and limited to help him make substantial changes in his attitudes and behavior.

We need not reiterate the counseling methods and techniques already discussed throughout this book, as many of those would be applicable to the adult with cerebral palsy. We believe that particular emphasis must be given, however, to the person's conceptual body and communicative behavior image, vocational adjustment and stability, and overall role in society.

Schontz (1970) reveals the profound effects of the disabled individual's denial of deep-rooted feelings concerning the self in relation to body image. Because our perception of how we communicate is intrinsic to our overall concept of self, it is necessary for the counseling therapist gently to encourage the client to identify objectively both acoustical and physical reality. Assuming that a trusting interpersonal relationship has been established, the client is more likely to be willing and motivated to explore ways in which communicative behavior can be improved or enhanced and the physical involvement that can be best adapted to daily functioning. To ignore the latter, in our opinion, would detract from maximizing the potential of the former, as communication is a manifestation of the totality of the individual. We further emphasize that direct work on the dysarthria and dysarthrophonia will help develop a more positive body image attitude.

Kolb and Woldt (1976) recommend Gestalt counseling techniques, in which fantasy and psychodrama are used to help the individual attend to parts of the body where sensation is blocked. They also believe that the disabled individual can best enhance interpersonal relationships through mutual body exploration with another individual in order to communicate on a purely sensory level.

Frequently, the fostering of extreme dependency in childhood will result in a lack of motivation and sense of alienation in adulthood, according to McDowell, Coven, and Eash (1984). They cite numerous references in the literature to support their contention. We see, in the case of Seth, however, that forcing independence can have similar effects. We must refrain, then, from making rigid generalizations in predictions of future outcomes, as each individual responds differently to early parenting influences. It is possible that Seth, for one, actually hungered for dependency precisely because he was *denied* opportunities for it in childhood. It appears to us that Seth needed to have early nurturing, loving, and caring, which would have allowed for some degree of dependency at first, and then gradually weaned in the direction of total independence.

Counseling should include the following toward helping the individual:

1. Establish realistic goals personally and vocationally in response to the present reality and ways in which the individual may effect changes in the environment to facilitate those goals.
2. Help the individual formulate his or her sexual identity, consistent with who that person *is* regardless of the physical disability, and explore ways in which positive relationships may be developed with others.
3. Help the individual recognize and confront the many obstacles society has placed in front of persons with cerebral palsy and ways in which these barriers may be circumvented. Awareness of the few positive changes society has made to ease the burdens of the person with a handicap also should be brought to light.
4. Help the individual discover the personal meaning of his or her life with due consideration to the positive role that may be played in relationship to the rest of society, and how changes on the latter may be effected.

Conclusion

We have only touched the surface of the complex psychodynamics operating in individuals with cerebral palsy and the counseling interventions that may facilitate positive change and growth. We do not wish to imply that the speech-language pathologist necessarily should be assigned or expected to assume the major role in such an intercession, but we do believe that it may be difficult to make the separation between the speech disorder itself and its effects on the individual. For this reason we must be prepared to function appropriately according to the reality with which we are confronted.

One note that demands reiteration is the recognition that persons with cerebral palsy are not characterized by distinctive psychological types. The family serves as the major source for investigating the direction and quality of the developing personality and growth pattern. But only through the aid of ongoing interdisciplinary management can persons with cerebral palsy find their proper place in society. It is also most fortunate that assistive technology and federal legislation developed during this past decade have radically changed the lives of persons with disabilities. As Scherer and Marcia (1993) indicate, such progress now enhances the attainment of the same educational, personal, and career goals as every other adult. We are reminded, though, that the personal issues and needs of persons with cerebral palsy still must be better understood by parents, educators, rehabilitation professionals, and employers.

Degeneratively Involved Individuals and Their Families

Despite the considerable diverse physical, physiological, neurogenic, and other qualitative differences among the various and wide range of degenerative disease with which medical investigators and clinicians from various disciplines must cope, there are significant commonalities relative to the psychological, social, and familial ramifications. Mindful of this premise, it would be appropriate initially to describe psychological characteristics unique to each of the major disease entities.

Alzheimer's Disease and the Other Dementias

To attempt any differentiation among the etiological, cognitive, linguistic, and neuropsychological characteristics of Alzheimer's disease (AD) and the "dementias" would be outside the scope and purpose of the present text. It should be noted, in fact, that several investigators and present medical practices appear to disregard categorization of the dementias and prefer a more unified approach mainly in terms of the reality of the progressively degenerative nature of the disease process and overall care of the patient (Katzman, 1986).

This is not to suggest that all dementias have a unitary neurophysiologic characteristic or heterogenity. The research clearly reveals definitive differences in subcortical and cortical substrates. Lovell and Smith (1997); Miller and Morris (1993); McPherson and Cummings (1997); Salmon and Bondi (1997) review many investigations in all of the dementias, including subcortical dementia, vascular dementia, Huntington's disease, Pick's disease, and Parkinson's disease (which presents a symptomatic picture demanding somewhat different attention by speech-language pathologists).

There is little question that the gradual loss of memory, cognitive regression, loss of touch with the immediate environment, and physiological degeneration common to both AD and the other dementias, in most cases becomes associated with varying degrees of fear, aggressiveness, depression, and disorientation. Eastly and Wilcock (1997) found in 52% of their 262 AD patients exhibition of some aggressive behavior. Ninety-one patients (35%) were verbally aggressive and 46 patients (18%) were assaultive to their caregivers in noninstitutionalized settings. Assaultive behavior was more likely to be associated with male patients.

Depression among those with dementia has been identified and described by many writers. Several have noted similarities in neuropsychological test performance between individuals suffering from depression and those diagnosed with subcortical dementia syndromes (Massman et al., 1992; King et al., 1991; and Wolf et al., 1987). A more thorough discussion of depression is hampered by the incidence of ischemic vascular dementia (IVD) in association with a CVA. Cummings and Sultzer (1993) report that depression is most commonly associated with lacunar infarcts and Binswanger's disease (a gradually progressive syndrome caused by ischemic injury to the deep white matter of the cerebral hemisphere). In a comparative study of IVD and AD in relation to neuropsychological and psychiatric factors, Starkstein et al. (1996) found IVD patients to be more emotionally labile but levels of depression were similar for both groups.

While we do not address possible dementia or cognitive deficits in the chapter on CVA, we need to assume that any counseling or family intervention would have to be adapted as deemed necessary by all concerned with rehabilitative efforts. In the present discussion, however, psychotherapeutic intervention must be dictated by a very different reality. For a comprehensive view on the psychology of dementia, the reader is advised to examine the work of Miller and Morris (1993), which provides valuable insights for professionals working with such patients and their families.

Parkinson's Disease

Distinctly different from the dementias just discussed, Parkinson's disease (PD) is the most common disease affecting the basal ganglia. Slowly progressive and neurodegenerative, it is characterized by cognitive, psychiatric, behavioral, movement, phonological, articulatory, swallowing defects, and at the extreme stage, possible dementia (Bondi and Tröster, 1997; Darley, Aronson, and Brown, 1975; Starkstein et al., 1996; and Murray and Stout, 1992). The last investigators found a solid relationship between PD and Huntington's disease (HD) relative to cognitive disabilities and the degeneration of comprehension. They also recommend that habilitation programs be encouraged to maximize quality of life potentials. It should be noted in this regard, however, that not all PD patients necessarily develop dementia (Rajput, 1992). From a neuropsychogenic perspective, depression is a common concomitant of PD as described by Bondi and Tröster (1997), but the nature, severity, and quality of the mood shifts do not necessarily reflect the quality of the motoric function and that depression may actually exacerbate cognitive function. What is not yet clear is the relationship between the behavioral and neurologic factors, relative to the involvement of the basal ganglia. This is a similar dilemma we faced with our earlier analysis of possible organic factors as they relate to emotional behaviors in CVA, TBI, and possibly AD.

Of crucial concern is that we avoid placing PD along with the dementias, since speech-language pathologists, depending on fee reimbursement, are more likely to intervene therapeutically with PD patients, for deficits in phonology, articulation, swallowing, and cognition. Of greater importance, from our perspective, is the role we must assume in assisting the family and the patient to cope, particularly when rehabilitative services no longer will be available.

Therapeutic Intervention

We have noted both markedly similar and different characteristics of the types of dementia but believe the nature of any therapeutic intervention involving counseling must be designed to fit the individual patient and his or her family. In the case of an institutionalized patient, our involvement is more complex, particularly if we must work with both family members and institutional staff.

Guidelines discussed in earlier chapters are helpful and we also include the guidelines proposed by Andrews and Andrews (1990), Burns (1996), and Woods (1996) as we include other instructions that fit more specifically with the population under current discussion:

1. On initial referral by the physician and consultation with that and other professionals, confirm your role with the patient and the family.
2. Meet with the patient and family members and, following your initial assessment, determine what appears to be the most pressing need of all, relative to your particular role.
3. Discuss tentative goals for both patient and family from a unified perspective, including direct input from family members.
4. Determine a flexible timeline encompassing your participation as provider and realistic costs as dictated by insurance reimbursement.
5. Depending on the information already gathered by the family, provide basic information regarding dementia and include bibliographic sources to which the family may turn. If computer astute, recommend use of the Web to connect to the United States Alzheimer's Association (www. aldo.org, as of the present writing), which will provide vast amounts of information. You can assist in helping the family sort out what is relevant for it.
6. Based on information gathered of the patient's emotional, social, educational, work, and family history, ascertain how these factors may play a role in the patient's present behavior.
7. Provide the family opportunity to express any feelings that appear on the surface. Be sensitive to emotional issues that appear to be withheld, particularly if family members still are in the midst of grief. It is better to use our ears more frequently than our mouths.
8. With respect to the preceding, be mindful there are no solutions, only means of coping and helping to enhance the patient's quality of life as best as possible.
9. Aid family members to relate to the patient with realism, appropriateness, and honesty,

knowing not to expect congruency or miracles in changed behavior. The adage we follow is this: Be yourself. Honor the patient as an adult, regardless of childlike behavior. Tune into "where the patient is coming from" rather than your own therapeutic agenda, and assist the family to do the same.

10. Employ cognitive strategies, such as memory exercises and activities of daily living (ADLs), only if appropriate, particularly if the patient is in the middle stages of dementia and receptive.

11. Some patients, in the early stages, may have a desire to attempt activities they may be unable to complete. We remember such a patient, who had spent several years with her spouse in Vietnam before this country's engagement and wished to complete writing her memoirs taken from voluminous notes. As a visiting home therapist, we integrated memory, organizational, and writing exercises along with supportive educational counseling regarding her request for frankness about the progression of her disease. The challenge for us was to be attuned to her disparate moments of lucidity and confusion. Her spouse also participated in our sessions and was able to carry on with the activities outside of formal therapy.

12. The therapist and family members need to be alert to any changes that occur relative to the progression of the disease and changes in behavior or attitude of other family members, then assist in any way. Ideally, the speech-language clinician will have the opportunity to provide input to the physician regarding patient depression or anxiety and inquire about the possibility of appropriate prescriptions.

13. Family support groups, including other families dealing with dementia, are a vital part of the ongoing adjustment each family member must make and a learning process for all the participants, including the therapist. The therapist, in fact, need not be the facilitator. It is better that the group be peer supportive and open-ended to allow for more meaningful sharing and expressing of feelings.

14. Any participation of extended family members, friends, or the patient's associates from work can enrich whatever daily thoughts and activities with which the patient may be engaged.

15. Finally, the overriding goal of familial intervention is not only flexibility as circumstances change but the continuing enhancement of the patient's dignity and quality of life, particularly if these are being endangered. Above all, the family needs to be *kept within the loop*, especially when other professionals are involved. Too often, particularly in nursing homes, the speech-language pathologist is put in the position of serving as an ombudsman. It is not our responsibility to assume such a role but we can certainly put the family in contact with such a person from the appropriate state agency.

Dysphagia

While dysphagia has been well documented in the late stage of AD, it has been difficult to ascertain when the eating changes occur, particularly when self-feeding begins to diminish (Priefer and Robbins, 1997). Dysphagia among residents of nursing homes often is associated with cognitive impairment. It is not atypical for aged individuals to refrain from eating and drinking, even when dysphagia may not be present (Steele et al 1997). In the treatment of the seriously and persistently mentally ill, Bazemore (1996) discusses the implication of dysphagia in these populations, which also suffer special medical problems and tend to have a shortened life span. Bores (1998) reports that one out of every three CVA patients demonstrate some swallowing disorder and the speech-language pathologist will need to include a regimen of measures to enhance the patient's swallowing function along with language therapy and psychsocial adjustment. The challenge for the therapist is to aid the patient in overcoming one more hurdle affecting his or her quality of life.

One of the myriad of problems suffered by the PD patient is the presence of dysphagia as it relates to the impaired head and neck posture, jaw rigidity, upper extremity dysmobility, and impulsive feeding behavior (Leopold and Kagel, 1996).

How the dysphagia therapist manages the dysphagic patient frequently will affect outcome in terms of continued success at deglutition. A natural consequence upon the advent of dysphagia is fear of choking, depression, frustration, anger, and in many cases rejection of food or liquid intake. The necessity for the introduction of a feeding tube obviously diminishes the patient's quality of life further. It is difficult, frequently, for the therapist to determine, through videofluroscopy alone, how effectively or ineffectively a patient swallows when we include the psychological factors just noted. As implied throughout the discussion of CVA, TBI, and AD, an added responsibility of the speech-language therapist is to assist any other personnel or family members in the management of the patient. It is particularly evident in the case of the dysphagic patient, who is at risk of aspiration pneumonia and must be sensitively and carefully guided in the feeding process.

Another group of dysphagic patients that draws our attention are those diagnosed with functional dysphagia. The present literature provides some evidence of such cases. Atkins and Lundy (1994) report the case of a 7-year-old who "could not swallow." While the child showed minimal response to behavioral, family, and play therapy, he rapidly improved with administration of alprazolam (antianxiety medication) before meals. Masters (1995) notes the need to discuss the possibility of sexual abuse, in that the choking symptom may be brought about by the child being forced to perform fellatio. Atkins and Pumariega (1995) believe functional or conversion dysphagia may persist despite psychotherapeutic intervention. They also address the influence of biological modifiers and advocate a multimodal approach to treating such traumatized children. Elinoff (1993) successfully used hypnosis to treat a 9-year-old child who presented with dysphagia that developed following an incident of choking on food. The problem was resolved following three hypnotic sessions. Schwartz (1995), in a practitioner's guide to biofeedback, offers strategies to treat functional dysphagia but does not explore its possible use for organically based dysphagia.

While antidepressant medication often is prescribed for CVA, TBI, AD, and PD patients with or without dysphagia, it may be done so by a family physician rather than a psychiatric specialist, who generally are more current in their understanding of the medication's interaction with the patient's other medications. These specialized psychiatrists also are more cognizant of the effects of the increasing number of antidepressants that become available. It often becomes the responsibility of the speech-language pathologist to be attuned, therefore, to any subtle behavioral changes that could affect swallowing function of the patient being treated. If the patient is not institutionalized, the therapist must maintain an ongoing communicative interaction with the primary care provider to ensure that proper feeding protocols are followed. In this sense, the therapist is a teacher as well as a supervisor. We should not assume that the therapist is manager of the patient's rehabilitation program unless that role is clarified in communicative interaction with the physician. Above all, only those clinicians who are confident in and have the appropriate skills necessary to aid the dysphagic patient should assume this task.

HIV/AIDS

The participation of speech-language pathologists in the care of HIV-related illness in children and adults has been recognized, particularly with regard to HIV-related speech, language, swallowing, and voice disorders (Scott and Layton, 1997). The psychological and social implications have received considerably more attention in the scientific literature of allied fields. For the present purposes, however, we can allude to only the psychological issues that may impinge on any services performed by speech-language pathologists.

Because of more effective medical and pharmacological interventions, individuals with HIV and AIDS are living longer, therefore the focus has shifted to the various rehabilitation practitioners who are asked to intervene (McReynolds, 1998). As speech-language pathologists, we need to work closely with other care providers and keep them informed of the nature and proccess of the procedures amicable to our expertise. Any counseling we perform needs to be in the context of the therapeutic strategies we employ (Johnston and Johnston, 1998;

Blechner, 1997). Issues that pertain to our own field of expertise, particularly as they relate to cognitive and neuropsychological functioning, are described by Kaplan and Sadock (1998) and the Dana Consortium on Therapy for HIV Dementia and Related Cognitive Disorders, USA (1996). It would be appropriate for us to consider many of the guidelines for the treatment of dementia, addressed earlier in the chapter.

Conclusion

Congenital and degenerative diseases extend far beyond those reviewed in this chapter. Stereotypic movement disorder, Creutsfeldt-Jacob disease, Pick's disease, amyotrophic lateral sclerosis, and multiple sclerosis are among those that may fall within the realm of our practices. While some present with symptoms different from those discussed, the speech-language pathologist versed in the subject will find many commonalities that can be addressed, not only from the standpoint of traditional therapeutic tools but also as counselor for the patient and family.

References

Andrews J, Andrews M. *Family-Based Treatment in Communicative Disorders: A Systemic Approach*. Sandwich, IL: Janelle Publications; 1990.

Anthony WA. A rehabilitation model for rehabilitating the psychiatrically disabled. *Rehabilitation Counseling Bulletin*. 1980;24:6–21.

Atkins DL, Lundy MS, Pumariega AJ. A multimodal approach to functional dysphagia. *J of the Am Academy of Child and Adolescent Psychiatry*. September 1994;33(7):1012–1016.

Atkins DL, Pumariega AJ. Functional dysphasia and sex abuse: Drs Atkins and Pumariega reply. *J of the Am Academy of Child and Adolescent Psychiatry*. March 1995;34(3):262.

Bazemore PH. Medical problems of the seriously and persistently mentally ill. In: Soreff M et al., eds. *Handbook for the Treatment of the Seriously Mentally Ill*. Seattle: Hogrefe and Huber Publishers; 1996:45–66.

Blechner MJ. Psychological aspects of the AIDS epidemic: A 15-year perspective. *Contemporary Psychoanalysis*. January 1997;33(1):89–107.

Bobath K, Bobath B. Cerebral palsy, part I: diagnosis and assessment of cerebral palsy; Part II: the neuro-devel-opmental approach to treatment. In: Pearson PH, Williams CE, eds. *Physical Therapy Services in the Developmental Disabilities*. Springfield, IL: Charles C Thomas; 1972.

Bond MW, Tröster AI. Parkinson's disease. Neurobehavioral consequences of basal ganglia dysfunction. In: Nuswsbaum PD, ed. *Handbook of Neuropsychology and Aging: Critical Issues in Neuropsychology*. New York: Plenum Publishing; 1997:216–237.

Bores J. Dysphasia: Swallowing disorders following a stroke. In: Sife W, et al., eds. *After a Stroke: Enhancing Quality of Life. Loss Grief and Care*. New York: Haworth Press; 1998:93–98.

Bradley DP. A study of parental counseling regarding cleft palate problems. *Cleft Palate Bulletin*. 1960;10:71–72.

Brantley HT, Clifford E. When my child was born: maternal reactions to the birth of a child. *J of Personality Assessment*. 1980;44:620–623.

Burns MS. Use of the family to facilitate communicative changes in adults with neurological impairments. In: JA Andrews, ed. *New Directions in Speech-Language Pathology: Systems, Context, and Change. Seminars in Speech and Language* 1996;17(2):115–122.

Buscaglia L. *The Disabled and their Parents: A Counseling Challenge*. Thorofare, NJ: Charles B. Slack; 1975.

Cummings JL, Sultzer DL. Depression in multi-infarct dementia. In: Starkstein SE, Robinson RG, eds. *Depression in Neurologic Disease*. Baltimore: Johns Hopkins University Press; 1993:165–185.

Dana Consortium on Therapy for HIV Dementia and Related Cognitive Disorders, USA. Clinical confirmation of the American Academy of Neurology algorithm for HIV-1-associated cognitive/motor disorder. *Neurology*. 1996;47(5):1247–1253.

Darley FL, Aronson AE, Brown JR. *Motor Speech Disorders*. Philadelphia: W. B. Saunders; 1975.

Diamond M. Sexuality and disability. In: Marinelli RP, Dell Orto AE, eds. *The Psychological and Social Impact of Physical Disability,* 2nd ed. New York: Springer-Verlag; 1984.

Drotar D, Baskiewicz A, Irvin N, Kennel J, Klans M. The adaptation of parents to the birth of an infant with a congenital malformation: a hypothetical model. *Pediatrics*. 1975;56:710–717.

Eastley R, Wilcock GK. Prevalence and correlates of aggressive behavior occurring in patients with Alzheimer's disease. *Int J Geriatr Psychiatry*. April 1997;12(4):484–487.

Eisenberg M, Gluechkauf R, Zaretsky H, Ehrman L. *Medical Aspects of Disability: A Handbook for the Rehabilitation Professional*. New York: Springer-Verlag; 1993.

Elinoff V. Remission of dysphasia in a 9-year-old treated in a family practice office. *Am J of Clinical Hypnosis*. January 1993;35(3):205–208.

Featherstone H. *A Difference in the Family: Life with a Disabled Child*. New York: Basic Books; 1980.

Gardner RW. Evolution of brain injury: The impact of deprivation in cognitive-affective structures. In: Sapir SG, Nitzburg AC, eds. *Children with Learning Problems: Readings in a Developmental-Interaction Approach.* New York: Brunner/Mazel; 1973.

Garrett MT, Myers JE. The rule of opposites: A paradigm for counseling. *J of Multicultural Counseling and Devpt.* 1996;24(2):89–104.

Gillete HE. *Systems of Therapy in Cerebral Palsy.* Springfield, IL: Charles C Thomas; 1969.

Goodstein LD. Psychosocial aspects of cleft palate. In: Spriesterbach DC, Sherman D, eds. *Cleft Palate and Communication.* New York: Academic Press; 1968.

Harper DC, Richman LC, Snider BC. School adjustment and degree of physical impairment. *J of Pediatric Psychology.* 1980:377–383.

Heller KW, Alberto PA, Meagher, TM. The impact of physical impairments on academic performance. *J of Developmental and Physical.* September 1996;8(3):233–245.

Hill R. Social stresses on the family: genetic features under stress. *Social Casework.* 1958;39:139–150.

Johnston DW, Johnston M, eds. *Comprehensive Clinical Psychology,* Vol. 8: *Health Psychology.* Oxford, England: Pergamon/Elsevier Science Ltd.; 1998.

Kaplan HI, Sadock BJ. *Kaplan and Sadock's Synopsis of Psychiatry: Behavioral Sciences/Clinical Psychiatry,* 8th ed. Baltimore: Williams and Wilkins; 1998.

Katzman R. Alzheimer's disease. *New England J of Medicine.* 1986:964–973

King DA, Caine ED, Conwell Y, Cox C. The neuropsychology of depression in the elderly: a comparative study of normal aging and Alzheimer's disease. *J of Neuropsychiatry and Clinical Neuroscience.* 1991;3:163–168.

Kolb CL, Woldt AL. The rehabilitation potential of a Gestalt approach to counseling severely impaired clients. In: McDowell WA, Meadows SA, Crabtree R, Sakata R, eds. *Rehabilitation Counseling with Persons Who Are Severely Disabled.* Huntington, WV: Marshall University; 1976:449.

Langlois JH, Stephen C. The effects of physical attractiveness and ethnicity on children's behavioral attributions and peer preferences. *Child Development.* 1977;48: 1694–1698.

Lefebvre A. The child with physical handicaps. In: Steinbhauer PD, Rae-Grant Q, eds. *Psychological Problems of the Child in the Family,* 2nd ed. New York: Basic Books; 1983.

Leopold NA, Kagel MC. Prepharyngeal dysphasia in Parkinson's disease. *Dysphasia.* Winter 1996;11(1):14–22.

Livneh H. On the origins of negative attitudes toward people with disabilities. In: Marinelli RP, Dell Orto AE. *The Psychological and Social Impact of Physical Disability,* 2nd ed. New York: Springer-Verlag; 1984.

Lovell MR, Smith SS. Neuropsychological evaluation of subcortical dementia. In: Nussbaum PD, ed. *Handbook of Neuropsychology and Aging: Critical Issues in Neu-*

ropsychology. New York: Plenum; 1997.

Lutz K. Counseling when there is a cleft palate. In: Hartbaner RE, ed. *Counseling in Communicative Disorders.* Springfield, IL: Charles C Thomas; 1978.

Massman PJ, Delis DC, Butters N, DuPont RM, Gillin JC. The subcortical dysfunction hypothesis of memory deficits in depression: neuropsychological validation in a subgroup of patients. *J of Clinical and Experimental Neuropsychology.* 1992;14:687–706.

Masters KJ. Functional dysphasia and sex abuse. *J of the Am Academy of Child and Adolescent Psychiatry.* March 1995;34(3):262.

McDowell WA, Coven AB, Eash VC. Special needs and strategies for counseling. In: Marinelli RP, Dell Orto AE, eds. *The Psychological and Social Impact of Physical Disability,* 2nd ed. New York: Springer-Verlag; 1984.

McPherson SE, Cummings JL. Vacular dementia: clinical assessment, neuropsychological features, and treatment. In: Nussbaum PD, ed. *Handbook of Neuropsychology and Aging: Critical Issues in Neuropsychology.* New York: Plenum; 1997.

McReynolds, CJ. Human immunodeficiency virus (HIV) disease: shifting focus toward the chronic, long-term illness paradigm for rehabilitation practitioners. *J of Vocational Rehabilitation.* June 1998;10(3):231–240.

McWilliams BJ. Psychological development and modification. *ASHA Reports No. 5.* Washington, DC: American Speech and Hearing Association; 1970.

———. Cleft patate. In: Shames GH, Wiig EH. *Communication Disorders: An Introduction.* Columbus, OH: Charles E. Merrill; 1982.

McWilliams BJ, Smith RM. Psychosocial considerations. In: McWilliams BJ, ed. *ASHA Reports No. 9.* Washington, DC: American Speech and Hearing Association; 1973.

Miller E, Morris R. *The Psychology of Dementia.* Chichester, England: John Wiley and Sons; 1993.

Mitchell DR. "Other people don't really understand": a survey of parents of young children with special needs. Occasional Paper No. 2, Project PATH, Hamilton, New Zealand: University of Waikato; 1981.

Murray LL, Stout JC. Discourse comprehension in Huntington's and Parkinson's disease. In: Huber SJ, Cummings JL, eds. *Parkinson's Disease: Neurobiological Aspects.* New York: Oxford University Press;1992:119–131.

Musgrave RH, McWilliams BJ, Matthews HP. A review of the results of two different surgical procedures for the repair of clefts of the soft palate only. *Cleft Palate J.* 1975;12:281–290.

Payton OD, Hirt S, Newton RA, eds. *Scientific Bases for Neurophysiologic Approaches to Therapeutic Exercise: An Anthology.* Philadelphia: David; 1977.

Perrin EC, Ayoub CC, Willett, JB. In the eyes of the beholder: family and maternal influences on perceptions of adjustment of children with a chronic illness. *J of Developmental and Behavior.* April 1993;14(2): 94–105.

Pisula E. Stress in mothers of children with developmental disabilities. *Polish Psychological Bulletin* 1998; 29(4): 305–311.

Priefer BA, Robbins J. Eating changes in mild-stage Alzheimer's disease: a pilot study. *Dysphasia.* Fall 1997;12(4):212–221.

Quine L, Rutter DR. First diagnosis of severe mental and physical disability: a study of doctor-parent communication. *J of Child Psychology and Psychiatry.* October 1994;35(7):1273–1287.

Rajput AH. Prevalence of dementia in Parkinson's disease. In: Huber SJ, Cummings JL, eds. *Parkinson's Disease: Neurobiological Aspects.* New York: Oxford University Press; 1992:119–131.

Richardson SA. The effect of physical disability on the socialization of a child. In: Gostin DA, ed. *Handbook of Socialization Theory and Research.* Chicago: Rand McNally, 1969.

Richman LC. The effects of facial disfigurement on teachers' perception of ability in cleft palate children. *Cleft Palate J.* 1978;15:155–160.

Richman LC, Millard T. Brief report: cleft lip and palate: longitudinal behavior and relationships of cleft conditions to behavior and achievement. *J of Pediatric Psychology.* August 1997;22(4):487–494.

Rutter M, Graham P, Yule WA. A neuropsychiatric study in childhood. *Clinics in Developmental Medicine.* 1970:35–36.

Salmon DP, Bondi MW. The neuropsychology of Alzheimer's disease. In: Nussbaum PD, ed. *Handbook of Neuropsychology and Issues (Critical Issues in Neuropsychology).* New York: Plenum; 1997.

Scheker LR, Cheser SP, Ramirez S. Neuromuscular electrical stimulation and dynamic bracing as a treatment for upper-extremity spasticity in children with cerebral palsy. *J. Hand Surg.* 1999;24(2):226–232.

Scherer J, Marcia S. *Living in the State of Stuck: How Technologies Affect the Lives of People with Disabilities.* Cambridge, MA: Brookline Books; 1993.

Schontz FC. Physical disability and personality. Theory and recent research. *Rehabilitation Psychology.* 1970;17: 51–59.

———. Six principles relating disability and psychological adjustment. In: Marinelli RP, Dell Orto AE, eds. *The Psychological and Social Impact of Physical Disability,* 2nd ed. New York: Springer-Verlag; 1984.

Schwartz MS. The frontier: old and new. In: Schwartz MS et al., eds. *Biofeedback: A Practitioner's Guide,* 2nd ed. New York: Guilford Press; 1995:840–890.

Scott GS, Layton TL. Epidemiologic principles in studies of infectious disease outcomes: pediatric HIV as a model. *J of Communication Disorders.* July–August 1997; 30(4):303–324.

Seidel VP, Chadwick OFD, Rutter M. Psychological disorders in crippled children: a comparative study with and without brain damage. *Developmental Medicine and Child Neurology.* 1975;563–573.

Shere E, Kastenbaum R. Mother-child interaction in cerebral palsy: environmental and psychosocial obstacles to cognitive development. *Genetic Psychology Monographs.* May 1966;73:255–335.

Shere MD. The socio-emotional development of the twin who has cerebral palsy. *Cerebral Palsy Review.* 1957;18:16–18.

Sigelman CK, Vengroff LP, Spanhel CL. Disability and the concept of life functions. In: Marinelli RP, Dell Orto AE, eds. *Psychological and Social Impact of Physical Disability,* 2nd ed. New York: Springer-Verlag; 1984.

Solnit AJ, Stark MH. Mourning and the birth of a defective child. In: *Psychoanalytic Study of the Child,* Vol. 16. New York: International Universities Press; 1961.

Spriesterbach DC. Counseling parents of children with cleft lips and palates. *J of Chronic Diseases.* 1961;13:244-252.

Starkstein SE, Sabe L, Petracca G, Chemerinski E, Kuzis G, Merello M, Leignarta R. Neuropsychological and psychiatric differences between Alzheimer's disease and Parkinson's disease with dementia. *J of Neurology, Neurosurgery, and Psychiatry.* 1996;61:381–387.

Starr P. Facial attractiveness and behaviors of patients with cleft lip and/or palate. *Psychological Reports.* April 1980;46:579–582.

———. Physical attractivness and self-esteem ratings of young adults with cleft lip and/or palate. *Psychological Reports.* April 1982;50(2):467–470.

Steele CM, Greenwood C, Ens I, Robertson C, Seidman, CR. Mealtime difficulties in a home for the aged: not just dysphasia. *Dysphasia.* Winter 1997;12(1):43–50.

Thurer SL. Women and rehabilitation. In: Marinelli RP, Dell Orto AE, eds. *The Psychological and Social Impact of Physical Disability,* 2nd ed. New York: Springer-Verlag; 1984.

Tiza V, Gumpertz E. The parents' reaction to the birth and early care of children with cleft palate. *Pediatrics.* 1962;30:86–90.

Versluys HP. Physical rehabilitation and family dynamics. In: Marinelli RP, Dell Orto AE, eds. *The Psychologcial and Social Impact of Physical Disability,* 2nd ed. New York: Springer-Verlag; 1984.

Weachter EH. Concerned of parents related to the birth of a child with a cleft of the lip and palate with implications for nurses. M.A. thesis. Chicago: University of Chicago; 1959.

Wolfe J, Granholm E, Butters N, Saunders E, Janowski D. Verbal memory deficits associated with major affective disorders: a comparison of unipolar and bipolar patients. *J of Affective Disorders.* 1987;13:83–92.

Woods RT. Psychological "therapies" in dementia. In: Woods RT, ed. *Handbook of the Clinical Psychology of Aging.* New York: John Wiley and Sons; 1996:575–600.

8

Psychological Considerations for Hearing-Impaired Individuals and Their Families

---

Part I.

The Psychology of Hearing-Impaired Children

Psychosocial Dynamics

The medical, educational, communicative, and audiological implications of hearing impairment in children are well known. But, the psychosocial factors that characterize hearing disorders in children have received little attention in the literature, particularly with respect to the services just noted. Blair and Berg (1982) first reported the insufficiency of supportive educational, social, and emotional services for these children and presented a strong case for the training of educational audiologists to serve them. Blair and Berg refute directly the contention "that the solution to hearing loss among children is simply wearing a hearing aid" (p. 541). More recent investigations support the contention that early intervention services are of utmost importance in serving the needs of hearing-impaired children and their families (Mauk, Barringer, and Mauk, 1995; Harris and VanZandt, 1997; Calderon, Bargones, and Sidman, 1998).

Children with hearing loss differ significantly among themselves in terms of many elements, including degree of loss, onset, etiology, intelli-

gence, presence of other physical problems, personal coping mechanisms, response by the family, and quality of habilitative management. In this chapter, our major attention focuses on the child's perception of self in relation to the hearing impairment and the influence of the family. We also consider how counseling strategies can be applied most effectively to aid the child and family in the overall adjustment to the problem.

Etiology

Although the causes of hearing impairment are predominantly organic, it should also be acknowledged that some children have what has been described as a "functional impairment" in which no organicity can be determined to explain discrepancies between audiometric results and observable behavior (Ventry and Chaiklin, 1962). Both congenital and acquired hearing loss are associated with heredity, toxins, disease, injuries, or varying combinations of any of these. Church et al (1997) and Church and Kaltenbach (1997), on reviewing human and animal research, found four types of hearing disorders associated with fetal alcohol syndrome: developmental delay in auditory maturation, sensorineural hearing loss, intermittent conductive hearing loss due to recurrent otitis media, and central hearing loss. The psychosocial ramifications cannot be differentiated on the basis of cause, however, as many individual factors will account for the way in which the child adapts to the problem. It seems more fruitful to distinguish psychosocial factors on the basis of congenital and acquired hearing loss.

Congenital Hearing Loss

By *congenital*, we mean that hearing loss is incurred either while the embryo is in utero or immediately at birth. Thus, to some varying degree, the infant is cut off from the major sensory avenue necessary for speech and language development. Among the probable causes might be a toxic reaction to a drug ingested by the mother during pregnancy, familial genetic pattern, viral infection such as rubella during the first trimester of pregnancy, or birth delivery complications. Although such factors serve as ready explanations, we cannot ignore the possibility that emotional stressors may trigger a physiological intolerance in the mother during pregnancy, consequently affecting the fetus. Presently, no empirical evidence supports such a hypothesis, but it could be a fruitful area for research. More important for us is an understanding of the psychological effects of genetic or other congenital hearing anomalies on the child and the family

The Relationship Between Central Auditory Processing Disorder and Attention Deficit Disorder

The incidence of audio processing (APD) and attention deficit disorder (ADD) in children has received considerable attention in the literature (Riccio, 1993), but the relationship between the two and the presence or lack of behavioral and language disorders and hyperactivity has made its study difficult. More confounding is whether or not they are mutually exclusive. The most recent research appears to be inconclusive (Cook et al., 1993; Riccio et al., 1994; Moss and Sheiffele, 1994).

Acquired Hearing Loss

Acquired hearing loss generally implies that the child had normal hearing at birth but, because of disease, physical, or (less often) psychological trauma, has lost the ability to hear. Conceivably, hereditary factors related to constitutional predisposition may play a role either directly or indirectly in the susceptibility to hearing loss. There are wider quantitative variations in degree of acquired hearing loss; and although psychological ramifications are present with congenital hearing loss, they are more complex and varied with acquired hearing loss, particularly if speech and language have already developed. The likelihood of combined congenital and adventitious factors, although less frequent, should also be considered.

Regardless of idiopathic origin, the effects on the child and the family are cause for particular concern.

Adjustive Responses of the Child

It is impossible to generalize about the adjustive responses of the child to hearing loss, whether congenitally or adventitiously acquired, as they would include a complex interplay of many factors. Among them are the severity of hearing loss, time of acquisition, familial and social influence and effects, nature and quality of educational and habilitative efforts, and unique personality and coping characteristics of the child. To present even a prototype example would force us to make generalizations that might distort an understanding of the problem. We prefer instead to discuss each of the major effects in terms of its special characteristics and allow the reader to formulate and apply his or her own perspective.

Effects on Speech and Language Acquisition

Time of onset of hearing impairment and loss is likely the major variable that determines the acquisition of speech and language. The child who has never had the benefit of sufficient auditory exposure to speech and language is unlikely, except under the most extraordinary circumstances, to develop these sufficiently to communicate normally in a hearing world. The child who is in the process of developing speech or language or who has already developed the skill is likely to retain the ability except under the most dire conditions, such as total loss. Even then, the possibility exists for retention of what has already been gained.

Of greater significance is that the child who has already acquired speech and language has had the benefit of developing ideational or cognitive processes appropriate to the living environment, whereas the child who is born deaf or hearing impaired is deprived of the opportunity to relate to the world cognitively. In the first case, a communicative relationship has already been established between parent and child, tapping at cognitive resources. When speech and language has not been learned, a crucial ingredient necessary for the parent-child relationship is lacking. Only through gesture and use of body language is it possible to establish a relationship, but in the case of profound hearing loss, this is mired in what Ramsdell (1960) describes as the "primitive level" of hearing. Only through the earliest and most intensive intervention efforts is it possible to ensure that the child will be in the mainstream of the communication world of the hearing, but even then, other variables will influence the outcome.

Effects of Psychosocial Development

In Chapter 5, we discuss the complex interactive relationship between psychosocial and speech-language development in normal hearing children. The ramifications of such a relationship in the case of deaf and hearing-impaired children are more extraordinary.

The child who is born deaf and deprived of the full verbal communicative interaction with the parents is prone to internalize thoughts and feelings, lacking the opportunity to experience the full range of sensory experiences necessary to relate to the parent and the environment. The deaf child usually is impulsive and socially immature, struggling to adapt in any way possible to the deficit. As Boothroyd (1982) has noted: "They perceive themselves as being acted upon more than acting and may compensate by developing rigid and manipulative behaviors" (p. 61). Hess (1960) writes of the tendency for these children to have a fantasy life that excludes awareness of the individuality of others and being unable to approach new situations in a flexible manner. Roberts and Hindley (1999) describe a complex interweaving of social, medical, and cultural factors related to the deaf child's communication, which in turn may be related etiologically or incidental to psychiatric disorder.

Because normal cognitive and speech-language development is likely to suffer in these children, it seems remarkable that many are able to adapt at all despite their isolation from a hearing environment. Perhaps, a good number of them learn to cope with their loss by utilizing other cues within their environment along with their own unique defense mechanisms. Appropriate and early professional intervention and support from knowledgeable parents certainly contribute further to the adjustment. We would go beyond the scope of the present text to encompass the complex and still controversial issues surrounding the habilitation, education, and position in society of the deaf child. Hindley (1997), however, presents a thorough review of the psychiatric aspects of hearing-impaired children with particular emphasis on the deafened or deaf child.

Children with a lesser degree of hearing impairment, although having the advantage of greater sensory exposure to others and their environment, also may suffer psychosocially. Those who incur hearing loss after having learned speech and language have to adjust to their changed circumstances, but they do so with varying degrees of frustration, anxiety, guilt, and inappropriate behavior. They, too, are struggling to adapt and, depending on the nature and degree of parental support and professional intervention, will learn to cope accordingly.

Consistent with the theme of this book, we hesitate to generalize how children will respond to their loss and the effort employed to help them. The many complex variables inherent in the interpersonal communicative process and the unique constitutional coping process of the child often determine the outcome. We should, therefore, not be surprised when we encounter profoundly deaf children who are less impaired or have already established speech and language. Indeed, "it may be easier to live with what one has never had than to live with what one has lost."

For adolescents, deafness or acquired hearing impairment have very special implications. Because the peer group often is the determining factor defining social competence, the hearing-impaired adolescent is vulnerable to social rejection, precipitating depression, withdrawal, or regression to a less mature emotional state. Christopher, Nangle, and Hansen (1993) review extensively procedures in social-skills training with adolescents, employing a behavioral approach that appears promising. For the individual who was born deaf, depending on earlier educational and habilitative intervention, adolescence is the crossroads for embarking on a path toward the world of the deaf, the world of the hearing, or a compromised adaptation to both. Regardless of degree of impairment, the entire adjustment is shaped by intellectual, family, and unique individual character factors as well as by the quality of previous educational and habilitative efforts.

Effects on Learning

The special educational needs of and minimal supportive services for school-age hearing-impaired children have been well documented (Blair and Berg, 1982). The effects of hearing loss on learning from birth to 5 years have received less attention and, as Culross (1985) notes, virtually no assessment instrument can adequately measure the educational potential and psychological abilities of preschool hearing-impaired children.

Lacking the necessary sensory avenue for learning speech and language, the deafened infant appears to seek out alternative ways of relating to the environment in order to learn. This shift to other sensory channels, which is described fully by Studdert-Kennedy (1976), is necessary for the child to integrate whatever information can be received. How deaf and hearing-impaired children handle this information is unclear, but it would seem logical that, with even minimal access to the auditory channel, a child has a greater potential for learning normally. We are certain of one thing: Even profoundly deaf children are capable of developing the symbolic system necessary for learning, but how well these children learn depends on inherent intellectual and external familial conditions.

On the high school level, learning takes on special significance for the deafened and hearing-impaired adolescent. Peer pressure, sexual urges, emotional lability, and self-esteem often are hooked into the person's perception of the hearing impairment. Too often, the disability may be used as an excuse to become reclusive, deficient in studying, or antagonistic to others or to drop out. Unfortunately, such behaviors often are interpreted by others not in terms of the implications of hearing impairment but as the acting-out behavior of a nonconforming teenager. What is misinterpreted is the young person's cry for equilibrium, emotional support, and practical assistance.

Reaction of the Family and Others

Like the parents of children born with cerebral palsy, cleft palate, or some other major physical impairment, parents of children born deaf go through a grief process. How they move through the process is dependent on several conditions, including the unique coping mechanisms of the family, the quality and degree of outside professional assistance, and the child's own adaptability to the blockage of the auditory channel. If deafness or impairment of hearing develops adventitiously, grief may be experienced but in a more varied or subtle manner. Again, much will depend on other variables. The reader will find a succinct and useful discussion of mourning as it applies to deafness in children in Boothroyd (1982). It will also be helpful to review the process as it is discussed in other chapters, in particular the adaptive process to child disability as identified by Shontz (1975).

More significant from our perspective are the specific effects of any degree of hearing impairment on individual family members, the marital relationship, and the overall family equilibrium.

Effects on Individual Family Members

Feelings of anger, bitterness, disappointment, frustration, and anger experienced by the parents in particular will vary greatly, depending on each parent's unique association with the child and personal emotional stability. To some extent, the degree to which each parent has fulfilled or is fulfilling his or her own life's goals will determine how well he or she will adjust to the child's disability.

Much, too, will depend, certainly, on whether or not one or both parents of deaf children are hearing impaired or deaf. We hesitate to generalize outcomes of such circumstances because of the uniqueness of all parents. Conceivably, it is as possible for deaf parents to provide the most educationally and habilitatively appropriate environment as it is possible for normal hearing parents to provide the least for theirs. Generally, though, the deaf child of normal hearing parents starts out with one major advantage: a potential auditorily rich and stimulating linguistic environment.

We are more familiar with adventitiously hearing-impaired youngsters in normal hearing families. The variety of effects of individual family members here are probably more infinite. Let us look at one such family.

The 11-year-old son had incurred a severe hearing loss three years previous to the referral, following a succession of serious middle ear infections and questionable medical management. Although very intelligent and sophisticated, the mother blamed herself for not having prevented the ultimate condition. Her marriage was relatively stable, but she felt unfulfilled as a woman and always considered her three children a burden even though there never had been any previous serious physical problems. Projecting her own guilt onto her severely deaf son, she felt compelled to dote on him and protect him from all life's stressors. She shopped for the best professional help she could possibly find but "never could find the right hearing aid for him." Her life had become a crusade that left little opportunity for her son to deal personally with his own struggles. Instead, the author was confronted with a fearful, dependent, uncommunicative youngster who had few friends and was barely getting by in school.

This description is just one of the many possible illustrations of the effects of a child's hearing impairment on one family member. It also is meant to illustrate the dynamic interplay between parent and child. Most important for us to understand is that parents do not necessarily pass through the various stages of the grief process in an orderly fashion or at any one time. As Boothroyd (1982) clearly indicates, "The mourning sequence can be replayed

several times in the parents' lives" (p. 64). We would add that any one stage may appear out of its classical sequence and may be manifest subtly or in combination with other stages. Therefore, an attitude such as denial by the parent may be expressed as a refusal to accept the hearing loss, the fitting of a hearing aid, modifying firmly entrenched behaviors, or any combination of these.

In any case, the child is affected either through overt or covert attitudes and actions by the parent. How readily the child falls victim to the unresolved anguish, rejection, and helplessness of the parent may be due in part, as indicated earlier, to the child's unique mode of coping or constitutional tolerance. Our task as caregivers is to assess the interplay of feelings, actions, and events to provide the best we have to offer professionally.

The way in which the family relates to the hearing impaired adolescent will have a profound influence on high school adjustment, "passage through puberty," individual self-esteem, and career or vocational choice. Regardless of time of onset of the hearing loss, the family will need to continue to nurture and enhance the child through all of the struggles typically associated with adolescence and those directly or indirectly associated with hearing impairment. To either reject or overprotect at this time will only make the child more rebellious or dependent and maintain the parental-infant bond. A gradual separation needs to happen, whereby the adolescent begins the process of functioning autonomously as an adult.

Effects on the Marital Relationship

The reality of hearing loss in the child is not the cause of marital dysfunction but can be the catalytic factor to disrupt what may have been a shaky marriage. Like the arrival of any child with either a physical or psychological disability, one or both partners may use the circumstance to inflict on the other blame, resentment, accusation, or recriminations that may appear to be related to their reaction to the child's disability but in fact are tied to their own unresolved marital problems.

Ironically, in some cases, although the traumatic occasion may be an excuse for both parents to inflict abuse on each other, it also could bring to the surface issues with which they previously had not been forced to cope. They may seek professional help for themselves, which ultimately will benefit their afflicted child. Unfortunately, this sequence of events is not the case generally. The parents are more likely to get further immersed in their own marital difficulty, which in turn can have a devastating effect on the child and the rest of the family.

Effects on Family Homeostasis

A psychologically healthy family can meet the multiple needs of a hearing-impaired child and, at the same time, cope with their own individual reactions. The members are not absolved from suffering stress or experiencing the various stages of the grief process. Family members can deal with the crisis by temporarily minimalizing their own personal ambitions, modifying their own role responsibilities to meet the needs of the hearing-impaired child, and cooperatively working together to minimize the effects of hearing impairment on the entire family (Hill, 1958). Some families are adaptable to change, genuinely affectionate with one another, and able to solve problems through congruent communications. At the core is a dynamic, creative, and loving marital relationship. We do not wish to imply that a functional family can satisfy all of these requirements or even that such an ideal family actually exists. But, as long as a family strives in the manner that is suggested, a hearing-impaired child will be a much more fortunate recipient.

In a more dysfunctional family, the equilibrium is disturbed in that the hearing-impaired child may deflect attention away from other conflicts. The child may displace the "identified" symptom in another family member from a previous familial conflict, thereby creating a situation in which the emotionality between the child and parent may become highly charged. If marital dysfunction has been present, the hearing impairment in the child may serve to submerge the conflict further by getting enmeshed in it. Parental attitudes and behaviors such as overprotection and overinvolvement are projected onto the child, who is now viewed as incompetent and made to feel "different." Thus, the true perspective of the hearing impairment is either lost or distorted.

The reader will recall from the earlier anecdote how the 11-year-old hearing-impaired child became the recipient of the mother's unresolved struggles. In that family, attention was first drawn away from the other children, one of whom became asthmatic, withdrawn, and uncommunicative. These behaviors however drew attention now to what the asthmatic child needed, thus becoming the identified patient. In this case, the father took on the major role of caregiver while the mother continued to dote on the hearing-impaired child. What originally was one family had in a sense become two families living in the same physical environment but in reality emotionally draining each other. The third child, striving to maintain some sense of family equilibrium, began to act out his resentment from being excluded from parental attention by reverting to infantile behaviors such as enuresis and tantrums.

The parents, realizing that all seemed to be collapsing around them, jeopardizing the entire family, sought counseling assistance in order to reestablish a healthy equilibrium.

Murphy (1979), in his introductory chapter to an excellent monograph on families of hearing-impaired children, alludes to the importance of family relationships in terms of family functioning and growth. Murphy implies that hearing impairment in the child cannot be separated from the entire interpersonal process that distinguishes the life of the family. He cites pertinent research concerning the father's role in assisting the hearing-impaired child and the need for more research relative to the father's as well as the mother's role.

Based on research and clinical work, Schlesinger and Meadow (1972), in their seminal text, "illuminate the relation between family patterns and social-intellectual-linguistic development in deaf children" (p. xi). They have applied the Eriksonian model of the eight stages of development to the understanding of the psychosocial development of the deaf from birth to death. For them, the chief handicap of early profound deafness is not bound only to the auditory deficiency but also to the communicative process within the family. In our view it is no less important to view the lesser hearing-impaired child in a similar manner. Calderon and Greenberg (1999) examine maternal and child adjustment as a result of the application of a stress and coping model to factors associated with having a school-aged child with hearing loss. They found that social support was an important predictor of maternal adjustment as well as a shield between current life stress and maternal adjustment. Maternal problem-solving skill also emerged as a potent determinant of child adjustment and a mediating factor between child's age and teacher rating of child adjustment. The authors conclude that parent and child outcomes can better be understood by a competency-based rather than a psychopathological perspective. Ducharme and Holborn (1997) established the efficacy of a social skills training program for hearing-impaired preschoolers, using stimulus exemplars and natural consequences to promote generalization of social interaction.

Counseling Strategies

Only in recent years have writers in the field of audiology stressed the need for counseling intervention for parents of hearing-impaired children (Stream and Stream, 1978; Murphy, 1979; Luterman, 1979; Sweetow and Barrager, 1980; Clark, 1982). Although these writers recognize that the role of the audiologist must be enlarged beyond the identification and assessment of hearing loss, hearing aid dispensing, and aural rehabilitation, they say little regarding the need for the child to be counseled as well. Also, in the otherwise excellent guidelines for counseling the family or parents, little has been written about the use of family therapy. We, therefore, need to examine all these procedures.

Family Counseling

Clark (1982) provides several excellent guidelines to assist in counseling parents of hearing-impaired children. We summarize them as follows:

1. *The intake procedure.* Present an opportunity for the audiologist to obtain a case history and determine the exact needs of the parents. An interpersonal relationship is established.
2. *The diagnostic interview.* Confirm the degree and quality of the hearing loss and provide only general information, so that the family will not be overwhelmed. Family members are given an opportunity to express their reactions.
3. *Subsequent counseling.* Provide more in-depth counseling so that the family can have a more complete understanding of the problem and of the habilitative-educational process. The counseling audiologist must provide enough time for the family to assimilate what it has *learned* and what it is experiencing.
4. *Fostering an interpersonal relationship.* Be open to the continuing concerns, feelings, and attitudes of the family. Nonjudgmental listening should be practiced by paying more attention to what the family needs and less to what the audiologist wants to discuss.
5. *Three major questions asked.* Following Luterman (1976, 1979), the parents are asked three types of questions: (a) The request for further information, (b) confirmation from the parents of the educational and habilitative procedure proposed by the audiologist, and (c) content questions with affectual components.
6. *Facilitating questioning by parents.* Provide an open atmosphere so that parents will not feel intimidated but free to ask anything they wish. An empathic and authentic attitude by the counselor is a must.
7. *Dealing with the grief process.* Be prepared to cope with the wide range of feelings inherent in mourning and helping the family understand that what they are experiencing is not abnormal.
8. *Shaping expectations.* Provide an honest picture of the implications of the hearing loss and a realistic assessment of what can be expected in the future.
9. *Ongoing opportunities for counseling.* Continued counseling may be necessary so that parents may work through their feelings and be given the opportunity to have more of their questions and concerns answered.

Provide Information

A study by Sweetow and Barrager (1980), who surveyed 154 parents of hearing-impaired children, draws our attention to the need for these parents to have much more information about hearing loss than they typically are given. Among the specific needs determined were these:

1. Translating "technical terminology into laymen's language."
2. Providing a means of communicating more effectively with their hearing-impaired child.
3. Providing a means for "contact with other parents of hearing impaired children."
4. Providing more written literature on the subject of hearing loss.
5. Providing "more specific information on educational sources."
6. Providing "more frequent referrals to external sources for assistance in emotional and financial support."
7. Answering the desire for "audiologists to take parents' observations and comments more seriously" (p. 847).

The comprehensive parent education program suggested by Dee (1981) is a practical and straightforward approach to helping these parents realize that their feelings are no different from those of others caught in a crisis.

Probably one of the most important considerations for the counseling audiologist to keep in mind when providing information is timing. It is necessary to be sensitive to the quantity and quality of information the parents can handle during the ongoing counseling relationship. The extent of their emotional reactions to the crisis will determine, in part, how much information they can process at a particular time. One effective way for the counselor to judge this is to check with their clients, on an ongoing basis, how much they feel they need to know. If the parents are helped to realize that they are free to ask questions at any time, the counselor will have a better sense of how much and what they need to know.

Provide Means of Coping

The counseling audiologist cannot solve the family's problems surrounding the hearing impairment of the child but can provide the family the necessary guidelines it needs to cope. We believe that the counselor's prime task is to help the parents become

as fully aware as possible of their own personal attitudes, beliefs, needs, and expectations before they can be in a position to help their child. They need to see themselves not as taking the hearing loss personally but viewing it essentially as belonging to the child. In this way they are better able to objectify the child's problem, gather a clear perspective of what *they* can do, and follow through with whatever educational and habilitative strategies are necessary.

This is no easy duty, because parents tend to want to assimilate their children's problems, the process of which, in our view, is likely a projection of their own unresolved feelings of guilt, resentment, and need for a perfect child and an absence of conflict. The counselor may find considerable resistance to exploring these aspects of parent-child relationships and must temper empathic understanding with gentle persuasion if parents are to change their firmly entrenched belief system. A judgmental know-it-all or condescending approach would be detrimental not only to the therapeutic process but to the eventual educational and habilitative outcome. However, if we, as counselors, can be conscious of these occasional professional slips in ourselves, then we are unlikely to do any irreparable harm.

Parents who are helped to relate to their hearing-impaired children in the way we are suggesting can better aid in developing the emotional and intellectual resources naturally available to children and thus ensure the most positive results.

Another task particularly important for the counselor is to be certain that the family knows exactly how to follow through with its own responsibilities toward the child and with the various other professional resources available. It is one thing to recommend that a hearing aid be fitted and another thing to make certain that it is appropriately used by the child. If recurring ear infections are the problem, the counseling audiologist may need to make certain that the child is checked out otologically.

We do not suggest that the audiologist alone should be the prime caregiving coordinator. Others, like the otologist, the speech-language pathologist, and the teacher, also might play a guiding role in helping the parents follow through with their responsibilities.

One of the most revealing results of the study by Sweetow and Barrager (1980) are the major concerns of the parents. When they were asked, "In general how would you like to see the role of the audiologist expanded or improved?" the three most common answers were

1. The audiologist should handle the hearing aids.
2. The audiologist should work more closely with the schools.
3. More information on educational programs and emotional support should be provided. (pp. 846–847)

From our perspective, the chief concern is that parents also know exactly where to go for assistance, know what to do, and do it. As professional caregivers, we must demand no less from ourselves. There is little question, too, of the effect of parental presence or absence on the psychosocial, linguistic and academic outcomes of deaf and hearing-impaired children. Calderon and Low (1998) found that children whose fathers were present had significantly better academic and language outcomes than those with no father present.

Family Therapy

Family therapy is a particularly relevant counseling procedure because it helps maintain the communicative interaction, which can readily be lost if the child is severely hearing impaired or deaf. Although typically the child may have difficulty in following the verbal interchanges, all attempts should be made to involve the child. If language has already been learned, amplification and speech reading will certainly enhance the communication process.

Family therapy is educational as well as therapeutic and helps remove the stigma of the "identified symptom or patient."

The Educational and Therapeutic Process

Consistent with the theme of this text, we believe family therapy to be a more thorough means of assisting the family to cope with many of the difficulties confronting it, and no less so for the hearing-impaired family. Although it could be argued that the affected child should not be subjected to

one more situation in which it feels cut off from communication and that traditional parent counseling will conveniently protect the child from being exposed to material that could be emotionally harmful, we suggest a different point of view.

The child, depending on the nature and degree of the hearing loss itself, already is likely to feel thwarted in understanding what is occurring in the immediate perceptual environment. Confused and bewildered, children may feel detached, isolated, and in some cases alienated from those around them, but the family therapy situation need not exacerbate these feelings. On the contrary, it could well enhance positive attitudes of belonging, self-identity, and self-worth merely by including the child in a process that at least will provide visual and perhaps some auditory input.

We also question the notion of shielding children from material to which they had already been exposed during daily family interactions. It is better that these elements be brought out into the open in the nurturing atmosphere of family therapy than allowed to fester in a milieu where communication is either closed or incongruent.

Family therapy is family counseling and more. It gives all family members an opportunity to learn, on differing levels, how to discover specific ways, with each other's assistance, to best contend with the reality of hearing loss. It also provides the right set of circumstances in which family members can assist themselves and each other to feel better, mature emotionally, and most important, make the best of what previously may have appeared to be an impossible situation. Also obvious is that hearing parents of deaf children who sign be skilled in signing as well, to readily facilitate the family therapy process.

Diminish the Impact of the Identified Symptom

We already discussed how the hearing impairment becomes the identified symptom in terms of family systems theory. Although hearing loss is a symptom in the ordinary sense of the word, it should not be used to represent aspects of underlying family dysfunction. That is, it must not be allowed to take on a meaning that is not inherent to the hearing loss itself. To do this, the family may be guided in several ways. Of overriding importance, though, is that the family be involved in the beginning of the rehabilitation process.

1. Help family members discover whatever areas of conflict interfere with healthy family functioning.
2. Help them understand the effects of hearing impairment as a family issue and not belonging to only one person per se.
3. Foster congruent communication among all family members, making certain that the hearing-impaired child has access to whatever communication aids are available.
4. Help each family member understand his or her unique role within the family and individual relationships with one another.
5. Help family members plan future goals for themselves as well as for the entire family.
6. Recognize differences in families regarding members' attitudes toward either a total, oral, or manual approach to speech and language.

These guidelines are not necessarily exclusive to the hearing-impaired family, but they must be used in the context of how the hearing impairment impinges on all family members. Moreover, because families with hearing-impaired children differ among themselves, the counselor needs to be careful not to formulate generalizations about the effects of hearing impairment, habilitative and educational goals, and prognostic signs unless they are relevant to the particular family being treated. In Great Britain, Roberts and Hindley (1999) demonstrate the importance of treatment strategies to be designed for psychiatrically disordered deaf children and their parents. The use of an interpreter skilled in family systems therapy naturally is essential.

Individual Counseling

It seems remarkable that, although the literature has given considerable attention to the value of parent counseling, virtually no emphasis has been placed on counseling the child individually. Can we assume that only parent counseling or family therapy will assist hearing-impaired children to use all of their emotional resources to enhance their edu-cational, social, and habilitative goals? We doubt it. In addition, no definitive experimental studies have been made to determine outcomes based on parent counseling or family therapy intervention.

We believe that individual counseling, either separate from or in conjunction with other strategies, can enhance the emotional, social, and educational life of the child. The particular procedure used will be determined by the age of the child, degree of impairment, communicative competence, and cooperation of the parents. The procedure can include play therapy, client-centered aural rehabilitation, or direct counseling.

Play Therapy

Play therapy for the hearing-impaired child is similar in many ways to play therapy with other communicatively disordered children, as discussed in previous chapters. To avoid redundancy, we describe only those aspects particularly pertinent to the hearing-impaired child:

1. Depending on the degree of hearing impairment, rapport may be established through basic signing, nonverbal body expression, amplification, or any combination of these. Use of puppets can be helpful here.
2. The free expression of feelings and verbal speech and language is encouraged, with the child encouraged to pay direct attention to the facial appearance of the therapist. Here, the therapist will need to be highly animated, to communicate recognition and reflection of feelings.
3. Make extensive use of sound toys as a means of communication, toward developing cognitive skills, and of enhancing whatever residual auditory acuity is present.
4. The parent should be encouraged to observe the sessions, preferably through a one-way mirror, to carry over into the home several of the skills being taught in therapy.

We have to realize that, although play therapy may stimulate the expression of emotional material, foster interpersonal communication, and enhance learning, it is not a panacea for habilitation. It is a procedure, however, that may be used in conjunction with the total management program. The therapist will need to determine its relevance, depending on the emotional needs of the child, cooperation of the family, and availability of other caregiving services.

Client-Centered Aural Rehabilitation

It is difficult to imagine the use of aural rehabilitation outside the process of client-centered counseling because they are both part of the interpersonal communicative process and mutually complementary. For instance, if one of the goals in therapy is to maximize the efficiency with which a child uses a hearing aid, it will be necessary not only to reinforce a positive attitude about its use but also to help the child break down barriers to its acceptance. The obstacles may include emotional conflict, poor self-esteem, embarrassment, denial, withdrawal from relationships with peers, unconsciously motivated destruction of the aid, or any combination of these. The reader obviously can add more forms of resistance based on individual clinical experience.

The effectiveness with which the hearing-impaired child learns to speech-read will be determined not only by perhaps an intuitive ability to use available cues within a communicative situation but also by the desire to learn from the environment. For the professional caregiver to rely only on the use of speech-reading techniques detached from the child's attitude or emotional state is neither realistic nor efficient. Here, too, it will be necessary to establish the optimum conditions under which the child can learn to speech-read regardless of the severity of the hearing impairment, and this includes the counseling process.

The problems for the deaf child are somewhat similar yet also quite different. Much already has been written concerning the integration of the deaf child within the community of the non-hearing-impaired and about the controversy surrounding the more than 100-year-old war over the oral versus manual approach. Although these are issues that go beyond the scope of this chapter, they are relevant to professionals who must counsel the deafened child.

Probably one of the chief challenges to professional counselors is to separate their own personal biases from the reality of the child's unique life circumstances and intellectual and educational potential. Counseling here becomes a process in which the counselor needs to learn what expectations are realistic for the child while the child must learn to develop maximum efficiency in communicating, regardless of the community within which the child ultimately may function. The counselor frequently may be faced with the dilemma of recognizing objectively that a vast potential for the child exists and should be acutely aware of the child's environmental circumstances that may impede that potential. Only then can some resolution be achieved.

Although we have no standards to assist us in case-by-case intervention, some generic guidelines may be useful regardless of degree and quality of hearing impairment:

1. *Assess the hearing along with the psychosocial status of the child.* It may be useful or necessary to have access to the services of a psychologist or psychometrist who is acquainted with the hearing problems of children.
2. *Educate the child about the hearing loss.* Too frequently, we educate the parents and assume somehow that the child will get the information through osmosis. Informative data need to be given to the child, geared to that child's age and intellectual level.
3. *Orient the child to the use of a hearing aid.* Fitting the aid is not enough. Teaching its use and care is meaningful only if we (a) allow the child to express his or her feelings about wearing it and respond empathically to possible resistance or concern, and (b) allow for possible resistance as an expression of real difficulties the child may be having with a particular aid and consider refitting if necessary.
4. *Have the child teach us what is needed to function more adequately.* We cannot assume that the age or naiveté of the child precludes awareness of obstacles to maximal use of residual hearing. We need to be open to whatever information is forthcoming from the child and place it in proper perspective with data we objectively gathered.
5. *Distinguish emotional issues associated with hearing loss from those unrelated to it.* This is no easy task for the counseling audiologist, because none of us behaves in a linear manner

but instead responds behaviorally to the sum of our experiences. What is necessary is that we discover those negative influences in the child's environment that at least appear to be unrelated to the hearing loss. These may include the effects of (a) being raised by one parent, (b) divorce, (c) extreme poverty, or (d) an emotionally disturbed family.

6. *Deal with emotional disturbance in the child.* Somewhat related to guideline 5, it may be necessary to refer the severely emotionally disturbed child for more extensive psychotherapeutic assistance, preferably to a professional who is well acquainted with the problems of hearing loss in children.

7. *Provide a supportive, empathic, and trusting therapeutic environment.* An environment in which the child feels free to express concerns regarding the loss of hearing and its many implications provides a valuable opportunity in which to apply our audiological knowledge effectively. Too often children view us as adversaries, united with parents against them, regardless of our best-intentioned efforts. Therefore, of considerable importance is that we relate to the child in the most genuine way possible rather than pose as individuals who "know what's best" for the child. This does not imply that we act the role of "buddy" but that we appear to the child, and the child appears to us, as distinct persons in our own right.

8. *Use special counseling techniques.* Consistent with the philosophy expressed throughout this text, we need to feel free to use whatever strategies with which we feel competent and that appear appropriate to a particular child. Among them are confrontation, self-disclosure, and contracting. In most instances, these will need to be connected to aural rehabilitation strategies, but always bear in mind that the child matters, not the technique.

Counseling or family therapy usually is thought necessary when hearing loss is first determined and during habilitative and educational planning. But, as the following anecdotal accounts illustrate, it may be important a considerable time after the onset of hearing loss and initial intervention. In fact,

it may be important on an intermittent basis throughout the child's early and pubescent years. Tsappis (personal communication, 1985) summarizes the psychological experiences of two congenitally hearing-impaired adolescents.

The first incident addresses the adolescent's increasing sexual awareness and various behaviors defining male and female social roles. During an annual visit to the Speech and Hearing Center, the mother of a 16-year-old youth reported that her son had recently discontinued hearing aid use and strenuously resisted and rejected parental efforts to encourage continued use of amplification. The young man had a moderate to severe, congenital, sensorineural hearing loss. He had been successfully using binaural amplification since approximately age 2. His speech and language and academic performance were excellent. He obviously had used two hearing aids consistently for 14 years with good results and no complaint. Consequently, his sudden rejection of amplification and resistance to parental support represented an important issue requiring resolution.

When questioned in the clinic about his rejection of hearing aids, all effort to obtain information were received with a shrug of the shoulders and a mumbled, "I don't know." Electroacoustic evaluation of the hearing aids indicated that they were functioning according to factory specifications, and audiological evaluation indicated no change in hearing when compared with prior test results. Following the structured hearing and hearing aid evaluations, we invited the young man to the hospital for a coke. Conversation drifted from school, recreation activities, and girls to automobiles. During this informal discussion, we learned the young man recently had obtained his driver's license and reported that during the course of his first driving date, his companion laid her head on his shoulder. The young lady's head provided a protective barrier at the pinna, which resulted in generating considerable acoustic feedback at his right hearing aid. The young lady did not know her escort wore hearing aids. Consequently when the feedback occurred she was quite startled. The young man reported that she practically jumped out the passenger door while the car was moving. She apparently huddled as close to the passenger door as she could and with a look of concern and confusion asked, "Did I hurt you?" In view of this report, it is not surprising that a young man, who had just obtained the greatest symbol of American independence and mobility and who was struggling to behave in a way that would identify and establish his masculinity, discontinued hearing aid use. The instruments were obviously directly responsible for causing considerable embarrassment during one of the most important evenings of his life. His attempt to explain what had occurred apparently did little to resolve his companion's concern at the time. We jointly agreed that anticipation of future events might dictate whether he should wear binaural or either monaural right or left instruments, depending on social circumstances.

The thought that such an event could be responsible for an adolescent's reluctance to continue to use required amplification was remote. Typically, considerable attention is directed to the adolescent woman's attitudes regarding physical characteristics, glasses, and hearing aids; however, as illustrated by the present event, little effort is directed toward dealing with adolescent men's attitudes.

The second incident involves a 13-year-old experiencing a severe to profound, congenital, sensorineural hearing loss. He also had been successfully wearing amplification since approximately age 2. Over the years, in typical fashion, he occasionally expressed to his parents his curiosity regarding the etiology of the hearing loss and his need to use hearing aids that were not required by his close friends. His parents had previously informed him that the loss was the result of maternal rubella occurring during the first trimester of pregnancy. Their descriptions were accurate and appropriate to his age at the time of the question. Over the years, the explanations offered were accepted with little or no ongoing dialogue, and family life proceeded as usual. At approximately age 13, following detailed discussion of the etiology of his hearing loss, his behavior toward his mother changed considerably. Responses to comments and questions regarding various family matters were abrupt and succinct. He generally began to avoid any verbal or social interaction with his mother, while generally maintaining his usual social routine with other family members. During a heated discussion, he confided to his parents that he "hated

his mother" because she and the illness she contracted while carrying him were directly responsible for his permanent affliction. The report obviously resulted in considerable parental concern.

We referred the family to a local psychiatrist with an excellent reputation. Our immediate opinion was that, since such feelings of parental hostility are known in the psychiatric community, therapy would be extremely beneficial. I expected that the youth's speech and language level would present no communication difficulties for the psychiatrist. Unfortunately, one and a half years of therapy and counseling did little to help the young man with his feelings of rage. In frustration, during that time, the parents sought help from various psychiatric and psychological professionals to no avail. At the end of the period, the family terminated therapy. The family problem and the young man's attitude toward his mother continued for approximately a year following the conclusion of therapy. Outward hostility toward his mother then diminished and eventually resolved. The family now enjoys the open, interactive relationships that existed prior to the overt onset and demonstration of anger. The problem apparently resolved as quickly as it began; however, the family was frustrated through the lack of assistance available that might have resolved the problem more quickly and avoided approximately three years of family disharmony.

These reports do not differ necessarily from those of normal hearing individuals whose anger is directed toward parents or who are coping with adolescence. They do illustrate the value of psychotherapy intervention even when it is resisted. Apparently, a child and family may "get better" despite it. The difficulties that can be expected in children with more profound hearing loss and limited oral language may be presumed to create even greater concerns for us.

Group Counseling

Whether a hearing-impaired child is in the educational mainstream or a self-contained classroom, group therapy can be a valuable adjunctive aid toward habilitation. Its value is probably greatest when it can be integrated along with aural rehabilitation that includes group amplification, auditory training, and speech reading. Among the psychological benefits to be gained are the following:

1. Recognizing and understanding that they are not alone as they experience their hearing loss.
2. Learning to discover their own unique ways to cope with their loss.
3. Sharing with each other methods those that had been useful and those that have not.
4. Depending on their age, learning how to adjust more effectively to special problems associated with adolescence, relationships with hearing peers, family relationships, and school studies.
5. Developing positive attitudes about themselves by learning how to maximize their potentials and minimize their liabilities.

Although it may not be possible to establish a set of guidelines that will determine the efficacy of having a particular child in group therapy, it would be more useful for the counseling audiologist to make a case-by-case decision, either independently or in consultation with other professionals. Most important is that the decision be based on what the child needs, the cooperation of the family, and the availability of resources. Furthermore, group therapy should not be viewed as a substitute for other management practices, and every effort must be made to provide those that will benefit the child most.

One final note should be added. Regardless of the group therapy counseling model used, every effort should be made by the counselor to establish a therapeutic process whereby the children learn to assist each other rather than become individually passive agents in a group. Although the counselor at times may lead, educate, reflect, clarify, and possibly even judge, the children themselves should be given the responsibility to work through with each other whatever problems are present and those that may arise.

Conclusion

Although children with hearing loss have many of the psychosocial concomitants associated with children having other communicative disorders and, in fact, may be afflicted with those disorders as well, many factors are unique to hearing impairment itself. We need to be cautious, however, not to generalize those elements to all hearing-impaired children nor neglect to recognize the possibility of phenomena atypical to these children.

Clinically, audiologists are familiar with the psychodynamic challenges these children present, but are also frustrated by the absence of solid experimental research to help them better understand the processes and to facilitate the delivery of their services. Audiologists are faced with no less a challenge when intervening with the hearing-impaired adult.

Part II.
The Psychology of Hearing-Impaired Adults

Psychosocial Dynamics

A major distinction between the psychosocial dynamics of hearing-impaired children and hearing-impaired adults is that the adults generally have had no hearing impairment for most of their lives. Although an individualistic approach is necessary to understanding their problems, as Orlans

(1985) has indicated, they present a singular combination typical to those whose hearing has been unimpaired during the substantial portion of their lifetime. More than that, however, they present us with the common problems of adults who must adjust to any radical change in their lives, regardless of the nature, quality, and degree of the disability or the event.

The central focus of this section is on age and etiological correlates and how the hearing-impaired adult is affected personally, socially, and vocationally. A further concern is the adjustment process related to the marital relationship, family functioning, and the effects on the children of hearing-impaired adults. Jerger et al. (1995), in reviewing current information about the epidemiology, etiology, pathogenesis, evaluation, and quality of life aspects of hearing loss in older adults consider how auditory peripheral and central mechanisms influence the social and emotional impact of the hearing disorder. They emphasize the significance of quality of life issues. This chapter addresses the last concept.

Etiology and Age

Among adults who become hearing impaired, it is important that we make several distinctions regarding age and etiology, so that we can better understand their adjustment to the loss and the counseling management that may follow. It should be further understood that we cannot always generalize adjustive responses nor the remediation needs on the basis of etiology or age alone, as many individual variations will dictate the course and progression of the overall rehabilitative process. The following anecdotes illustrate what we mean.

Mr. P, an auto mechanic, began losing his hearing in his late twenties and wore a hearing aid until he went totally deaf at age 55. Over the years he had learned speech reading but most of it was self-taught. Although he and his family, a wife and grown son and daughter, were unprepared for a total loss, their essential mutual love, caring, and trust sustained them all during the traumatic final year of hearing. Family therapy was initiated to help them through this adjustments process but was discontinued after three sessions because they were capable of letting go of their previous hope for arrest of the gradual hearing loss. Mr. and Mrs. P also were able to begin plans for making other changes in their lives. These consisted of preparations for Mr. P's early retirement, an intensive program of aural rehabilitation, and an extended motor home tour throughout the United States.

We are not suggesting that the family did not suffer the anguish typifying the trauma of total hearing loss, but the mental health that characterized the family was a key factor to their overall adjustment and positive planning for the future. Although the year-long program of aural rehabilitation helped him to understand only 30% of normal speech, he felt ready to "move on to other things in my life."

Twelve years following his traumatic loss of hearing, Mr. P volunteered for the most highly developed electronic cochlear implant, which even without speech-reading cues helps him to understand about 40% of normal speech. Using both, he now hears well enough to carry on normal conversations.

It should be understood that Mr. P's decision to volunteer for the research project involving cochlear implantation was not based on a personal search for the proverbial Golden Fleece but a willingness to help otologic and audiologic researchers in their quest to enable thousands of other totally deaf people to hear normal speech.

Another anecdote concerns Madge T, a single, attractive, well-groomed 35-year-old practicing courtroom attorney who, as a result of otosclerosis, ultimately acquired a moderate bilateral hearing loss. Resisting efforts to be fitted with a hearing aid, she denied that the loss warranted aid and continued courtroom work despite admonitions by trial judges to pay more attention to what was being said during trial proceedings. Curiously, even without aid, she should have been able to function at least adequately in the courtroom, albeit with concentrated attention, but her high degree of anxiety prevented even that. Rather than confronting the reality of her life situation, she took fewer and fewer cases, depleting whatever savings she had to maintain the style of living to which she had been accustomed.

Although psychotherapy was instrumental in uncovering deep-seated struggles related to her self-concept and adequacy as a woman trying to function in an essentially male-oriented profession, she continued to resist her psychiatrist's advice to purchase the aid with which she had been adequately fitted.

After several months she terminated psychotherapy and sought further otologic-audiologic assistance. Soon she relinquished the notion that further surgery would be of any benefit to her and was now open to further counseling from her audiologist. Although he had recommended that it would be useful for her to return for further psychiatric assistance, she preferred instead to work through her "blocks," as she put it, with her audiologist.

During the first few months of counseling she agreed to wear intermittently the aid she had finally purchased and, with continued therapeutic support, empathy, and at times confrontation, was wearing the aid consistently after one year.

These two illustrations are examples of etiological, psychological, environmental, and individual factors that constitute adjustment to hearing loss by adults. It is useful, however, to consider how together age and etiology play a significant role in the adjustment process and to be aware that the premorbid attitudes and affectual state of the individual also determine the reactive response to the hearing loss.

Traumatic Hearing Loss and Age

Generally speaking, the occurrence of traumatic hearing loss at any age during adulthood is likely to cause far more upheaval in that person's life than we would expect with gradual impairment, regardless of age. This is not to suggest that the psychosocial consequences for the latter necessarily would be any less profound in specific cases.

It readily can be understood that any drastic change brought about by external forces will test the unique adjustment resources of an individual. If the trauma occurs in conjunction with other disabling conditions associated with such events as a gunshot wound to the head, automobile accident, fall, or toxic poisoning, we would expect the adjustment process to be far greater and more complex.

For the young adult who is typically entering the stage of developing a career, establishing primary relationships, and becoming a self-directed individual, the reaction to a traumatic loss of hearing may stalemate him or her from achieving any one or combination of these goals. What the audiologist must differentiate are the effects of the individual's reaction to the loss from the direct effects of the loss itself on the wide range of possibilities in that person's life. Obviously, the combined effects also require a considerable degree of counseling expertise if the impaired individual is to embark in a new or modified direction.

In middle adulthood, traumatic hearing loss produces somewhat different consequences. Here, the individual already is practicing a particular profession or occupation, has likely established a family, and has already adopted a particular self-identity. Depending on the strength and the quality of these, the individual may be able either to find a way to cope with the loss or lose personal perspective in the form of self-doubt, self-recrimination, resentment, and anger. Although the latter also may characterize the younger adult, the older adult may be experiencing a midlife crisis that in no way is related to the traumatic loss of hearing but could certainly influence it now.

Here, the combined effects may influence and distort either the real implications of the loss itself or the individual's personal response to it. The task for the audiologist will be to help the individual sort through the personal issues that either directly or indirectly relate to the hearing loss.

In older adulthood, depression frequently appears and, with the occurrence of traumatic hearing loss, is likely to be intensified, particularly if the individual also is suffering from other physical or psychological incapacities or if it occurs in conjunction with other physical problems. The adjustment of the individual to the many problems associated with aging in general has been well documented (Breslau and Haug, 1983). Any drastic alteration of physical capabilities like traumatic hearing loss, however, also is likely to magnify such issues as dependency on children, fear of death, general helplessness, loss of self-esteem, and lack of purpose or meaning in life. Perhaps already feeling alienated from the environment, as similarly aged friends and family members die, the individual is cut off further, dramatically, from the world.

The overwhelming effects of traumatic hearing loss in the aged population probably present to the counseling audiologist the greatest challenge of all. It will be necessary to sort out all of the effects of the loss and the circumstances with which the client must struggle.

Hearing Loss with Gradual Onset

The counseling audiologist is more likely to be confronted with hearing loss as it develops gradually in the adult. Here, too, however, the variables of etiology and age play a significant role, although the process of progressive hearing loss presents with somewhat different implications. That is, the process allows the individual to adjust more slowly and perhaps more thoroughly to the overall loss, but the psychosocial effects may not necessarily be any less profound in individual cases.

Young adults whose hearing losses are due to middle-ear, cochlear, retrocochlear, or brain-stem dysfunction may not necessarily differ affectually in terms of the pathology itself, but more likely in terms of the degree of loss. Like the young adult whose loss has been precipitous, the individual is apt to feel some degree of self-imposed alienation from hearing peers. The person may resist wearing a mechanical device that may call attention to itself. Whereas a precipitous loss of hearing may be cause for the individual to take immediate remediation measures, the individual whose loss is gradual may adapt a wait and see attitude in hopes the loss will either remit or disappear.

Rousey (1971) suggests that occasionally the grief response to a hearing loss may unconsciously characterize feelings of sexual inadequacy. Such feelings should not be interpreted literally but rather be conceptualized in terms of interpersonal relationships, particularly in the case of hearing-impaired young adults.

In middle adulthood, personal and life responsibilities typically become more numerous and complex. The individual certainly is not immune to the effects discussed previously, but if family, professional, and social conditions have already been stabilized, the person is more likely to adapt to hearing loss. No longer striving like the younger person to achieve a sense of identity, place, and position in life, the older person is apt to have the advantage of an environmental support system that may mollify the effects of hearing loss. Obviously, not all hearing-impaired older adults fit such categorization; therefore, the counseling audiologist must be wary of overgeneralizing.

Older adults with gradual onset of hearing loss characterize the largest population with whom the audiologist is likely to deal. The effects of presbycusis, resulting in gradually decreased acuity for pure tone signals speech recognition, have been well documented (Hayes, 1984). Less is known of the presbycusic effects on the psychosocial aspects of the population, although Alpiner (1979) and Orlans (1985) paint a comprehensive picture of the current knowledge on the subject. It cannot be assumed that, because the hearing impairment is gradual, the effects are any less profound for the person. It is important, then, that we look at the specific adjustive responses that are made.

Adjustive Responses of the Adult

Although the adjustive responses of adults with hearing impairment may vary, depending on age and etiological factors, specific effects relate to self-esteem, emotional stress, and adjustment in the work environment. In a paper examining the role of social support and environmental and perceptual variables in explaining variations in behaviors in a sample of 240 hearing-impaired adults, Frankel and Nuttall (1984) found considerable levels of distress among their sample. The authors argue for the necessity of increased intervention by health care services and increased social support. The adjustive responses of the older adult are particularly noteworthy.

Effects Related to
Self-Esteem and Emotional Stress

We recognize that the individual response to hearing impairment depends on a number of variables, including the environmental, social, and psychological characteristics of the person. To discuss these within the context of specific psychological theories would take us beyond the scope of this text. We believe it is useful to describe the effects within a generic framework instead.

To begin with, the prior emotional status and coping capabilities of the individual determine, in part, how the hearing loss will be experienced and how adjustment will occur. One further significant factor is the degree to which and the quality with which the individual already has shaped his or her personal life. The individual who has been functioning in a healthy and productive manner is better prepared to cope with the distress caused by hearing impairment and more likely to take constructive steps toward rehabilitative management. Also, the individual who copes realistically with the loss and is future oriented is less likely to suffer the extreme of grief characteristic of those whose lives have been unfulfilled and wrought with emotional conflict. Therefore, we should not be surprised when we encounter some individuals who are devastated emotionally by their even mild or moderate loss while others with more severe losses appear to adapt quite well. One illustration of a very particular response is provided by the work of Jaworski and Stephens (1998), who investigated self-reports by hearing-impaired adults, related to silence as a face-saving strategy. They found, among a sample of 100 subjects, avoidance or termination of speaking in problematic and face-threatening situations when communicating with hearing individuals.

Effects in the Work Environment

Related to the discussion, the individual who suffers hearing impairment may need to make certain adjustments within the work environment to maintain the lifestyle to which he or she is accustomed. In rare cases, this means transferring to a new environment or vocation.

In the anecdote given earlier, Mr. P never considered a change of occupation, although as he began to lose his hearing, it was recommended that he wear ear defenders while working in the noisy environment of an auto repair shop. The degree to which such an environment contributed to the onset of his loss is irrelevant to our present discussion, but it should be noted that Mr. P was quite diligent in his efforts to protect his ears as often as practically possible.

More significant was the fact, that even with virtually complete loss of hearing, Mr. P continued in his occupation with the same firm. Although he certainly needed to make some adjustments, such as relying more on auto repair manuals than on fellow worker input, in his own personal way, he also educated his work supervisor and other workers in means by which they could help him. These included having them speak to him directly, but naturally, and expecting them to treat him not as disabled but different.

In the case of Madge T, the adjustment in the work environment was not so simple. Even while wearing her aid in the courtroom and during client consultation, she continued for some time to be self-conscious, anxious, and preoccupied. Viewing herself as disabled, she felt insecure in taking on the difficult cases by which she had always felt delightfully challenged. Instead, she relied more on legal matters that involved less face-to-face interaction and courtroom work. Frustrated by what she considered uninteresting and dull cases, she seriously contemplated giving up her profession, although her aided hearing in no way interfered with her ability to function as she had previously. Only her negative self-perception was creating a self-fulfilling prophecy of a failure. Fortunately, after a year and a half of counseling from an audiologist, she began to take on the kinds of cases she had always enjoyed and ironically became interested in the legal problems of the disabled.

What is most important to understand from these case illustrations is that it is necessary to distinguish between the objective realities and requirements of any particular work environment and the perceptual attitudes of the hearing individuals toward self in relation to that work environment. In a very real sense, hearing loss to some degree may be as severe as we choose to make it.

Special Problems of the Older Adult

The adjustive responses of older adults to their hearing loss may be quite similar to those of the younger adult, but there are differences, some of which we discussed earlier. Older adults who have not reconciled themselves to the aging process or who have not adjusted to the many upheavals associated with old age, like the death of a spouse or friends, forced retirement, or frequent illnesses, may be less apt to accept the hearing impairment, aural rehabilitation management, and the wearing of a hearing aid. This is not to infer that they necessarily are emotionally disturbed or have not lived creative, useful, and productive lives. What may be evident is that their life patterns have become essentially fixed and, rather than make any changes, even if these apparently are for "their own good," they would rather "make the best of it" with no external assistance.

These adjustive responses might be clinically described as defense mechanisms, which serve to protect the person from the effects of what is being experienced, and may be a means by which conflict is handled. They can be useful or counterproductive for the person, which can be determined only by an overall psychosocial assessment of the individual. As evidenced by the research of Anderson et al. (1995), their sample of 68 elderly hearing-impaired adults who had been fitted with hearing aids revealed relationships among measures of coping, dispositional optimism, dysphoria, and health. The clusters identified included high copers, copers with moderate psychological and somatic complaints, and low copers.

Probably the greatest influence on the adjustive responses of older adults are elements associated with family relationships.

Reaction of the Family

Hearing impairment in adulthood affects not only the individual but those with whom that person relates daily. Surprisingly, scant research is available to describe the effects on the marital relationship, overall family functioning, and the children and other family members. Little is known of how the stress brought on by hearing impairment affects everyone and interpersonal relationships. Oyer and Oyer (1985) contribute considerably to our understanding of adult hearing loss and the family, but as they point out, few scientific experiments have studied the relationship between the two.

In terms of family systems theory, we are certain of at least one thing: The adventitious development of hearing impairment in an adult family member will disrupt the functioning of the family. The degree and quality of the dysfunction, however, depend on previous family functioning and the emotional stability of each member.

Effects on the Marital Relationship

We cannot assume that acquired hearing impairment in one person will automatically affect a marriage, even if marital problems existed prior to onset. If a healthy and creative marriage has existed, the hearing impairment actually may help bring both parties even closer together. Should marital difficulties increase, timed with the onset of hearing impairment, it is likely that a preexisting marital conflict may have been present but concealed. The hearing impairment may activate the original conflict, not necessarily to reveal it but to obscure it further under pretense of the hearing loss. We illustrate this.

Les and Diane had been married 30 years and had a relationship that was barely tolerable. Childless, they used each other to inflict their own personal, unresolved inner turmoil without ever coming to terms with the true essence of the relationship requiring love and trust.

Les, an avid hunter and disdainful of any ear protection, sustained a moderate to severe bilateral hearing impairment due to acoustic trauma. Refusing to wear the hearing aid that was fitted and likely would have helped him, his relationship with Diane deteriorated further in the form of mutual recriminations. Diane ridiculed him for being childish about refusing to wear the aid and felt angry and frustrated whenever he did not hear her. Her sarcasm, which had always been present, did not abate but became more volatile. Les, on the other hand, was infuriated with the increased intensity of her voice and her "bitchiness." Although previously, they had done many things separately, they now spent even less time together. Whatever time they did spend together often consisted of arguments surrounding his stubbornness and her judgment about his hearing impairment. Neither was able to relinquish the projections and the defenses that had built up over the lifetime of the marriage, nor did they desire a divorce.

This anecdote illustrates how extreme marital dysfunction may sometimes distort the incidence of hearing impairment. Based on a model by Jacobson and Bussod (1983), we would say that the way in which a couple copes with hearing impairment in one partner will be determined by the distortions in each person's perception of the other. The degree to which these perceptions are based on the perceiver's own unresolved conflicts rather than on the actual qualities of the other person will determine the wideness of the discrepancy and the amount of distress over the hearing impairment.

Effects on family equilibrium

Recall from the discussion of family systems theory that, although a communication disorder symptomatizes one individual, it does not imply that individual to be the actual "identified patient," who serves as a scapegoat for the family as a whole. For example, if the mother acquires a hearing impairment and is unable to cope adequately with it and there are preexisting unresolved family or marital conflicts, the stage may be set for another family member to take the burden of the problem or the attention away from the hearing impairment. This person now represents the true "identified patient."

We said that family patterns of interaction are directed toward maintaining the status quo, the equilibrium with which the family is familiar. Therefore, if family anxiety is aroused by the advent of a hearing impairment to unbalance the scale, at least one family member becomes "identified" as the person instrumental in regaining homeostasis for the entire family.

Ideally, if the wife and mother is able to manage constructively the consequences of her hearing impairment with open support from the rest of her family, in particular her husband, no other family member will need to assume the burden or become an identified patient. Thus, she becomes responsible for maintaining family equilibrium by the nature of her positive efforts. Most important is the necessity to separate the issue of hearing impairment from other, unrelated family issues. Only when the former is submerged by the latter do the real problems begin to surface.

Effects on Adult Children

Grown-up children of older adults with hearing impairment may play a significant role in assisting their parents to cope with the loss. A significant variable in this interaction is the quality of the parent-child relationship. A relationship in which mutual respect and support have been present will be the most effective in helping the hearing-impaired older person adjust to hearing loss. The implied assumption is that an open communication system has existed in which each person has been able to relate to the other as an individual in his or her own right. Age differences are of no consequence, because at least, they can acknowledge each other's intelligence, capabilities, knowledge, emotional attitudes, and points of view.

These are not individuals enmeshed in unresolved parent-child struggles or caught up in parent-child role reversals. Should the parent resist efforts either to wear an aid or participate in an aural rehabilitation group, it does not mean that the son or daughter should adopt a hands-off attitude but rather should communicate his or her personal feelings of opposition to the parent's stance. At the least, a dialogue can be initiated in which mutual attitudes and feelings can be expressed, acknowledged, and respected, even if some judgments are made. Most important is the mutual agreement that the parent must make the ultimate choice regardless of the consequences.

More frequently, the children of older or elderly parents with impaired hearing feel they must assume the burden of their parents' problem. The guilt they often experience when the parent is disinterested in receiving professional help is not so much related to their failure to convince the parent of the necessity but more likely related to having failed the parent previously in other matters. An example of this might be the elderly mother who feels that her son has made too little effort to visit her more often since her husband died. Indeed, she may resent his intrusion now because "he's never been there for me when I've needed him anyway." Certainly her own present negative attitude toward him and professional assistance or the wearing of an aid is connected to unresolved parent-child issues that probably belong to earlier times.

Also, some children essentially are disinterested in their parents' hearing impairment and feel that anything asked of them, like arranging for transportation to an aural rehabilitation group, is an imposition. Here, too, the issue is not the present negative response to the parent but a manifestation perhaps of long-standing resentments, anger, and bitterness characteristic of their essential relationship.

Such reactive responses by children frequently are evident when the parents are confined to a convalescent hospital or nursing home. Audiologists who consult in such institutions are quite familiar with families who do not follow through with recommendations regarding a change of ear mold, keeping fresh batteries on hand, or visiting more frequently.

Clearly, children of elderly parents with hearing impairment are affected in various ways, and although we might be tempted to categorize their behavioral responses, we must view them selectively and individually. In doing so, we are in a better position to determine how we can intervene psychotherapeutically, if necessary.

Counseling Strategies

We believe that, for any aural rehabilitation program for hearing-impaired adults to succeed, some form of counseling intervention must be included. This seems obvious, as aural rehabilitation, like counseling, is a communicative process in which the individual is assisted to relate more effectively with others by enhancing whatever hearing abilities are present. In addition, it seems unlikely for a person who has not adjusted emotionally to the impairment to derive much from an aural rehabilitation program that relies merely on a curriculum or on specific techniques.

The professional caregiver must decide first, however, which overall counseling strategy is appropriate, realistic, and potentially meaningful for the client. Second, it must be determined if counseling is to be used within the aural rehabilitation session or as an adjunctive procedure. Unfortunately, there is no objective or empirical evidence to assist us in that decision; the counseling professional must rely on whatever data the audiological evaluation has revealed and on information gathered during initial interviews with the client or the family.

Each of the major counseling strategies described has its own intrinsic value and, although they could be suitably combined with some clients, we address each separately.

Family Therapy

Generally, family therapy is an appropriate procedure if the hearing impairment has induced a crisis in the family. Either the actual patient, another member who has become the "identified patient," or both may provide the justification for such intervention. If family therapy is to have any chance of success, however, the family must be motivated at least to participate in the process. Participation does not necessarily ensure a success, because typically family members will resist the therapist's attempts at change. It is necessary, however, for the therapist to help the family stay focused on how the hearing impairment has activated other dysfunctional elements within the family and to deal with these as they surface.

Hearing Loss as a Family Issue

In family therapy, the hearing loss is treated as a symptom that has affected the entire family. In this sense, family therapy is quite different from traditional therapy models. The hearing-impaired individual is urged to share deeply held feelings with other family members, and they are encouraged to do likewise. The importance of this approach is highlighted by the fact that the hearing impairment itself may be interfering with normal family communication, and it will be necessary for individual or collective attempts to be found to modify or eliminate that interference.

The father who shuts himself off from other family members, however, may be doing so not because of his hearing impairment but for different reasons. The hearing loss could be used as an unknowing excuse to conceal other unresolved personal or family issues. Such issues need to surface if the hearing impairment is to be placed in its proper perspective.

Similarly, if another family member is having more difficulty in adjusting to the hearing impairment than the father, the underlying feelings and attitudes must be determined. These, in fact, have less to do with the actual impairment than with that person's essential relationship with the father. It does not mean that the person necessarily becomes the "identified patient" because of symptoms serving the family as a whole, unless the person's actions are used to protect other family members or conceal other family issues. The family therapist may have to work separately with that person and the father to determine the essence of their relationship.

If the person's behavior or attitude is used to obscure other family issues, the family therapist will need to promote a more functional family structure, in which the hearing impairment is placed in a realistic and objective perspective. The family of a hearing-impaired individual will need to discover, with the assistance of the family therapist, its own mode for coping with hearing loss in one member and for dealing with contaminating family issues.

Special Therapeutic Problems of Aged Parents

We have said that defensive attitudes on the part of older hearing-impaired individuals are a means of self-protection and a way of coping with hearing loss. In families where these individuals live with their grown children, such attitudes get enmeshed in other issues concerning not only the relationship with their children but also their self-concept, adjustment to old age, and loss of other functions.

More often than not, unfortunately, older parents have little choice in living with their adult children. Either because of other physical disabilities, loss of a spouse, or severe economic conditions, the older parent may feel guilty about disrupting his or her children's lives or being a burden and simultaneously feel resentful about dependency on them.

The therapist's first task in such family circumstances is to help the hearing-impaired person separate out feelings regarding the loss and its appropriate management from other emotional issues. The second task is to help the children understand that their well-intentioned judgment about what should be done to help can be counterproductive. Although we still consider the problem of hearing loss a family one, the affected parent's responsibility is to take charge of the predicament and do what is personally deemed best.

Important, too, however, is that the children be given the opportunity to express their own feelings and for the hearing-impaired parent to acknowledge the validity of their children's attitudes, even if these should differ from his or her own. Regardless of differing opinions or attitudes, the loss should remain the major focus of attention. Of course, if

other underlying emotional issues or conflicts are observed to be operating, they must be distinguished from the hearing-impairment issue and dealt with independently, if necessary.

The value of family therapy in these circumstances is that a valuable opportunity is provided for family members to understand and appreciate each other differently and enhance interpersonal relationships in a way that may never have been possible without the occurrence of the hearing impairment. Family therapy may not be the solution to all the relevant issues. But, at least, it allows for the maintenance or establishment of the personal integrity of each individual, regardless of other rehabilitative services deemed important or appropriate.

The hearing-impaired adult must make the ultimate decision regarding further remediation for the impairment. To deny that person the power to do so would, in Schlesinger's (1985) view, imply that the individual does not have "the cognitive competence, psychological skills, instrumental resources and support systems needed to influence his or her environment successfully" (p. 105).

Individual Counseling

Of all the counseling strategies, individual counseling is likely to be the most appropriate for adults with hearing impairment. Its relevance is determined by the degree to which the individual is adjusting to the loss and motivated toward being helped by amplification (if deemed necessary) and aural rehabilitation. In fact, it is best employed within the context of the audiological evaluation, the hearing aid fitting, and the aural rehabilitation process.

It is particularly important, however, that the audiologist be sensitive to the emergence of emotional attitudes or issues that do not relate directly to the hearing impairment. The individual can be gently encouraged to seek more intensive psychotherapeutic assistance if the problems cannot be dealt with professionally by the audiologist. Such referral, however, could be self-defeating, if the "helper" is uninformed about the consequences of hearing impairment and practices a "medical model," which, according to Schlesinger (1985), sees the hearing-impaired person as "ill or incapacitated" (p. 111).

We tend to agree somewhat with Schlesinger's view, based on the research of Coates, Renzaglia, and Embree (1983) that considerable evidence exists to suggest "that well meaning helpers may often do more harm than good" (p. 110). Silbergeld's (1983) examination of the negative effects of psychotherapy also is pertinent. We believe, however, that the potential benefits of counseling far outweigh its negative effects. (Further discussion of this issue is found in Chapter 9.)

Above all, the hearing-impaired client's attitude toward counseling must be respected, even if it means rejection of the process. The audiologist may have to be satisfied with providing information, even if it should fulfill only basic technical purposes, such as accommodation to amplification or care and use of the aid. Speech reading, too, in such cases, may have to be treated solely as an educational process.

Moreover, it must be understood that many hearing-impaired adults learn to adapt to their loss without the client-centered counseling we would advocate for other hearing-impaired individuals. So, we need to examine what our criteria should be and several counseling intervention guidelines.

Criteria for Intervention

The individual who has been traumatized emotionally by the hearing loss and who has no external support from others is likely to welcome the input of an empathic, understanding, and caring audiologist. Likewise, the individual who is struggling to reconcile the known benefits from amplification with preconceived notions of the stigma attached to hearing aid use might be motivated to "talk out" the conflict if unable to make a decision.

Some hearing-impaired individuals initially are unwilling to discuss their feelings of depression or explore the implications of their loss but, because they derive nonjudgmental support from their audiologist, may in time risk revealing very personal feelings they have been concealing. Oftentimes the aural rehabilitation process itself arouses feelings of frustration, struggle, or despair; and clients welcome the opportunity to ventilate their concerns, particularly if the modified approach is not identified as counseling per se.

Sometimes, the spouse or another family member seeks counseling assistance because he or she is unable to cope effectively with the hearing-impaired individual's continual self-pity, withdrawal, depression, and refusal of counseling assistance. Although family therapy might be the treatment of choice in such instances, it is of little value without the participation of the hearing-impaired person. Nonetheless, counseling at least can assist the spouse in coping more effectively at home and may indirectly help the other person as well.

Any decision by the audiologist to intervene psychotherapeutically must be based on the unique situational circumstances of the client with careful attention to individual client needs. It is impossible to generalize the effect of hearing loss on any one individual; therefore, the audiologist must view each case separately and be flexible enough to vary the therapeutic or educational approach as seems appropriate.

Guidelines for Client-Centered Intervention

Counseling begins once the individual has been informed of the degree and nature of the hearing loss following otological and audiological examination. Depending on the adaptive capabilities of the client, it may continue throughout the entire aural rehabilitation process, which includes learning to live with amplification. For the most part, counseling here is nothing more than effective communication therapy.

1. *Learning the facts about the loss.* Knowledge is enlightening but also painful. Once the reality has been objectified by means of the differential assessment, the worst fears are either realized or reduced. As information is provided, the client must have the opportunity to respond both affectively and cognitively. It may be difficult for the client to process all the information at once; so, care should be taken to impart information gradually and, if necessary, to repeat it in subsequent interviews, to avoid overload.

2. *Providing a therapeutic environment for the interpersonal relationship.* Such an environment is one in which the audiologist can admit to the client that some questions—like "How long will it take me to adjust to my aid?" "Will my hearing get worse?" "What if speech reading doesn't help me?" or "Will others get used to me and my hearing loss?"—cannot be readily answered. But every attempt is made to be supportive of the client's concerns and understanding of even irrationally expressed attitudes. Being defensive or providing the client a false sense of security should be avoided, so that the individual can gradually learn to adopt a realistic attitude toward the hearing impairment.

3. *Helping the client become his or her own agent of change.* A major goal in therapy is to encourage clients to take control of their own lives relative to the hearing loss, use of amplification, and the maximizing of the opportunities to use the environment in the fullest way possible. The client is helped to recognize that there is a choice between wallowing in self-pity and depression and learning to live with the hearing impairment. The therapist also must realize that resistance to such a choice is natural and vacillation is likely. Therefore, a confrontive approach should be used gently and caringly.

4. *Facilitating hearing aid use.* Orientation to the most effective use of amplification should be individualized so that the client will know what it can and cannot do. The frustrations and the delights associated with its use in varying situations should be reported and mutually analyzed. Modification of settings, change of ear molds, internal adjustments, even substitution of another aid may be necessary to maximize its use. Any resistance expressed to wearing the aid requires continued therapeutic attention. The user, nevertheless, has to make the ultimate decision, even if that decision is contrary to the wishes of the rest of the family.

5. *Integrating counseling with speech reading.* Frequently, attempts at learning to speech read are fraught with frustration and intermittent failure. Conceivably, the client may be preoccupied with other matters that interfere with concentration. These other concerns will need to be aired and resolved so that the client will focus on the primary task at hand. Should the speech-reading process itself be difficult to master, the client must learn to realize that it is natural for some comprehension in speaking situations to be lost. Sometimes speech reading can be formally structured as part of the counseling dialogue itself and thereby serve comprehension and affective needs simultaneously. More important for the client to realize is that speech reading can be learned but that it requires considerable diligence and effort to develop the skill.

6. *Dealing with depression and withdrawal from social interaction.* During the adjustment period, the client will experience wide shifts of mood and tend to feel cut off from others. He or she may isolate himself or herself either as a means of coping or as a defense to fend off further anxiety. The client should recognize that such behavior is not unnatural and even that his or her wish not to discuss feelings is acceptable. Indeed, some clients feel that they must reconcile their feelings with their loss through independent soul-searching in spite of the "rescue" efforts by the therapist. It is better that clients feel free to engage the therapist at their own discretion rather than be prodded to disclose everything being experienced. If the client's depression should encompass all daily life situations, the therapist at least can indicate what he or she personally is perceiving and experiencing from the client and thereby indirectly motivate the person to share more.

7. *Making the environment more conducive to listening.* Sometimes clients must be helped to assert themselves more to create an environment whereby listening is better facilitated. It may include such things as requesting an amplified telephone for the office, educating fellow workers about the importance of speaking directly to him or her, or transferring to another job activity within the firm. At home, it means that the client will modify the listening environment by urging reduction in ambient noise from varying sources or improving the acoustics of the home. Generally, it means mastering control of the environment rather than becoming a victim of it.

8. *Treating hearing loss when it is used or exaggerated as an expression of underlying psycho-*

logical conflicts. Occasionally, clients ostensibly will commit themselves to a regimen of aural rehabilitation but, at the same time, sabotage efforts to make substantial gains. Mia, a 30-year-old Vietnamese woman with a severe to profound bilateral hearing loss acquired during her childhood in Vietnam, was making only minimal progress in an intensive aural rehabilitation program that included speech reading, auditory training, and speech and language training (for her foreign dialect and speech conservation). She also was enrolled in an English as a second language class. During actual clinical work, she was very cooperative and usually met the criteria for all of the tasks undertaken. Bilateral amplification was apparently also quite beneficial. But, little was carried over from session to session, so her therapist was unable to increase the complexity of the tasks. Mia lived with American-born Victor, two years younger than her, who apparently had taken on a "Pygmalion" or "Henry Higgins" role in their living-together relationship. Only after several months of therapy was it learned that Mia had been living under considerable pressure from Victor to conform to his expectations and practice her clinical assignments beyond any reasonable presumptions. Sensitive to Mia's need to talk about her relationship with Victor, the therapist provided clinical time for Mia to express feelings of resentment, anger, and hostility toward Victor. He had been adamant in refusing joint counseling, viewing Mia's overall problems as her own, but he made a modest attempt to reduce the pressure at home. Most revealing, after several weeks of counseling, was that Mia had been unwittingly using her lack of progress to strike back at Victor and his paternalistic and dictatorial authority. Only through continual counseling did Mia arrive at a point where she could assert her independence and separate her hearing, speech, and language needs from her emotional relationship with Victor.

9. *Learning to accept a different self-image.* The degree to which a hearing-impaired adult is able to adjust his or her perception of self in relationship to the loss is determined in part by the quality of that individual's previous emotional health

and stability. For a client to move toward a more realistic attitude, it is necessary first for the therapist to help the person separate the objective reality of the loss from other issues that had been unresolved prior to the loss. The therapist also can aid the client to have positive and realistic expectations that he or she can perform successfully with a hearing loss, which in turn will lead to a positive outcome. Bandura (1977) describes this treatment concept as self-efficacy, which is quite different from the concept of outcome expectancy, whereby the individual only *believes* that a particular behavior will result in a particular outcome. Self-image is related to self-efficacy in the sense that, if the client's perception of self as a hearing-impaired person is negative, then there is a greater likelihood that he or she will have lower expectations about communicating with others. Therefore, a positive outcome is less likely because of the implied self-fulfilling prophecy, which says that what a person expects often will happen.

The guidelines we present are not meant to characterize any one counseling approach but should reflect the personal and professional position of the therapist. They also should be followed within the context of the client's unique circumstances and personal needs. Above all, if the client resists what the therapist is attempting to accomplish, then it is important that other goals, strategies, or theories be generated in the hope that they may be better accepted.

Group Counseling

Among the elderly in particular, group counseling as part of the aural rehabilitation process appears to be the treatment of choice. Throughout the United States, more and more senior citizen centers, often in conjunction with university or hospital speech-language and hearing programs, are offering space and personnel to developing ongoing rehabilitation services. These are not meant to replace traditional therapeutic services but to augment them in very practical ways for the senior citizen with a hearing impairment. They are intended to serve as social support networks, self-help opportunities, and citizen participation possibilities to help reduce the alienation, depression, and worries older people experience in relation to their hearing loss and other physical ailments.

Although group counseling certainly can be beneficial for any age group, we have chosen to concentrate on its practicality for older clients. We outline several major advantages:

1. *Peer support.* Nothing is more lonely for an individual than to feel that he or she is the only person suffering from the effects of hearing impairment. The opportunity to share with one another experiences, troubling concerns, and fears can help reduce feelings of vulnerability, incompetence, and helplessness. The peer counselor needs to allow for the greatest latitude in the communicative interpersonal relationships as they develop and serve as an information provider and feeling clarifier. The counselor also must be sensitive to the differing coping strategies each of the group members use and allow for the confrontations each makes on the others. The individual who refuses to wear an aid because of its intermittent discomfort is likely to be more responsive to another member who also has had the experience than to the counseling audiologist "who really doesn't understand what I'm going through."

2. *Enhancement of speech-reading skills.* There is no better situation in which to practice speech-reading skills than one that closely approximates the real world of the clients. Regardless of the difference between the safe, protective, and supportive milieu of group counseling and a non-caring, unconcerned, or rejecting environment outside of therapy, the counselor can readily simulate situations or communicative interactions that are similar and have created difficulties for the members.

3. *Opportunities for coping with other issues.* A frequent concomitant benefit of group counseling is the opportunity for the members to explore with one another concerns that are separate from the hearing loss or only indirectly related. It is difficult to imagine, however, that the hearing impairment does not impinge on every aspect of the individual's life, to some degree, at least. Consider, for example, relationships with grown children, managing retirement, loss of a spouse, getting older, other physical problems, and living out the remaining years creatively and productively. For the counselor, the task may appear formidable but need not be, so long as he or she does not attempt to carry the burden of clients' concerns or act as rescuer.

4. *Cost-effectiveness.* Considering the drastic increases in the cost of medical and ancillary health services over the last 20 years and the inability of the older population to afford such services, group counseling can be a welcome opportunity to minimize the costs somewhat. In adddition, local and state governments or charitable agencies are more likely to give financial support for such cost-efficient services but only through public and professional lobbying and educational efforts.

5. *Citizen participation.* Group counseling also may motivate its members to take a more active role in their community as they begin to recognize more clearly that their loss of hearing can become an opportunity for self-growth and for helping others. An excellent example of this is the founding of the Self-Help for Hard of Hearing People (SHHH) organization in 1979 by Stone (1985). This organization has given many hearing-impaired adults a new meaning for their lives as well as having become the advocate for hearing-impaired people in industry and government.

Based on the work of Trychen (1986, 1988), Abrahamson (1991) developed a program that deals with the psychological and social impact of hearing loss on the individual and his or her family. The program encourages independent, active management of communication-related problems as they relate to the family. The program includes environmental management, principles of behavior, use of assistive devices, stress management, cognitive management, and coping. Using an adult education class model, spouse participation is an integral part of the program.

Conclusion

The psychological ramifications of hearing impairment in adults of all ages present the audiologist a challenge that cannot always be met by virtue of their previous traditional training. Although others in the psychotherapeutic helping professions serve an important and often significant role in caregiving for the hearing-impaired adult, the audiologist in particular most frequently shares center stage with the client. Consequently, it is imperative that the audiologist develop counseling skills that can be facilitated by his or her own natural intuitive abilities, interpersonal communication and clinical competence, and professional commitment.

References

Abrahamson J. Teaching coping strategies: a client education approach to aural rehabilitation. *J of the Academy of Rehabilitative Audiology.* 1991;24:43–53.

Alpiner J. Psychological and social aspects of aging as related to hearing rehabilitation of elderly clients. In: Henoch MA, ed. *Aural Rehabilitation for the Elderly.* New York: Grune and Stratton; 1979.

Anderson G, Melin L, Lindberg P, Scott B. Dispositional optimism, disphoria, health, and coping with hearing impairment in elderly adults. *Audiology.* March–April 1995;34(2):76–84.

Bandura A. Self-efficacy: toward a unifying theory of behavioral change. *Psychological Review.* 1977;84:191–215.

Blair JC, Berg FS. Problems and needs of hard-of-hearing students and a model for the delivery of services to the schools. *ASHA.* 1982;24:541–546.

Boothroyd A. *Hearing Impairments in Young Children.* Englewood Cliffs, NJ: Prentice-Hall; 1982.

Breslau LD, Haug MR, eds. *Depression and Aging—Causes, Care and Consequences.* New York: Springer-Verlag; 1983.

Calderon R, Bargones J, Sidman S. Characteristics of hearing families and their young deaf and hard of hearing children. Early intervention follow-up. *Am Ann Deaf.* October 1998;143(4):347–362.

Calderon R, Greenberg MT. Stress and coping in hearing mothers of children with hearing loss: factors affecting mother and child adjustment. *Am Ann Deaf.* March 1999;144(1):7–18.

Calderon R, Low S. Early social-emotional, language, and academic development in children with hearing loss: families with and without fathers. *Am Ann Deaf.* July 1998;143(3):225–234.

Church M, Eldis F, Blakley BW, Bawle EV. Hearing, language, speech, vestibular, and dentofacial disorders in fetal alcohol syndrome. *Alcoholism: Clinical and Experimental.* April 1997;21(2):227–237.

Church MW, Kaltenbach JA. Hearing, speech, language, and vestibular disorders in the fetal alcohol syndrome: a literature review. *Alcoholism: Clinical and Experimental.* May 1997;21(3):495–512.

Christopher JS, Nangle DW, Hansen DJ. Social-skills interventions with adolescents: current issues and procedures. *Behavior Modification.* July 1993;17(3):314–338.

Clark JG. Counseling in a pediatric audiologic practice. *ASHA.* 1982;24:521–526.

Coates D, Renzaglia G, Embree M. When helping backfired: help and helplessness. In: Fisher JD, Nadler A, eds. *New Directions in Helping*, Vol 1. *Recipient Reactions to Aid.* New York: Academic Press; 1983.

Cook JR, Mausbach T, Burd L, Gascen GG. A preliminary study of the relationship between central auditory processing disorder and attention deficit disorder. *J of Psychiatry and Neuroscience.* May 1993;18(3):130–137.

Culross RR. Adaptations of the pictorial self-concept scale to measure self-concept in young hearing-impaired children. *Language, Speech and Hearing Services in the Schools.* April 1985;16:132–134.

Dee AD. Meeting the needs of the hearing parents of deaf infants: a comprehensive parent-education program. *Language, Speech and Hearing Services in the Schools.* 1981;12:13–19.

Ducharme DE, Holborn SW. Programming generalization of social skills in preschool children with hearing impairments. *J of Applied Behavior Analysis.* Winter 1997; 30(4):639–651.

Frankel BG, Nuttall S. Illness behavior: an exploration of determinants. *Soc Sci Med.* 1984;19(2):147–155.

Harris LK, VanZandt CE. Counseling needs of students who are deaf and hard of hearing. *School Counselor.* March 1997;44(4):271–279.

Hayes D. Hearing problems in aging. In: Jerger J, ed. *Hearing Disdorders in Adults.* San Diego, CA: College-Hill Press; 1984.

Hess DW. Evaluation of personality and adjustment in deaf children using a modification of the make-a-picture story (MAPS) test. Ph.D. dissertation. University of Rochester; 1960.

Hill R. Social stresses on the family: generic features of families under stress. *Social Casework.* 1958;39:139–150.

Hindley P. Psychiatric aspects of hearing impairments. *J Child Psychiat* [London: Cambridge University Press]. 1997;38(1):101–117.

Jacobson NS, Bussod N. Marital and family therapy. In: Henson M, Kasdin AE, Bellack AS, eds. *The Clinical Psychology Handbook.* New York: Pergamon Press; 1983.

Jaworski A, Stephens D. Self-reports on silence as a face-saving strategy by people with hearing impairment. *Int J of Applied Linguistics.* 1998;8(1): 61–80.

Jerger J, Chmiel R, Wilson N, Luchi R. Hearing impairment in older adults: new concepts. *J Am Geriatr Soc.* August 1995;43(8):928–935.

Luterman D. The counseling experience. *J of the Academy of Rehabilitative Audiology.* 1976;9:62–66.

———. *Counseling Parents of Hearing-Impaired Children.* Boston: Little, Brown; 1979.

Mauk GW, Barringer DG, Mauk PP. Seizing the moment, setting the stage, and serving the future: toward collaborative models of early intervention services for children born with hearing loss and their families: 1. Early identification of hearing loss. *Infant Toddler Intervention.* December 1995;5(4):367–393.

Moss WL, Sheiffele WA. Can we differentially diagnose an attention deficit disorder without hyperactivity from a central auditory processing problem. *Child Psychiatry and Human Development.* Winter 1994;25(2):85–96.

Murphy AT. The families of handicapped children: context for disability. In: Murphy AT, ed. *The Families of Hearing Impaired Children. Volta Review.* 1979;81:265–278.

Orlans H, ed. *Adjustment to Adult Hearing Loss.* San Diego, CA: College-Hill Press; 1985.

Oyer HJ, Oyer EJ. Adult hearing loss and the family. In: Orlans H, ed. *Adjustment to Adult Hearing Loss.* San Diego, CA: College-Hill Press; 1985.

Ramsdell D. The pscyhology of the hard of hearing and the deafened adult. In: Davis H, Silverman SR, eds. *Hearing and Deafness*, rev. ed. New York: Holt, Rinehart and Winston; 1960.

Riccio CA. Comorbidity of central auditory processing disorder and attention deficit disorders in children. *Dissertation Abstracts International.* 1993;54(6-A):2101.

Riccio CA, Hynd GW, Cohen MJ, Hall J, et al. Comorbidity of central auditory processing disorder and attention deficit hyperactivity disorder. *J of the Am Academy of Audiology.* July–August 1994;33(6):849–857.

Roberts C, Hindley P. The assessment and treatment of deaf children with psychiatric disorders. *J Child Psychol Psychiatry.* February 1999;40(2):151–167.

Rousey C. Psychological reactions to hearing loss. *J of Speech and Hearing Disorders.* 1971;36:382–389.

Schlesinger HS. The psychology of hearing loss. In: Orlans H, ed. *Adjustment to Adult Hearing Loss.* San Diego, CA: College-Hill Press; 1985.

Schlesinger HS, Meadow KP. *Sound and Sign.* Berkeley: Univeristy of California Press; 1972.

Shontz FC. *The Psychological Aspects of Physical Illness and Disability.* New York: Macmillan; 1975.

Silbergeld B. *The Shrinking of America: Myths of Psychological Change.* Boston: Little, Brown; 1983.

Stone HE. Developing SHHH, a self-help organization. In: Orlans H, ed. *Adjustment to Adult Hearing Loss.* San Diego, CA: College-Hill Press; 1985.

Stream RW, Stream KS. Counseling the parents of the hearing-impaired child. In: Martin FN, ed. *Pediatric Audiology.* Englewood Cliffs, NJ: Prentice-Hall; 1978.

Studdert-Kennedy M. Speech perception. In: Lass NJ, ed. *Contemporary Issues in Experimental Phonetics.* New York: Academic Press; 1976.

Sweetow RW, Barrager D. Quality of comprehensive audiologic care: a survey of parents of hearing-impaired children. *ASHA.* 1980;22:841–847.

Trychin S. *Relaxation Training.* Bethesda, MD: SSH Publications; 1986.

———. *So That's the Problem.* Bethesda, MD: SSH Publications; 1988.

Ventry IM, Chaiklin JB. Functional hearing loss: a problem in terminology. *ASHA.* 1962;4:251–254.

9

The Use of Power in the Therapeutic Relationship

Analysis and Description of the Concept of Power

If we are to take Webster's definition of *power* as an "ability to act; capacity for action or being acted upon; capability of producing or undergoing an effect; . . . the possession of sway or controlling influence over others; also a person . . . invested with authority or influence or exercising control," then it is readily apparent we are applying the broadest perspective to the use of power in the therapeutic relationship in speech-language therapy.

Backus (1960), in her provocative study of psychological processes occurring in the client-therapist relationship in speech-language therapy, reminds us that we place so much emphasis on rational thinking that we neglect our feelings and intuition and are insufficiently aware of the creative power within us. She goes on to state:

> We have thought so largely of the "rescuing power" for our lives as coming from events, things, and persons in the outside world. Thus when we *are* aware of feelings welling up from levels deeper than consciousness they are more often the negative ones. Moreover, what is unconscious in us is unknown and we usually fear what is unknown. Psychic energy is indeed power to be respected and under certain conditions even to be feared. To be feared, however, should mean to be reckoned with creatively rather than to be ignored through further repression. (p. 507)

Implicitly, then, we can view power as operating along a continuum representing both positive and negative aspects. Unfortunately, we cannot always be certain or in agreement as to *what* is positive or negative, as that will depend on *who* makes the inference. Take, for example, the phrase *the use of power for the greatest good of the client*. We are immediately confronted with the task of defining the nature of power as it may be used for a particular purpose. We also must define what is meant by *good*, because that depends on the value judgment of who is *doing* and who is *receiving*. We perhaps can answer this dilemma by exploring first the motives behind the use of power.

Motives in "Helping"

On the surface, it would appear that, in the helping relationship, the helper, the speech-language pathologist or audiologist, initiates a process whereby the client will be relieved of his or her communication impairment. Beneath this altruistic aim, however, lies the very complex hidden agenda of the therapist, who on one level may enter the profession of speech-language pathology or audiology for money, satisfaction with the substantive nature of the field, or the pleasure derived from helping someone else, and on a deeper level for satisfying ego needs of power, validating oneself, or solving one's own problems. No value judgment should be implied here, because our own nature and uniqueness determine the course we follow in our professional and personal lives. That our motives indeed have hidden meanings urges us to explore these factors so that we can enhance our own personal and professional growth as well as that of our clients.

Guggenbühl-Craig (1971), a Jungian psychiatrist, introduced the thesis that, in their desire to help, members of the helping professions also can psychologically damage their patients or clients. Although he refers in his writings more specifically to the physician, priest, teacher, psychotherapist, and social worker, speech-language pathologists and audiologists could be included in this group. He suggests that negative and positive motives get activated in helping. In one sense, the helper is highly motivated to do all that is possible for the client but, at the same time, may be imbued with a sense of self-importance and reflect an attitude of professional omnipotence. The helper then gets caught up in what Guggenbühl-Craig describes as a "lust for power" over the client. This becomes most evident when the helper recognizes behavior by the client to be self-defeating or perhaps destructive. In attempting directly to change the behavior and overcome the client's resistance to change, the helper's power is demonstrated. The helper rationalizes its use to enforce what is "right and good for the client." This is not to suggest that the helper is harming the client per se. These actions, in fact, might be quite beneficial to the client. But the reality is that the helper is unwittingly pretending to act selflessly. The more imbued the helper becomes with the ability to "know what's best," particularly when the client's behavior is positively changed, the greater the likelihood of making uncritical and questionable decisions later.

Nothing, however, can deaden our professional sense more than the sweet smell of therapeutic success. It lulls us into a state of complacency, and if we later are confronted with unexpected and difficult challenges from our clients, we are apt to rely on what has worked before. This is particularly evident if the new material is threatening to our own egos. When caught unaware we may tend to defend ourselves with the one arsenal we know is at our disposal—our professional power—and thereby

possibly obscure the issues. Heller (1985), in his extensive study of the power relationship between the client and therapist, describes in great detail how power can enhance the therapeutic relationship, client confidence, and hope or be used to induce client powerlessness and the imposition of the therapist's values. Heller is careful not to condemn dynamics of power but to analyze and unravel its elements as it is used in psychotherapy.

Applying a transactional analysis (TA) model as developed by Eric Berne, Hornyak (1980) describes how "games" are used in the interpersonal relationship in speech-language therapy, as a manifestation of "hidden agendas," which result in ulterior transactions between people. On the social level, the person may be doing or seeking one thing, but on the inner or psychological level, the person may be doing or looking for something else. Because two persons are involved, the transaction first takes on the aspect of a "con" that is fed by the other person, who is also operating with a hidden agenda, referred to as a "gimmick." As Hornyak states,

> The two players now transact with each other until a crisis point or climactic moment occurs in which the relationship between the two players suddenly changes. This is called the switch and is followed by a state of confusion, called the crossup, in which both players try to figure out what has happened and determine why their relationship has changed. This is followed by a payoff for each player. Payoffs are familiar feelings such as despair, anger, hopelessness, or elation. (p. 86)

We would agree that the communicative interaction between therapist and client is obscured and further contaminated by hidden motives, as implied by Hornyak's analysis. Yet we must also take into account that the therapist and client do not start out on the same level, as assumed by a TA interpretation. The client, from the onset, is in the inferior position, whereas the helper is in the position of authority or power. Therefore, it is the *helper's* major responsibility to initiate and maintain a constructive transactional process.

In our view, the helper uses power as a means for self-protection. Carl Jung (1968) explains this self-protection to be within all of us and related to the "shadow side of our unconscious." That is, we are not always aware, or do not always have a conception, of why we behave the way we do. This unknowing part of ourselves is characterized by our unrealized potentials, undiscovered fears and conflicts, and the part of ourselves we resist looking at. That is, the "shadow" represents thoughts, feelings, and attitudes that, although unknown to us, characterize much of our daily behavior and interactions with others. For example, if the client, during the early phase of the therapeutic relationship, asks for justification of the fee being charged, the therapist may either deal with this issue in an objective, mature, way, fully conscious of his or her own personal attitude toward money, or may react in a subjective, defensive manner, unaware of the deep-rooted attitude stirred. Unwittingly, the therapist may be concealing personal material that is threatening, and this behavior subsequently is characterized by a need to dominate the relationship as a means of self-protection. This gets translated into a demonstration of power over the client in which the therapist is in a safe, superior position to maintain control over the client and the therapeutic situation.

Projection and the "Shadow Side"

Certainly, we would be loathe to admit that we actually derive pleasure or comfort from feeling superior to our clients and that we are egotistical or self-serving. That we have chosen a humanitarian profession, often characterized by frustration, nebulous outcomes, and sadness, suggests that the choice may derive from our own unresolved or even resolved struggles. We are not always in complete control of our psyches, conscious of all our motivations and needs, or immune to the pain and struggles of our clients. We indeed are affected by our clients.

In our attempts to help, we actually could be resisting our own negative impulses, which in some way may be associated with attitudes and behaviors of our clients. Such resistance generally is connected to projections (which we define as the casting out on another person the ideas and impulses that belong to us), oblivious to the real person with whom we are relating. This is where power may be negatively expressed. Our unawareness of many of our inner struggles distorts the possibility of a completely objective appraisal of our clients. Judg-

ments, therefore, may be made, not in accordance with what the client truly needs, but in terms of what the helper needs. The more material our clients evoke, the greater is the possibility for our "shadow side" to be activated in conjunction with our increased use of negative power.

We are not questioning our conscious intention here but only the ramifications of our own unrealized expectations and attitudes that may be connected to our personal inner struggles. As Guggenbühl-Craig describes it, "There is a perpetual split between conscious values and the power of the shadow which would like to destroy those values." According to Jung, it takes considerable moral effort to become conscious of our "shadow," because it means looking at those parts of ourselves we do not like. Although this is essential for self-knowledge, we resist because of the painstaking work involved. Although it is possible for us to assimilate aspects of our shadow into our conscious personalities, certain features defy assimilation because they are too frightening to acknowledge and therefore usually are connected to projections.

We recall a graduate student who admittedly could not work effectively with her client because "he is so hard to like." This, in effect, isolated the therapist from her client. To objectify who that client really was meant that the therapist had to be willing to explore deeply within herself what she was projecting onto her client. Obviously, this client represented some things the therapist could not face within herself. Fortunately, in this case, the student was determined to discover what was so disturbing to her about her client and ultimately was able to admit to herself that he reminded her of certain things she "detested" in herself. Interestingly, once she brought this revelation to consciousness, she not only began to relate more positively to her client but also began to feel better about herself as a person and as a therapist. The student, unsurprisingly, has since developed into a highly competent and mature speech-language pathologist.

This example notwithstanding, we should be leery of making the generalization that one instance of self-revelation is all it takes to become an objective therapist. The student now saw the opportunity and the need to learn more about herself, albeit with considerable effort and courage.

Dynamics at the Onset
of the Therapeutic Relationship

The initial sessions in speech-language therapy are critical in that they determine, in part, how the client-therapist relationship will evolve and the direction the therapy process will take. We must bear in mind that the course of therapy will be determined in part not so much by what the therapist *does* but who that person *is*. Jung's theory of personality type is relevant to our discussion here (Campbell, 1971).

Jung believed that, although there are basic differences in the way people use their perception and judgment, this does not mean that people are necessarily right or wrong, bad or good. It does mean, however, according to Myers (1962), that "people differ systematically in what they perceive and the conclusions they come to" and "as a result [they] show corresponding differences in their reactions, in their interests, values, needs, and motivations, in what they do best and in what they like best to do" (p. 1).

Jung's theory is particularly important when we consider the effects of power as it emerges in the therapeutic relationship. That is, we must understand that the way power is used by the therapist is on the basis of how that person judges and perceives the client within the reality of the therapeutic situation. The use of negative or positive power is not to be viewed as good or bad, right or wrong, but merely as the manifestation of complex interpersonal dynamics within the therapeutic environment.

The Purpose of Therapy

Crucial to the development of the relationship and the progression of therapy are the conscious purposes first established by both the client and the therapist. The client desires to improve the ability to communicate. The therapist is viewed as the expert who will remove the problem so that the client will be able to communicate like everyone else. The therapist, too, has a conscious purpose—to help the client develop a more normal way of communicating. On the surface at least, there appears to be congruence between the client's and

therapist's goals, but the reality is quite different, as we shall see.

Purpose of the Client

Beneath the overt expectation or intention to communicate more effectively are unconscious motives that contain expectations of which neither the client nor the therapist may be aware. Unwittingly, the client also desires to be free of all other of life's problems as well. Therefore, the therapist easily could be assigned the role of "savior" by the client. For example, the aphasic adult, aside from desiring full language recovery, may unconsciously seek resolution of premorbid marital difficulties through the empathic therapist. In doing so, the client tends to relinquish control over personal choice-making possibilities, putting the therapist in the position of making a choice to either welcome or reject the opportunity. If the therapist chooses the former, the "savior" role expectation of the client is strengthened and perhaps guaranteed. If, however, the therapist chooses to deal only with language issues, the client's purpose is incompletely satisfied. We discuss the implications of this later.

Purpose of the Therapist

Meanwhile, the therapist has the conscious purpose of helping the client develop a more normal way of communicating. Conducive to this goal is the conscious aim to use predetermined strategies that are believed by the therapist to be appropriate to the presented problem. The way in which these strategies are employed also depends on the philosophical orientation of the therapist, be it behavioral, humanistic, directive, or nondirective, or combinations of these. Consciously or unconsciously, the therapist also may wish to help the client resolve other personal issues related directly or indirectly to the main problem. Regardless of the goals, the therapist attempts to enlist the client's help in improving or modifying the communication disorder.

On a conscious level at least, we might say that the therapist is using power appropriately. But as we have already noted, the unconscious shadow side also may be operating. On one level, the therapist may be caught between the desire to be the expert who will help this "poor fellow" and the realistic unwillingness to take on the perhaps frustrating burden of helping the client make changes in other aspects of living. On a deeper level, though, the decision is influenced by the therapist's own unconscious needs, whicht may emerge at the onset of therapy as projections, which in turn will determine the nature of the therapeutic alliance.

The Therapeutic Alliance

We have seen that the therapist's initial conscious intention may be to enlist the client's help in improving the latter's communicative ability. The client's conscious intention is to have the therapist solve the communication problem. The two intentions are not necessarily incompatible as long as it is made clear from the outset what is expected of the client, why practice is important, and what the therapy will focus on. If these are acceptable to the client, there appears little likelihood of an ensuing power struggle. If, on the other hand, these intentions are not first clarified by the therapist, a power struggle could emerge. The client may find it very frustrating and believe it unimportant to practice outside of formal therapy. Meanwhile, the therapist believes outside practice to be crucial for any change to take place and cajoles the client into practicing. Not only is the stage set for the development of a parent-child relationship, as described by Berne (1964), which can interfere with client growth, but also for activation of unconscious elements in the client that can sabotage the therapeutic process.

The relationship takes on greater complexity if the client expects and hopes to rely on the therapist to find solutions to all his or her problems. Here, the therapist would be taking on the projections of the client and may find it difficult not to be affected by them. The therapist, in fact, may enforce power and prominence as a result of having his or her own unconscious tapped.

Guggenbühl-Craig describes the intensification of the power struggle between therapist and client as a "game of sorcerer-and-apprentice." The client expects and hopes to find the all-powerful sorcerer who will answer everything. How much "magic" or

power the therapist exerts on the client, of course, depends on the degree to which the therapist has recognized and acknowledged the "shadow" personally and the projections that emanate from it.

But even the "magical alliance" cannot tolerate the effects of other underlying issues. For example, the client may resist the home assignments because they interfere with other urgent needs. The client's wife may be an impatient person who will resist taking on the role of "therapy aide." She could do so, but grudgingly, and the client recognizes it. Here, again, the therapist's projections intrude into the therapeutic relationship. Puzzled by the client's apparent uncooperativeness and stubbornness, the therapist readily generalizes that the client essentially is negative toward his rehabilitation. If the therapist has had previous experiences with negative clients, personal preconceived attitudes now appear. The situation is made more complicated by the spouse's psychosocial processes, and the struggle between client and therapist becomes acute. It can become so powerful that it may obstruct therapeutic success and destroy the entire therapeutic process before it can begin.

The Power Struggle in Ongoing Therapy

We now need to look more closely at how the complex interpersonal relationship manifests itself in ongoing therapy and the communication process.

The Conflict Between Conscious and Unconscious Intentions

It has been seen that, in a clinical relationship, the client's and the therapist's conflicting intended goals may be obscured or distorted by unconscious motives, which in turn may create a power struggle. This may not be apparent at first, but through the ongoing relationship, the conflict between conscious and unconscious intentions begins to emerge.

Hood (1974) describes the difficulty with which the client faces change and growth, because of fear of the unknown and defense to challenge or threat. The therapist, according to Hood, must be in tune personally to be sensitive to the client's needs. If not, an incongruence will develop between the parties, resulting in friction, denial, and defensiveness. The therapist now must deal not only with the client's hidden agenda but with his or her own as well, so that the interpersonal interaction can be relatively free of contamination.

The therapist's task, nonetheless, is to establish a hierarchy of procedures that the client must follow to ameliorate the identified speech-language disorder. The therapist now is in the seat of power. As long as the client cooperates (making the clinician feel successful), all will be well. This is not to imply that the client will not benefit. The client, obviously, also wants to eliminate the speech-language problem, but at what cost? Clients must put themselves at the "mercy" of the therapist, which could trigger elements associated with the shadow, thereby making them vulnerable in terms of self-concept. In this way, clients lose power as new patterns of behavior are adopted that may appear very foreign.

The client must put complete faith in the therapist, but is that possible? Not if more powerful unconscious forces contribute to the client's vulnerability. Not if it means the client no longer can use the disorder, such as stuttering, to define or justify a current mode of personal existence. Moreover, if the client has become overly dependent on the therapist, the opportunity to take greater responsibility for the problem and its solution will be hindered. Hood reminds us, too, of "the inability of the client to accept present and changing roles, status and relationship conflicts, and to give up using [the disorder] as an ego-protecting mechanism" (p. 51).

The Therapist's Role

Defining the therapist's role in the therapeutic relationship is probably the most complex, challenging, and deceptive aspect of speech-language therapy procedures, in that it assumes we can objectively decide what that role should be. As Perkins (1974) notes, "The intervention of one person, the therapist, in the life of another, the client, is sufficiently sanctified when done in the name of therapy that motives, reasons, and effects are rarely examined" (p. 369). Alluding to the therapist's hidden agenda, Perkins asks us to consider our values, motives,

therapeutic orientation, professional responsibilities, and training with respect to our clinical intervention. Most relevant in our view is the choice, conscious or unconscious, that the therapist makes in the pursuit of improving defective communication. Let us examine several of these possible choices.

As Benign Dictator

At one extreme, the therapist may choose to assume the role of benign dictator, legislating every step the client must take to communicate more effectively, discounting "extraneous" material (elements such as the client's unconscious connection between sexual and communicative adequacy) and charismatically intimidating the client into accepting what the therapist believes is best. The therapist justifies this approach by reason of education, ability, and previous success. Not only is the therapist the "expert," but the judge and jury as well, who will insist that the client conform to the therapeutic regimen established.

Here, the therapist's use of negative power comes into full play. The more the client conforms to the therapist's prescription, the more impressed the therapist becomes with a personal image as healer and the less likely to recognize personal underlying motives. If the client questions or resists certain intervention strategies, the therapist views this as childlike and asserts power as a parent. In either case, the therapist deprives the client of responsibility for the problem and may destroy the very process that would ensure communicative success; that is, the development of a process through which the client must learn to take charge and cope when the therapist no longer is present.

The client's realization of success in speaking and independence is not a threat to the therapist's conscious goal but to the unconscious motives that characterize the therapist's shadow side and represent individual life struggles. These may consist of the need for control and dominance that compensate for feelings of self-doubt and inferiority and placate strivings for self-worth. The client also responds on the conscious level, unaware of the dominant unconscious motives that characterize his or her own shadow side. These may consist of a need to always be in control, for total independence, and for complete self-sufficiency, perhaps compensating for more deeply rooted feelings of low self-esteem. What results is a dual intra-interpsychic conflict represented as a struggle for power.

It would be difficult for the therapist we describe to acknowledge, in response to the client, that "there, but for the grace of God, go I." Certainly, such an admission would not be permissible for that person, and moreover would serve no purpose. What is of chief importance to the benign dictator is that, as long as the communication disorder is improved, nothing else is relevant as far as speech-language therapy is concerned. If that is so, then perhaps we are only technicians who should limit ourselves to the surface aspects of communication and refrain from involvement in meaningful interpersonal relationships in therapy.

As Benign Supertherapist

At a different point on the continuum is the therapist who feels qualified (though may not be) to cope with all the client's conflicts and problems associated directly, indirectly, or not at all with the speech-language problem. This person is the benign supertherapist, who, being in the power position as helper, attempts to intrude into the client's unconscious world and takes on the responsibility of facilitating not only effective use of speech and language but also changes in all aspects of the client's life. For this therapist, it is not enough to deal only with symptomatic features of, say, a functional voice disorder. The therapist is interested in making the client aware not only of the etiological factors associated with vocal dysfunction but of other dysfunctional aspects of that person's life. Here is a situation where the client's conscious intention to "correct my voice problem" is given secondary importance by the clinician, who believes that permanent vocal change can come about only through the analysis of the client's personality and emotional attitudes.

We characterize this approach as negative use of power by the therapist. Even if the client accedes to the therapeutic desires of the therapist, the unconscious motives of each are activated. And if there is an immediate conflict between the client's and ther-

apist's conscious motives, the conflict is further intensified. The therapist interprets the client's appropriately realistic resistance as a refusal to face the facts. The therapist cannot recognize that, perhaps, irritation felt toward the client is related to deep-seated insecurity about personal therapeutic competence or, deeper yet, related to unresolved conflicts over strict parental controls in the therapist's own childhood. The client, in turn, is threatened by possible exposure of personal material with which she or he has not dealt or of which that person is unaware. For the client, the therapist also may represent a parental figure to whom the client may still be bonded.

The ensuing power struggle may result in any one of several possibilities. The therapist ultimately dominates, coercing the client to accept "what is good for her (or him)." The client then acquiesces, discounting the validity of her or his early conscious intention. Or the client resists, this lack of cooperation interpreted as unwillingness to work on the voice problem. Or the client chooses to terminate therapy, labeling the therapist "one of those Freudian kooks" and blocking off any desire to change the vocal behavior or look beyond the vocal symptoms. Any subsequent encounter with another therapist is likely to be viewed with perhaps natural overcautious concern, which could inhibit therapy based on a different orientation.

The therapist, too, ultimately is affected by whatever course therapy takes. Forced to confront the many challenges, inner and outer, to personal "expertise," a self-protective professional barrier is erected to fend off threats by other clients. In doing so, the therapist consolidates individual power, further abrogating objectively conceived conscious intentions.

As Sophisticated Therapist

Even the more sophisticated psychotherapeutically oriented therapist may be treading on territory well obscured by the client's major conscious intention and fall victim to personally established intellectualization. Considering, as an example, the adult aphasic client, the therapist may lose sight of the more pressing functional linguistic needs of the client. Astute as the therapist's assessment of the client's psychosocial state may be and competent in the subsequent psychological counseling of the patient or family, the risk is run of raising issues that may actually impede linguistic progress.

Several years ago, we created a therapeutic situation whereby a 55-year-old right hemiplegic, apraxic, and aphasic woman was provided the opportunity to ventilate long-repressed feelings of resentment toward her husband. Although unrelated to her stroke, her anger and depression replaced any desire to focus attention on her apraxic use of language. Nonetheless, after five months of psychotherapeutic counseling twice a week, she had achieved a level of better than minimal functional communication. During the fourth month of therapy, she expressed misgivings about not "working on language exercises." When these were introduced, however, she elected to continue talking about her "empty marriage" and "thoughtless husband." (It should be noted that both she and her husband had adamantly refused family therapy.) Also during the fourth month post onset, she began to have consistent attacks of diarrhea immediately prior to her therapy session. Toward the end of the fifth month of therapy, she confirmed her personal physician's and our private analyses by stating insightfully and linguistically perfectly, "I guess I don't want to let go of all my shit." Unsurprisingly, she chose to terminate therapy rather than delve further into the "emptiness of my 30 years of marriage." She refused, also, any therapy limited to traditional strategies, as these too she felt would "get my head working again."

This clinical anecdote illustrates that, although the immediate functional linguistic needs of the patient were not necessarily neglected, the therapist was in a sense "seduced" by the clinical challenge of dealing with a classic dysfunctional marital relationship. Disregarding the stirrings of his own shadow side, his negative power was awakened in his attempt to prove his hypothesis. An early decision was made to satisfy our "professional expertise," thereby encouraging an ambivalent client to discuss long-repressed issues for which no real solutions could be attained during speech-language therapy. Had she been willing to delve more deeply into her own shadow side, she might have achieved a more meaningful awareness of herself and begun to consider other options open to her. Had we been fully in tune with our own shadow, regardless of the client's level of awareness, the employment of purely traditional speech-language treatment strategies might have been efficacious and justified.

It should not be presumed, however, that the client would have continued therapy. Given this particular client and special environmental circumstances, it is conceivable that no therapeutic strategy ultimately would have been successful, despite the functional level of communicative competence actually achieved. Confronted with a moral dilemma, we made a choice based on our experience and level of self-awareness. That the client, too, made a choice to terminate therapy suggests how tenuous therapeutic relationships are and emphasizes again the significance of the human factor in all of us.

As Benevolent Therapist

Typically, we would be more familiar with the helper who can be described as the benevolent therapist. Although use of undesirable power may not be expressed to the degree in the previous examples, it may be exercised in a more subtle manner and yet contain elements that can be manipulative.

Take, for example, the stuttering client whose conscious intention to become fluent is congruent with the therapist's conscious intention. A behavioral approach in conjunction with client-centered counseling has been initiated and mutually acceptable. Therapy in fact may proceed with the client carrying out successfully the fluency contracts that have been mutually agreed on. The client also may feel free to reveal in therapy elements that heretofore had been hidden unconsciously. Because these elements relate to the stuttering behavior, the therapist listens and attempts to understand. The client, highly responsive to the therapist's empathic attitude, now feels freer to share more or may use the occasion to avoid pertinent issues by discussing social niceties. But, this intrudes on therapeutic contract time directly related to fluency improvement.

What may be occurring is either the germination of resistance to more difficult contract work or the emergence of a need to discuss anxieties concerning stuttering and other related issues. In any case, the therapist's previous attitude of composure is disrupted. The therapist may respond initially by gently persuading the client to stay with the contract or may allow the client to continue exploring other concerns. If the former is pursued, the therapist may meet with greater resistance by the client and then have to cope with personal feelings of guilt for having forced the issue. If, on the other hand, the therapist accedes to the client's wishes, the client may feel compromised and that he or she is not accomplishing "all that I should be doing."

Regardless of the choice made, the therapist's shadow side is evoked and the therapist may begin to feel frustrated, angry, or helpless. The therapist's projections now are manifested by the manner in which control over client and therapist power are displayed. The therapist feels overwhelmed by the client's ambivalent attitudes and is unable to separate his or her own feelings of powerlessness from the struggles of the client. If the therapist refrains from coercion and continues to go along with the client, he or she may be denying a growing anger or frustration. If the therapist dictates the course therapy must follow, the initial agreement with the client has been nullified. In a sense, the therapist feels "damned if I do and damned if I don't." Either way, power is used negatively. The client no longer is the subject of real concern because the therapist becomes bound up in personal psychic struggles. (Naturally, such therapists would deny this preoccupation and appear to most observers to be in full control of the clinical situation and their clients.)

Even if we were to predict that the likelihood of a positive therapeutic outcome would depend on everything in therapy progressing by the book, we would have to ask the question, "Whose book?" And if a prescriptive therapy model is dictated initially, the further question arises: "Can it be followed?"

As Powerless Therapist

On the continuum where the therapist relinquishes all apparent power, there certainly would be little hope or reason for any improvement in the communicative impairment being treated. Ideally, we might assign such a label as *powerless therapist* only to novice student therapists who would be receiving the best in professional supervision. (The delicate issue of supervisory power and its use is familiar to many students as well as former students, but we do not discuss it at this time. Perhaps the reader who is both therapist and supervisor may uncomfortably identify with several issues presented in this chapter. If so, let the shoe fit as it may.)

The client receiving therapy from a powerless therapist would be confused and bewildered by his or her lack of intention or power. In transactional analysis terms, the therapist may take on the role of "Child" to get approval from the client, who is projected as the "Parent." In doing so, the therapist wills all control of the therapeutic situation to the client. But, this may be characeized as a form of manipulation that has evolved from the therapist's shadow side and could be considered an aspect of negative power unconsciously used. The result would be therapeutic chaos, driving the client to seek someone more competent. Should the client choose to remain in the therapeutic situation, satisfying client power needs, the therapeutic process also is unlikely to have a positive outcome.

Ridiculous and unimaginable as the powerless therapist example may seem, it may not be as infrequent as we would wish and does point up the inevitable interplay of unproductive unconscious intentions when conscious motives are allowed to be distorted.

Use of Positive Power

The use of power, in and of itself, is not necessarily destructive, and the illustrative examples given are not meant to imply absolute and distinct therapeutic conditions or rigidly categorize therapists. As therapists, we not only vary our roles according to the clients with whom we work but also our clinical behavior for any one client. Thus, it is likely that the distinction between the types of therapists we describe may begin to blur. Obviously, although we may always strive for perfection as therapists, we cannot expect to succeed all the time. It is not surprising, then, if we see a little bit of each type of therapist in all of us.

Ideally, what we hope to learn, however, is that the therapist who guides and yet is flexible to the client's needs will provide a therapeutic environment where the client can grow and change within his or her greatest potential. We refer to the therapist who does not take on personally every negative response by the client but uses the response constructively to help the client. That is, the therapist is able to separate personal ego concerns from those of the client, uncontaminated by psychological projection. In so doing, the therapist must be able and willing to assume the challenge of the client's projections, fully aware of the power assigned as a natural consequence of the therapeutic role. The therapist also must be conscious of how dramatically the power element may change during the therapeutic process, aware of the subtle nuances that may challenge the therapist's therapeutic role and authority.

We do not suggest that the ideal therapeutic relationship should be free from any power struggle. Such struggles are common and natural to all interpersonal relationships, particularly the therapeutic relationship. They well could serve as catalysts for positive change in the client, enabling the latter to confront issues that heretofore may have inhibited progress. They also provide opportunities for the client to assume more responsibility for change, taking power into his or her own hands and gradually weaning him- or herself away from dependency on the therapist.

In Chapter 1, on counseling, we discuss transference and countertransference and their effects on the therapeutic process. It is readily apparent that such dynamics are intrinsic to projection, but when viewed objectively by both client and therapist, they can be put to productive use for the mutual benefit of all, by raising self-awareness and contributing to personal growth.

The Challenge to the Therapist

Our therapeutic task is formidable. It entails, first of all, our willingness and action to search within ourselves to discover those unconscious elements that constitute personal anxieties, struggles, biases, and unresolved conflicts. This certainly can be difficult and emotionally painful; our natural tendency

is to resist looking at those aspects of ourselves that threaten us. Nonetheless, it behooves us to attempt to understand what the personal shadow components mean and how they enter into and intrude upon the therapeutic relationship.

Perhaps the most difficult task of all is for us to be willing to maintain a constant vigil over our shadows. We cannot assume that once we have been enlightened by a new self-discovery that we now can "work it all out with the client" and be done with it. Our personal shadow world is in constant flux, always revealing newer and perhaps more threatening features as we move through life's experiences. Thus it becomes more apparent to us with each new professional experience to rest on the laurels of success and to discount opportunities to look within ourselves during the therapeutic process. In fact, the more comfortable we feel as therapists, the greater is the danger of being intoxicated by our own power. As Guggenbühl-Craig aptly puts it, "He cannot, like the biblical Isaac, spend just one night wrestling with the angel to win his blessing. His struggle for the blessing must last a lifetime" (p. 155).

Finally, we must recognize that, as long as we are human as well as professionals, we can never be perfect in all of our behavior and that we always will err, depending on certain circumstances. But, we must realize that we also have within us the power to choose to continue to err or to change our actions so that our clients can derive the full benefit not only of our professional expertise but also our humanness as well.

Research Considerations

In this chapter, several theoretical issues are raised and a number of assumptions implied. To put these to experimental testing presents a prodigious task, one with which researchers of the Jungian orientation have had to struggle. We, nonetheless, believe that some attempt, difficult as it may be, can be initiated to support the conjectures made.

It appears to us that one of the most crucial questions we must answer is, How can we objectively analyze what occurs during the interactional therapy process? Collaterally, what do we wish to measure? A linguistic discourse analysis, alluded to in Chapter 1, would not provide us with the necessary objective analysis of the affectual and attitudinal features discussed here. Labov and Fanshel (1977) explore the goals and techniques of psychotherapy through precise analysis of linguistic forms used by the therapist and client during 15 minutes of one session—hardly sufficient to generalize to other clients, therapists, and circumstances. Bandler and Grinder (1975) apply transformational grammar clinically in their analyses of psychotherapy, translating surface structures into deep ones systematically, but fail to provide any penetrating analysis of underlying motives, much less any sufficient understanding of the affectual interactional process. Weintraub (1981) demonstrates the possibility of defining and measuring several speech characteristics apparently related to psychological defense mechanisms in the psychotherapeutic process. He developed a system of verbal behavior analysis that is highly sensitive to nuances of style among various groups of individuals sharing deviant styles of thinking and behavior. Flanagan (1954) developed the Critical Incident Technique, consisting of a series of procedures for making direct observations of human behavior. It has been demonstrated to be highly effective in measuring typical performances in various occupational settings; in measuring proficiency, motivation, and leadership; and in counseling and psychotherapy.

Flanagan and Weintraub's investigations would be fruitful avenues of research to follow in formulating objective analyses of the interactional process in speech-language therapy. With the aid of a computer-based data collection, it would be possible to correlate many variables simultaneously in the analysis of syntactic, semantic structures. It should be understood, however, that present computers will not solve the inherent variables associated with measurable categories of verbal expressions. We would be naive, also, to hope that scoring systems on computers could be sensitive enough to lead toward validation of Jung's concept of shadow or unconscious processes per se. It is hoped, however, that we could be provided with an effective base for understanding the complex dynamics of manipula-

tive functions both positive and negative in speech-language therapy.

Conclusion

In this chapter, we attempt to describe the complexity of the interpersonal relationship in speech-language therapy relative to the way power becomes manifest in that relationship. We see that, when elements of our psyches coincide with those of our clients, there is the possibility that deeply unconscious motives, represented by our shadow side, may dominate and perhaps endanger the therapeutic process. When this occurs in us, as therapists, we easily may lose sight of what our clients genuinely need and, in doing so, may exert negative power over them. We illustrate several ways in which power is used by therapists with different psychological traits and how adult clients may affect and be affected by the helping process. Although child clients were not discussed, it should be readily apparent that they would be vulnerable to the clinician's power and thus a greater challenge to the therapist's struggle for objectivity.

As Pickering (1984) suggests, in a revealing study of interpersonal communication in speech-language pathology supervisory conferences, supervisors and students "appeared to lack knowledge about how to analyze the interpersonal dimension of therapeutic relationships." Pickering further adds that "client change will need to be complemented by an emphasis on process-oriented, transactional, and existential-phenomenological issues" (p. 195). We would concur and thereby encourage our profession to take steps toward facilitating and understanding the complex dynamics underlying the interpersonal relationships in speech-language pathology.

A final note is in order. Despite the necessity for being conscious of all of the psychological factors related to power that impinge on the therapeutic relationship, we need not be ashamed of the pride we feel when we indeed help our clients communicate more effectively. The "good" we do, in fact, says much for the essential emotional health of speech-language-hearing professionals and the clinical competency with which we practice. We conclude with the question: "Why not enhance our skills and ourselves even further?"

References

Backus O. The study of psychological processes in speech therapists. In: Barbara DA, ed. *Psychological and Psychiatric Aspects of Speech and Hearing.* Springfield, IL: Charles C Thomas; 1960.

Bandler R, Grinder J. *The Structure of Magic I: A Book about Language and Therapy.* Palo Alto, CA.: Science and Behavior Books; 1975.

Berne E. *Games People Play: The Psychology of Human Relationships.* New York: Grove Press; 1964.

Campbell J, ed. *The Portable Jung.* New York: Viking; 1971.

Flanagan JC. The critical incident technique. *Psychological Bulletin.* 1954;51:327–358.

Guggenbühl-Craig A. *Power in the Helping Professions.* Irving, TX: Spring; 1971.

Heller D. *Power in Therapeutic Practice.* New York: Human Sciences Press; 1985.

Hood SB. Clients, clinicians and therapy. In: Emeerick LL, Hood SB, *The Client-Clinician Relationship.* Springfield, IL: Chas. C. Thomas; 1974.

Hornyak AJ. The rescue game and the speech-language pathologist. *ASHA.* 1980;22:86–89.

Jung CG. *Analytic Psychology: Its Theory and Practice (The Tavistock Lectures).* New York: Pantheon; 1968.

Labov W., Fanshel D. *Therapeutic Discourse: Psychotherapy as Conversation.* New York: Academic Press; 1977.

Myers IB. *Myers-Briggs Type Indicator Manual.* Palo Alto, CA: Consulting Psychologist Press; 1962.

Perkins WH. *Speech Pathology: An Applied Behavioral Science.* St. Louis, MO: C. V. Mosby; 1974.

Pickering M. Interpersonal communication in speech-language pathology supervisory conferences: a qualitative study. *J of Speech Hearing Disorders.* 1984;49:184–195.

Weintraub W. *Verbal Behavior: Adaptation and Psychopathology.* New York: Springer-Verlag; 1981.

Appendix

Recommended Training Requirements for Marriage and Family Counseling

It should be obvious from the theme and substantive nature of this book that most traditionally trained speech-language pathologists and audiologists obtain little or no academic and clinical training to counsel effectively with the communicatively impaired or their families. Although the American Speech-Language-Hearing Association has professed the importance and desirability for counseling expertise in its members, there has been minimal evidence of university curriculums in support of communication disorders to satisfy that requirement. Even though some programs offer courses in parent counseling, psychodynamics, and counseling theory and practice, and further recommend that electives be taken in psychology, counseling, and social work, most graduates feel ill-prepared to cope effectively with the psychological needs of their clients and families.

The dilemma for most programs is that they already are overburdened by professional demands for further course offerings in such subject matter as dysphagia, head injury, linguistics, and specialized diagnostic test instrumentation. Academicians in the profession certainly can add several other courses to the list.

We do not wish to suggest that current programs be drastically altered to fit the philosophical position offered in this text, although many programs throughout the country are being modified continually to satisfy new and unmet needs of the profes-

sion. We do recommend that the following suggestions and rationale be considered and that they at least be openly debated. It will be evident that several ideas are already implemented and should add greater validity to our proposal.

1. Undergraduate students in communicative disorders programs should be encouraged to take as many elective units as possible, in such courses as introduction to psychology, abnormal psychology, personality theory, and learning theory. It is assumed that the student will be required to have a varied liberal arts background in general studies that would allow for inclusion of these courses.

2. It should be possible to include coverage of the psychology of the various communicative disorders discussed in introductory courses. Coverage should be limited to the most elementary psychological principles because the novice student generally is confounded sufficiently with the complexities surrounding the various communicative disorders.

3. Many programs provide clinical experiences for undergraduates that are essentially observational in nature. We consider it important for these students to have opportunity to observe master clinicians who are skilled in the techniques of counseling communicatively disordered individuals and their families. In those programs where

undergraduates are expected to perform clinically, they can be introduced to counseling practices, but only under the strictest supervision by a master clinician skilled in psychotherapeutic techniques. (Unfortunately, at the present time, probably few university or college instructors feel comfortable or trained enough to take on this responsibility. This is all the more reason for intensive psychotherapeutic training at the doctoral level.)

4. Assuming undergraduate students will have the aforementioned experience, the transition to more complex psychodynamic principles and practices can be made more readily, assuming, of course, that the graduate program in communicative disorders is prepared to offer such courses. We realize that master level programs in either speech-language pathology or audiology are highly specialized and that faculty often are frustrated by the inability to cover everything they consider important. The feasibility of including the psychodynamic features associated with the various disorders, however, is strengthened by the coverage of the disorders in a more highly specialized manner.

5. To complement any specialized course work that can be offered as electives in counseling itself, graduate students should have frequent exposure to as many clinical opportunities as possible in order to practice counseling skills, when appropriate. Again, it must be presumed that the students will be supervised at least 50% of the time at first, depending on the counseling competence level of the student.

6. Graduate students should be encouraged to enhance their counseling skills by enrolling in courses outside the major department. These recommendations are not intended to delay graduation as long as the school or university allows an interdisciplinary policy whereby the student would be permitted to take a core of courses on a post-master's level, without having to reenroll formally at the institution.

7. A key indicator that marks the successful counselor is a background that includes an extensive and intensive clinical practicum in counseling therapy. We hesitate to recommend a specific number of clinical practicum hours but suggest instead that the student be allowed, following mutual agreement with the counseling supervisor, to take a practicum test after an externship of no less that 200 client contact hours. In California, the State Board of Behavioral Examiners requires that students must have a minimum of 3,000 supervised clock hours before they can be eligible for licensing as a marriage, family, and child counselor. No less than 1,500 hours of experience shall be gained subsequent to the granting of the qualifying master's or doctor's degree. For those applicants who enroll in a qualifying degree program on or after January 1, 1995, no more than 750 hours of counseling and direct supervisor contact may be obtained prior to the granting of the qualifying master's or doctor's degree. They also must take an oral and written examination.

We do not suggest that individuals who counsel their communicatively disordered clients should be required to be licensed as marriage, family, and child counselors, as long as they do not breach the ethical boundaries of dealing only with the problems associated with the communicative disorder itself. We would urge, however, that they pass a competency exam in the use of counseling skills before they be allowed to counsel.

We recognize the complex philosophic and administrative problems inherent in such a recommendation and, therefore, would encourage the American Speech-Language-Hearing Association and state organizations to make a thorough study of the issue. Certainly there are those individuals who, having been certified and licensed as speech-language pathologists or audiologists, also qualify for licensing as marriage, family, and child counselors. We are acquainted with several such individuals who are duly licensed in the state of California. As for the *practicing* speech-language pathologist, the following guidelines may be helpful:

1. Students enrolled in doctoral programs should have ready access to an elective core curriculum that provides sufficient learning in counseling theory and practice, particularly if these competencies have not been satisfied for their predoctoral degrees.

2. Many opportunities are available for those already certified and licensed as speech-language pathologists or audiologists to gain access to counselor training in universities, institutes, independent seminars and workshops, or professional conferences, so that they be better prepared to serve a counseling role in their professional settings.

3. Speech-language pathologists and audiologists typically have satisfied several competencies in counseling by virtue of their academic background. In fact, before 1978, the California State Board of Behavioral Examiners accepted a master's degree in communicative disorders as satisfying most academic requirements for the marriage, family, and child counseling license. The board now requires that persons desiring this license hold a doctoral or a master's degree that contains no less than 48 semester or 72 quarter units of instruction. The instruction shall include no less than 12 semester units or 18 quarter units of course work in the areas of marriage, family, and child counseling and marital and family systems approaches to treatment.

To qualify for a license, an applicant must be qualified in all the following areas:

1. The major theories of a variety of psychotherapeutic orientations directly related to marriage, family, and child counseling and the marital and family systems approaches to treatment.
2. Theories of marriage and family therapy and how they can best be utilized to intervene therapeutically with couples, families, adults, children, and groups.
3. Developmental issues and life events from infancy to old age and their effect on individuals, couples, and family relationships. This may include course work that focuses on specific family events and the psychological, psychotherapeutic, and health implications that arise within couples and families, including, but not limited to, childbirth, childrearing, childhood, adolescence, adulthood, marriage, divorce, blended families, stepparenting, and geropsychology.

4. A variety of approaches to the treatment of children.
5. No less than six semester or nine quarter units of supervised practicum in applied psychotherapeutic technique assessment, diagnosis, prognosis, and treatment of premarital, marital, family, and child relationship dysfunctions.

While many states have their own regulations governing counseling and use of family therapy, many of them are similar to these requirements.

For a more complete description of licensing requirements, see

Board of Behavioral Science Examiners Regulation and Laws and Regulations Relating to the Practice of Marriage, Family, and Child Counseling, Licensed Clinical Social Work, and Licensed Educational Psychology

State of California Department of Consumer Affairs; August 1999:1–93.

Available from:

State of California Department
  of Consumer Affairs
400 R Street, Suite 3150
Sacramento, CA 95814-6240.
Website: http://www.bbs.ca.gov

Index

DATE DUE

DEMCO 13829810